T0110511

The Cambridge Illustrated History of Surgery

Written in a lively and engaging style, by a medical author and teacher of great renown, this book provides a fascinating and informative introduction to the development of surgery through the ages. It illustrates some of the key advances in surgery from primitive techniques such as trepanning, through some of the gruesome but occasionally successful methods employed by the ancient civilisations, the increasingly sophisticated techniques of the Greeks and Romans, the advances of the Dark Ages and the Renaissance and on to the early pioneers of anaesthesia and antisepsis such as Morton, Lister and Pasteur. Heavily illustrated in colour, The Cambridge Illustrated History of Surgery is the only serious choice for a reader wanting a lively and informative single-volume introduction to surgical history.

The Cambridge Illustrated History of Surgery

Harold Ellis, CBE, FRCS

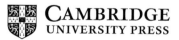
CAMBRIDGE
UNIVERSITY PRESS

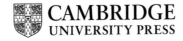

Shaftesbury Road, Cambridge CB2 8EA, United Kingdom

One Liberty Plaza, 20th Floor, New York, NY 10006, USA

477 Williamstown Road, Port Melbourne, VIC 3207, Australia

314–321, 3rd Floor, Plot 3, Splendor Forum, Jasola District Centre, New Delhi – 110025, India

103 Penang Road, #05–06/07, Visioncrest Commercial, Singapore 238467

Cambridge University Press is part of Cambridge University Press & Assessment, a department of the University of Cambridge.

We share the University's mission to contribute to society through the pursuit of education, learning and research at the highest international levels of excellence.

www.cambridge.org
Information on this title: www.cambridge.org/9780521720335

© H. Ellis 2009

This publication is in copyright. Subject to statutory exception and to the provisions of relevant collective licensing agreements, no reproduction of any part may take place without the written permission of Cambridge University Press & Assessment.

First edition published 2001 by Greenwich Medical Media
Second edition first published 2009
5th printing 2015

A catalogue record for this publication is available from the British Library

Library of Congress Cataloging-in-Publication data
Ellis, Harold, 1926–
    The Cambridge illustrated history of surgery / Harold Ellis. – 2nd ed.
      p. ; cm.
    Rev. ed of: A history of surgery / Harold Ellis. 2001.
    Includes bibliographical references and index.
    ISBN 978-0-521-89623-8 (hardback) – ISBN 978-0-521-72033-5 (pbk.)
    1. Surgery–History.   I. Ellis, Harold, 1926– History of surgery.   II. Title.
    III. Title: Illustrated history of surgery.
    [DNLM: 1. Surgery–history.   WO 11.1 E47c 2009]
    RD19.E43 2009
    617–dc22   2008039645

ISBN   978-0-521-89623-8   Hardback
ISBN   978-0-521-72033-5   Paperback

Cambridge University Press & Assessment has no responsibility for the persistence or accuracy of URLs for external or third-party internet websites referred to in this publication and does not guarantee that any content on such websites is, or will remain, accurate or appropriate.

....

Every effort has been made in preparing this book to provide accurate and up-to-date information which is in accord with accepted standards and practice at the time of publication. Although case histories are drawn from actual cases, every effort has been made to disguise the identities of the individuals involved. Nevertheless, the authors, editors and publishers can make no warranties that the information contained herein is totally free from error, not least because clinical standards are constantly changing through research and regulation. The authors, editors and publishers therefore disclaim all liability for direct or consequential damages resulting from the use of material contained in this book. Readers are strongly advised to pay careful attention to information provided by the manufacturer of any drugs or equipment that they plan to use.

To Wendy, and to our children and grand-children

Contents

Preface

This book presents, I hope, a fairly succinct overview of the story of surgery. The first chapters deal with the development of the subject from its earliest days, then the great watershed in the mid-19th century, with the discovery first of anaesthesia and then of antiseptic surgery. This is followed by the extraordinary explosion in progress which took place in the decades after Lister. Later chapters deal with specific fields of surgery, starting with, perhaps appropriately, the surgery of warfare, since over the centuries so many advances in the subject were made on the field of the battle. Further chapters then deal with orthopaedics, breast surgery, stones in the bladder, the thyroid and the parathyroid glands, surgery of the lungs, heart and blood vessels, organ transplantation and, finally, a look into the present and the future.

I have to confess that my personal interests and my own heroes have crept heavily into the text and into the illustrations. I do not apologise for wandering off here and there to describe the characteristics and accomplishments of men that I have come to admire as I have read of their contributions to the science and art of surgery.

The opportunity to prepare a second edition has allowed me carefully to revise and amplify the text, add a section on the story of Caesarian section and to bring up to date, as far as is in my power, the final chapter on the present and future. New illustrations have been added and some old ones replaced with colour versions.

I hope that this new edition will bring as much pleasure to its readers as its writing has been to the author.

Harold Ellis

Acknowledgements

I have many people to thank for their help with this book. I must mention in particular Tina Craig and her staff at the library of the Royal College of Surgeons of England, Miss Elizabeth Allen, George Qvist Curator of the Hunterian Museum at the Royal College of Surgeons, William Edwards, Keeper of the Gordon Museum at Guy's Hospital, and Susan Smith, photographer to the Department of Anatomy at the Guy's Campus.

The following gave immense assistance with references and illustrations: Mr. Paul Aichroth FRCS, London; Dr. Roger Alberty, Portland, Oregon; Mr. A.A. Attewell, Florence Nightingale Museum, London; Dr. Stewart Bath, Launceston, Tasmania; Prof. Christopher Buckland-Wright, London; Dr. Richard Carter, Indian Wells, California; Dr. Frank Clifford Rose, London; Prof. Jean-Jacques Duron, Paris; Mr. Jules Dussek FRCS, London; Mr. H.H.G. Eastcott FRCS, London; Dr. Stanley Goldberg, Minneapolis; Mr. John Goodfellow FRCS, Oxford; Dr. Ira Kodner, St. Louis; Prof. Gabriel Kune, Melbourne; Dr. John Mathews, London; Dr. Andrew Olearchyk, Cherry Hill, New Jersey; the late Mr. Roger Parker FRCS, Reading; Dr. Carole Rawcliffe, University of East Anglia; Mr. David Rosin FRCS, London; Dr. Mark Silverman, Atlanta; Mr. Mathew Welck MRCS; Dr. Ray Wiley MBE FRCS, Toronto.

The Officers of the following Institutions: The American College of Surgeons (Miss Marian Rapp and Miss Kate Early); German Historical Institute, London (Miss A. Robrecht); Royal College of Physicians (Miss C. Fowler); Royal College of Physicians and Surgeons of Canada (Mr. M. Thibault); Royal College of Radiologists (Miss H. Beckitt); Royal College of Surgeons of Edinburgh (Prof. D.L. Gardner); Royal Humane Society (Miss Diana Coke); Worshipful Company of Barbers (Mr. I.G. Murray); The Cultural Attachés of the Embassies of Denmark, Italy, Portugal and Sweden in London; The photographic department at Guy's (Mr. Mark Simon); The library of the Royal College of Obstetricians and Gynaecologists (Mr. Stephen Cook).

Above all, I thank my daughter-in-law, Mrs. Katherine Ellis, for her meticulous secretarial help and for her ability to understand my cockney accent on the Dictaphone.

Further Reading

The author can recommend the following books to those who wish to find further information on the History of Surgery:

Cope Z: *A History of the Acute Abdomen.* London, Oxford University Press, 1965.

Hurt R: *The History of Cardiothoracic Surgery from Earliest Times.* London, Parthenon Publishing Group, 1996.

Medvei VC: *A History of Endocrinology.* Lancaster, MTP Press, 1982.

Murphy LRT: *The History of Urology.* Springfield Ill., Charles C Thomas, 1972.

Rutkow IR: *Surgery, an Illustrated History.* St. Louis, Mosby, 1993.

Singer C Ashworth E: *A Short History of Medicine.* London, Oxford University Press, 2nd edition, 1962.

Wangensteen OW, Wangensteen SD: *The Rise of Surgery.* Minneapolis, University of Minnesota Press, 1978.

Zimmerman LM Veith I: *Great Ideas in the History of Surgery.* New York, Dover Publications, 1967.

Surgery in prehistoric times

The word 'surgery' derives from the Greek cheiros, a hand, and ergon, work. It applies, therefore, to the manual manipulations carried out by the surgical practitioner in the effort to assuage the injuries and diseases of his or her fellows. There seems no reason to doubt that since Homo sapiens appeared on this earth, probably some quarter of a million years ago, there were people with a particular aptitude to carry out such treatments. After all, there is an innate instinct for self-preservation among all mammals, let alone man, so that a dog will lick its wounds, limp on three limbs if injured, hide in a hole if ill and even seek out purging or vomit-making grasses and herbs if sick.

We are talking about times many thousands of years before written records were kept and, indeed, evidence of disease or injuries to soft tissue of that period has long since rotted away with the debris of time. Palaeopathologists (students of diseases in the long distant past) have, however, uncovered abundant evidence in excavations of ancient skeletons that fractures, bone diseases and rotten teeth tortured our oldest ancestors. Of course, animals were also subject to all sorts of diseases. Indeed, a bony tumour was obvious in the tail vertebrae of a dinosaur that lived millions of years ago in Wyoming. Other excavations also reveal that injuries were inflicted by man upon man (Figures 1.1, 1.2) and, as we shall see, that broken bones were splinted and skulls operated upon.

We can make a reasonable guess at what primitive healers may have done from studies carried out by anthropologists and ethnologists (students

of primitive tribes) who, at around the beginning of the 20th century, carried out detailed studies of communities as far apart as West and Central Africa, South America and the South Pacific who had never had contact with 'modern' man. It is surely reasonable to surmise that treatments found in such communities, often amazingly similar in very different parts of the world, might well match the care given by our prehistoric ancestors in man's fundamental instincts of self-preservation. The assumption might be wrong but it would require a great deal more research before a distinction between 'modern' primitive and prehistoric medical and surgical treatments could be made. It goes without saying that these early studies are immensely valuable to us today since few if any primitive communities nowadays remain untainted by Western civilisation.

Injuries inflicted by falls, crushings, savage animals and by man upon man, demand treatment; among primitive tribes in the aforementioned studies, open wounds were invariably covered by some sort of dressing. This might take the form of leaves, parts of various plants, cobwebs (which may well have some blood-clotting properties), ashes, natural balsams or cow dung (Figure 1.3). Indeed, even in recent times, the use of dung as a dressing for the cut umbilical cord in West African village babies still took place and was responsible for many cases of 'neonatal tetanus' – lockjaw in babies – from the tetanus spores that are almost invariably present in faeces.

Among the Masai of East Africa, wounds were stitched together by sticking acacia thorns along

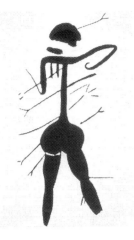

Figure 1.1 A warrior pierced with eight arrows. Drawn from a rock painting in eastern Spain, and probably the first portrayal of wounding.
Reproduced from Majno G: *The Healing Hand*. Harvard University Press, 1975.

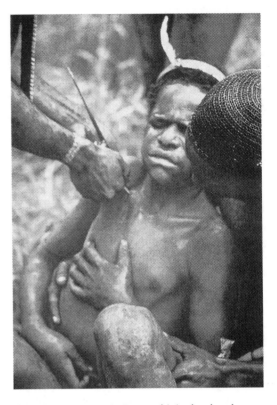

Figure 1.3 A warrior in Borneo, hit in the chest by an arrow, is treated by a healer. This photograph was taken some 30 years ago.

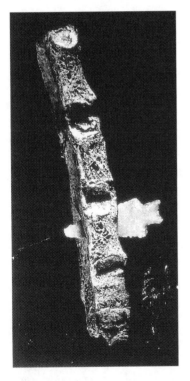

Figure 1.2 A flint arrow head embedded in the human sternum. From the Chubut Valley, Patagonia. Musée d'Homme, Paris.

the two edges of a deep cut and then plaiting the thorns against each other with plant fibre. In both India and South America termites or beetles were employed to bite across the edge of the wound whose lips were held together by the surgeon. The bodies of the insects were then twisted off, leaving the jaws to hold the laceration closed, remarkably like the metal skin clips employed in operating theatres today. Splints of bark or of soft clay (which was then allowed to set) were used to immobilise fractured limbs, and such bark splints have been excavated from ancient Egyptian burial sites (Figure 1.4).

Apart from dealing with wounds and fractures, early surgeons carried out three types of operative procedure, namely cutting for the bladder stone, circumcision and trephination of the skull. Cutting for the stone is such a fascinating and important topic in the history of surgery that it merits a chapter of its own (see Chapter 12).

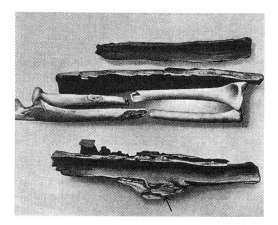

Figure 1.4 Fractured forearm bones with bark splints, from Egyptian excavation and dated about 2450 BC. Note the blood-stained lint dressing (arrowed), the oldest specimen of blood.
From Majno G: *The Healing Hand.* Harvard University Press, 1975.

Circumcision

Circumcision might well be claimed to be the most ancient 'elective' operation and was practised in Ancient Egypt by assistants to the priests on the priests and on members of Royal families. There is remarkable evidence for this carved on the tomb of a high-ranking royal official which was discovered in the Sakkara cemetery in Memphis and is dated between 2400 and 3000 BC (Figure 1.5). This represents two boys or young men being circumcised. The operators are employing a crude stone instrument. While the patient on the left of the relief is having both arms held by an assistant, the other merely braces his left arm on the head of his surgeon. The inscription has the operator saying 'hold him so that he may not faint' and 'it is for your benefit'.

The ancient Jews may have learned the art of circumcision during their bondage in Egypt and, indeed, circumcision is the only surgical procedure mentioned in the Old Testament, the practice of circumcision among Jews being attributed to Abraham. In the book of Genesis (17;1–2), probably written about 800 BC, we read: 'This is the covenant

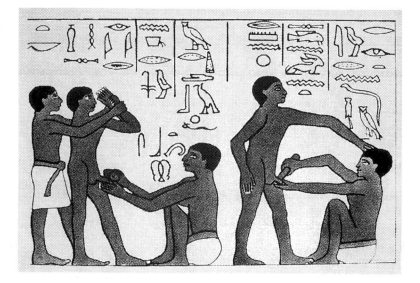

Figure 1.5 Drawing of a tomb carving of a circumcision scene. Sakkara cemetery at Memphis, Egypt, c. 2400–3000 BC.

between me and you and your seed which you must obey; all males among you shall be circumcised.' Again, in the second book of Exodus, Zipporah, the wife of Moses, 'took a sharp stone and cut off the foreskin of her son'.

Early ethnological studies revealed that circumcision was practised very widely among primitive communities, including those of equatorial Africa, the Bantus, Australian Aborigines and in South America and the South Pacific, as well as being traditional among Jews, Muslims and Copts. We can only guess at its origins, perhaps as a fertility or initiation rite or possibly for cleanliness or hygiene. Its traditional basis is confirmed by the fact that in many communities, even though metal instruments were available, the operation was still performed with a flint knife.

Trephination of the skull

Undoubtedly the most extraordinary story in the history of surgery is that, long before man could read or write, as long ago as 10000 BC, surgeons were performing the operation of trephination or trepanning – boring or cutting out rings or squares of bones from the skull – and, just as remarkably, their patients usually recovered from the procedure.

Although the words 'trepanation' and 'trephination' today are interchangeable in common practice, trepanation comes from the Greek trypanon, meaning a borer, while trephination is of more recent French origin and indicates an instrument ending in a sharp point, so that this implies using a cutting instrument revolving around a central spike. Trepanation thus connotes scraping or cutting, while trephination describes drilling the skull, as in modern neurosurgical operations.

Different techniques of trepanation in ancient times, and in recent primitive communities, involved scraping away the bone, making a circular groove so that a central core of the bone would loosen, boring and cutting away the bone, or making rectangular intersecting incisions in the skull (Figures 1.6, 1.7).

This story begins in 1865 when a general practitioner, Dr Pruniers, who was also an amateur archaeologist, discovered in a prehistoric stone tomb in Central France a skull which bore a large artificial opening on its posterior aspect. With it, he found a number of irregular pieces of bone which might have been cut from another skull.

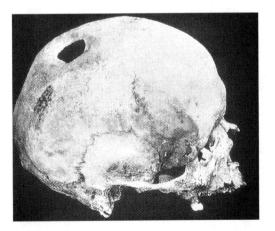

Figure 1.6 Trephined skull, from an Anglo-Saxon skeleton excavated in East Anglia.

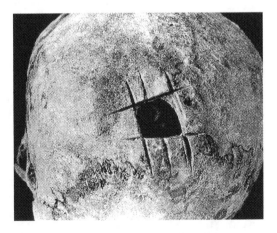

Figure 1.7 Trepanned skull from ancient Peru. The operation has been performed by means of a series of incisions placed at right angles to each other.

He postulated that the skull had been perforated so that it might be used as a drinking cup. Soon after this, a number of other holed skulls were found in other parts of France and Professor Paul Broca (1824–1880), a distinguished French physician, suggested that these openings were the result of an operation of trepanation and that the instrument employed was a flint scraper. Broca suggested that survivors of the operation were endowed with mystical powers and that, when they died, portions of their skulls, especially those that included a part of the edge of the artificial opening, were in great demand as charms.

Following these discoveries, thousands of such specimens have been discovered from many parts of the world: the United Kingdom (Figure 1.6), Denmark, Spain, Portugal, Poland, the Danube Basin, North Africa, Palestine, the Caucasus, all down the Western coastline of the Americas and, especially, in Peru (Figure 1.7), where more than 10000 specimens have been excavated.

Two questions immediately come to mind: why was the operation performed, and how? In many cases it seems that trephination was carried out on patients following a head injury. We can see an obvious fracture line on many specimens, often coinciding with, or near, the site of the trephine defect. We can be sure that many such patients recovered because numerous specimens show clear evidence of healing of the fracture and of the edges of the trephined defect. The frequent use of stone clubs and sling stones among ancient warring Peruvians may account for the large numbers of specimens recovered from that country; in one collection of 273 skulls from Peru, 47 had been trephined in from one to five places. We can only guess at the frequent use of trephination in skulls with no obvious evidence of injury. In many of these, indeed, the operation had obviously been performed several times at intervals. Intractable headaches, epilepsy or an attempt to confer mystical powers on the subject are all possible motives, and there seems little doubt that the fragments of bone removed were themselves often regarded as possessing magical powers.

Of course, the operation was performed without the benefit of anaesthesia, although authorities have surmised that an extract of the coca plant might have been used by the ancient South American practitioners. The instrument would originally have been a sharpened flint or piece of obsidian, (a hard black laval stone), fastened by cord to a wooden handle. These were later replaced by a copper or bronze blade. Techniques varied from place to place: a circular cut through the skull bone, a series of circular drill holes which were then joined together, or triangular or quadrangular cuts through the skull bone. Professor Broca, who we have mentioned above, using an ancient flint instrument, showed that he could produce such a defect in a skull in 30 to 45 minutes. Even more remarkably, in 1962, Dr Francisco Grana of Lima operated on a 31-year-old patient, paralysed after a head injury, and evacuated a blood clot from beneath the skull using ancient Peruvian chisels to trephine the bone. The patient recovered.

Our knowledge of prehistoric trephination would remain mainly a matter of conjecture if it were not for the fact that the operation was still being performed by primitive races in some widely separated parts of the world, the South Pacific, the Caucasus and Algeria, at the end of the 19th and in the early 20th century. From New Guinea and the surrounding islands of Melanesia many skulls have been collected which show perforations very similar to those found in stone age specimens. Writing in 1901, the Reverend J A Crump noted that in New Britain the operation was only performed in cases of fracture, which was a common injury in tribal warfare. The instrument employed was a piece of shell or obsidian and the wound was dressed with strips of banana stalk, which is very absorbent. The mortality was about 20%, but many of the deaths resulted from the original injury rather than from the operation itself. In other islands, the operation was performed to cure epilepsy, headache and insanity, while in New Ireland, an island north of New Guinea, a large number of natives had undergone trephination in youth as an aid to longevity. In The Lancet of 1888 there is an account of the practice of trephining in the Caucasian province of Daghestan, on the borders of the Caspian Sea. Here it was carried out for head injuries and it is interesting that it was the aggressor who was obliged to pay the surgeon for the operation. In 1922 Hilton-Simpson published a book about his four visits to the Aures Mountains in Algeria, where he was able to study the work of local surgical practitioners. Here knowledge was passed from father to son and the surgeons carried out splinting of fractures, reduction of dislocations, circumcisions and lithotomy for stones in the bladder. Trephination was commonly performed, always as a treatment of some form of head injury. The operation comprised the removal of a circular portion of scalp with a cylindrical iron punch heated red-hot and then cutting an opening in the skull by the use of a small drill and a metal saw. Great care was taken not to damage the underlying coverings of the brain, the dura mater.

The question that remains unanswered is how was it that this sophisticated neurosurgical operation came into being so long ago, in such widely separated centres, in communities that surely could have had no possible contact, indeed even knowledge of each other? This is a question that will continue to be debated but will probably never be answered.

Cutting for the stone

This, the third and perhaps most interesting, of these 'primitive' procedures, deserves a chapter of its own, (see Chapter 12).

2

The early years of written history – Mesopotamia, Ancient Egypt, China and India

Mesopotamia

Civilisation as we recognise it today, with cities, organised agriculture, government and a legal system, dates back some 6000 years to the Valley of the Nile and the adjacent land of Mesopotamia between the Tigris and Euphrates. Above all, man learned to write, and translations (an extremely difficult task) of carvings on stone, statues and tombs and writings on baked clay from Mesopotamia and papyri from ancient Egypt give us a much clearer idea of what medicine and surgery must have been like in those times.

The Tigris flows for 1200 miles from the mountains of Armenia to the Persian Gulf. The Euphrates, even longer, runs roughly parallel to its twin. These unpredictable rivers may overflow their banks as the Armenian snow melts in Spring and floods vast areas of land – probably the basis of the story of the Flood in Genesis, a story repeated in much ancient folk lore. At around 4000 BC there arose in this region the highly developed civilisation of Sumeria, with city states of Kish, Lagash, Nippur, Uruk, Umma and, best remembered of all, Ur. In these cities dams were built, surrounding fields irrigated, taxes levied and a picturograph script invented, which was somewhat similar to that developed in Egypt. This primitive writing developed into a script that could be incised onto clay tablets. On clay it is easier to produce lines rather than curves, and the wedge shape of the script gave its name to cuneiform writing, which comprised some 600 signs.

Great kings arose, such as Sargon of the city of Akkad (around 2350 BC), who subjugated the whole of Sumeria and Hannurabi (around 1900 BC), who established his capital at Babylon. In time, Babylon was conquered by Tiglath-Pileser, king of the northern neighbour Assyria, with its capital at Nineveh around 1100 BC. The power of Babylon remained until, in 539 BC, it gave way to the rise of the Persian Empire.

The medicine of Mesopotamia was primarily medico-religious. Practitioners were priests and were ruled by the strict laws included in the code of King Hannurabi. This code, carved on a black stone about eight feet high which was discovered at Shush in what is now Iran in 1901, can be seen today in the Louvre Museum in Paris. At its top can be seen the Emperor Hannurabi receiving the laws from the sun god Shamash (Figure 2.1). His code details family law, the rights of slaves, the penalties for theft and the rewards for success and the severe punishment for failure on the part of the surgeon. We have evidence from these writings that surgical conditions such as wounds, fractures and abscesses were treated. Thus we read:

If a doctor heals a free man's broken limb and has healed a sprained tendon, the patient is to pay the doctor five shekels of silver. If it is the son of a nobleman, he will give him three shekels of silver.

If the physician has healed a man's eye of a severe wound by employing a bronze instrument and so healed the man's eye, he is to be paid ten shekels of silver.

If a doctor has treated a man for a severe wound with a bronze instrument and the man dies and if he has opened the spot in the man's eye with the instrument of bronze but destroys the man's eye, his hands are to be cut off.

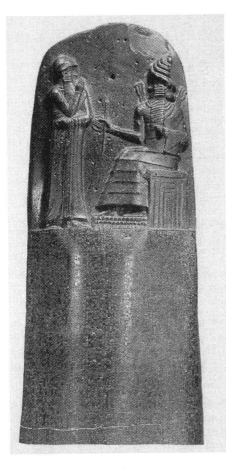

Figure 2.1 The code of King Hannurabi.
Louvre Museum, Paris.

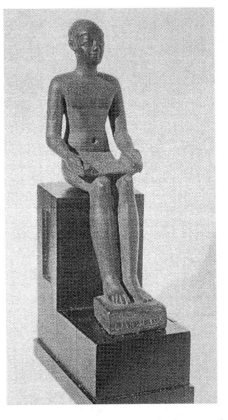

Figure 2.2 Imhotep (c. 2900 BC), the first named physician.
Louvre Museum, Paris.

It was obviously a dangerous profession in those days!

If it were not for Hannurabi's code of laws, all memory of surgery in Babylon, nearly 4000 years ago, would have been lost. Surgery as a craft was hardly worth mentioning; only when it became of interest to the law was it engraved in stone.

Ancient Egypt

The influence of Sumerian civilisation upon that of Egypt is a subject of interesting and continuing debate, but certainly as long ago as 4000 BC there was a well organised governmental system in the Nile delta. With it came the development of the pictorial writing of hieroglyphics and the discovery that writing material could be prepared from the papyrus reed, a more convenient medium than clay bricks. Around 2900 BC lived the first famous individual whose name has come down to us in medicine, Imhotep, vizier to King Zoser. An administrator, politician and builder of the great stepped pyramid of Sakkarra, still to be seen today, he must also have been distinguished as a physician, although we know nothing of his medical contributions. He was worshipped for many centuries after his death as god of medicine (Figure 2.2).

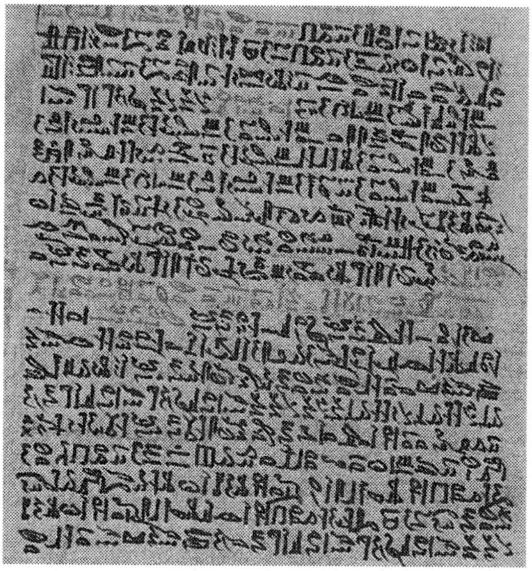

![The Ebers papyrus]

Figure 2.3 The Ebers papyrus.

A number of medical papyri have come down to us which are of great interest. The Ebers papyrus was found in a tomb at Thebes in 1862 by Professor George Ebers and is now preserved in the University of Leipzig (Figure 2.3). It consists of 110 sheets and contained 900 prescriptions. As a calendar has been written on the back of the manuscript, the date of its writing can be fixed with reasonable accuracy at about 1500 BC. However, there is good evidence to show that much of it has been copied from other works many centuries before. The writings are sprinkled with incantations, which suggest that the remedies were given with the intention of driving out the demons of disease. Amulets were also advised; these often consisted of images of the gods and were to be hung around the neck or tied to the foot. A whole variety of drugs are mentioned, including castor oil, which was used as a purgative. All sorts of animal substances were used, including the fat of various animals and bile. Medicine in ancient Egypt would appear to have been of an empirical or magical variety.

Of even more interest to us in our study of the early history of surgery was the discovery by a

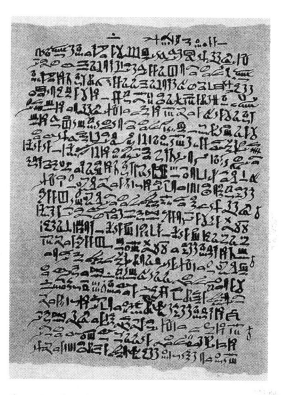

Figure 2.4 The Edwin Smith papyrus.

young American egyptologist named Edwin Smith of another papyrus at the same place as the Ebers papyrus. It remained in Smith's possession until his death in 1906, when his daughter gave the papyrus to the New York Historical Society. The complex task of translation was entrusted to Professor James Breasted. The Smith papyrus (Figure 2.4), like the Ebers papyrus, dates from about 1550 BC, but Breasted demonstrated that it was undoubtedly a copy of much more ancient text, since it used Egyptian words that were no longer current at that time. It comprises 48 case reports which commence with the top of the head and proceed systematically downwards – nose, face, ears, neck and chest – and then mysteriously stop at the spine. Having described the physical signs of the patient, the surgeon goes on to decide on the outlook of the case. If the prognosis is good, or if there is a chance of success, treatment is then advised. If hopeless, then the

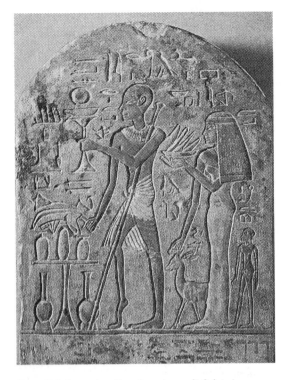

Figure 2.5 An ancient Egyptian stone relief showing a patient with obvious poliomyelitis. Note the shortened right leg with muscle wasting and talipes deformity, together with the crutch.

patient should be left to his inevitable fate. This guarded attitude was widespread in antiquity, when there was rich reward for recovery of your wealthy patient but grave risk of punishment in the case of failure.

The description of a patient with a dislocated jaw and its treatment is very similar to that which can be found in a modern textbook:

If you examine a man having a dislocation of his man-dible, should you find his mouth open, and his mouth cannot close again, you should put your two thumbs upon the ends of the two rami of the mandible inside his mouth and your fingers under his chin and you should cause them to fall back so that they rest in their places.

Equally clear are the instructions concerning a fracture of the upper arm:

If you examine a man having a break in his upper arm and you find his upper arm hanging down separated from its fellow, you should say concerning him – one having a break in his upper arm. An ailment which I will treat. You will place him prostrate upon his back with something folded between his two shoulder blades; you should spread his two shoulders in order to stretch apart his upper arm until the break falls into place. You shall make for him two splints of linen and you apply one of them to the inside of the arm and the other to the underside of the arm. You shall bind it with ymrw (an unidentified mineral substance) and treat it with honey every day until he recovers.

From these writings it appears that the only surgical conditions treated, just as our evidence from Babylon suggests, were wounds, fractures, dislocations and abscesses. The exception is that circumcision was performed, presumably by priests, as part of a religious ceremony among the nobility (see Figure 1.5).

From the earliest days of Egyptian civilisation, belief in reincarnation meant that members of the royal family and nobility had their bodies preserved. Initially, this was merely done by drying the corpse in sand, but over the centuries increasingly sophisticated techniques of embalming were developed. As a result of our examination of these preserved bodies, a great deal has been learned of the diseases of ancient Egypt. These include congenital deformities such as club foot, dental decay, arthritis, bone tumours and fractures. Some of these injuries, indeed, show treatment by quite sophisticated splinting (see Figure 1.4). Models in tombs and wall carvings demonstrate a variety of diseases, including poliomyelitis, spinal kyphosis and achondroplasia (Figures 2.5, 2.6 and 2.7).

China

The Chinese traced their history back to six emperors. Shen Nung was the inventor of agriculture, Huangt Ti of ships, the bow and arrow, music and writing, Fu Hsi founded the arts of hunting and fishing, the emperors Yao and Shu established the calendar and administration, while the emperor Yu controlled the floods of the Yellow River. According

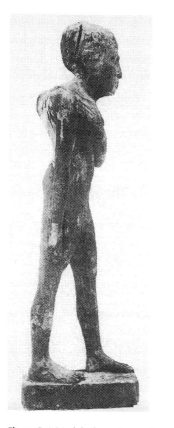

Figure 2.6 Model of a patient with a kyphosis, probably tuberculosis.
Cairo Museum.

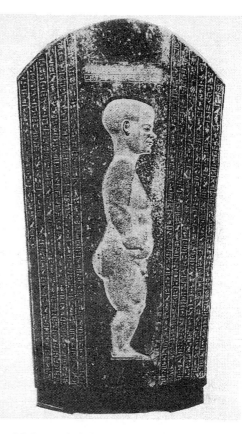

Figure 2.7 Stone relief of an achondroplastic.
Cairo Museum.

to Chinese tradition, these rulers lived between 2852 and 2205 BC. To what extent these kings were legendary inventions will probably never be established but certainly, by the second millennium BC, thousands of bones since excavated were inscribed with characters in a script not fundamentally different from the Chinese picture writing of later periods.

Over these thousands of years, China remained more or less in isolation and it is not surprising that a system of medicine developed there that was quite different from its Western counterpart. It was based on the Taoist philosophy of life; a kind of world spirit, the Tao, permeated all growth and decay and was an interplay between two forces, Yang and Ying. Yang was hard, male, creative and dark, hot and dry, in contrast to Ying which was light, soft, receptive, feminine, cold and moist. Health depended on harmony between these opposing forces. Disease represented disharmony. Treatment had its goal in the restoration of harmony by stimulating Ying or Yang so that balance would be regained and health restored. Life force, composed of Ying and Yang, flows through channels in the body which are related to points on the skin. By assessing the patient's symptoms and by careful palpation of the pulses, the medical practitioner could determine which part was diseased, which channel affected and which force was

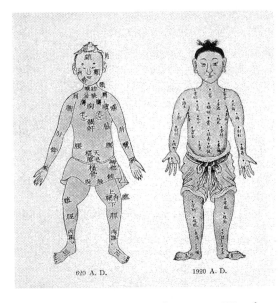

620 A. D.   1920 A. D.

Figure 2.8 Chinese acupuncture diagrams, A D 630 and 1920.
From William Osler: *Evolution of Modern Medicine*. New Haven, Yale University Press, 1921.

responsible. From earliest times the phenomenon of the pulse in the different parts of the body fascinated Chinese physicians and the pulse became the most important sign by which internal processes of the body could be determined. Even the pulse of a pregnant woman could be used to diagnose the sex of the expected child: 'When the pulse of the left hand is rapid, without fading, the woman will give birth to a male child'. The segment of the pulse at the right wrist gave information concerning the state of the lungs, that of the left side on the condition of the heart. A second segment of the right wrist indicated whether the spleen and stomach were affected, while another on the left wrist determined the state of the liver and bile or whether the condition was being caused by an excess of Ying or Yang. Palpation of the pulses, and comparison with the physician's own was an elaborate ritual which might take several hours. The modern doctor is taught to recognise the rate of the pulse, its force and various irregularities that may

occur; how much more sophisticated the Chinese physicians could have been is a matter for speculation although the prolonged contact between doctor and patient must surely have been a source of comfort to the latter.

By stimulating appropriate parts of the skin, Ying and Yang could be restored to harmony and the patient to health. This stimulation could be carried out either by burning the powdered leaves of the mugwort, a procedure called moxibustion, or by using needles (acupuncture). This form of treatment has been continued for thousands of years and has enjoyed a recent vogue in the alternative medicine of the West (Figure 2.8).

In addition, Chinese medicine employed the use of herbal remedies, and this was widely developed. In the 16th century, a 52 volume compendium entitled Classification of Roots and Herbs was published by a government official, Li Shih-Chou; this catalogued no less than 1892 medications, many of which extended back into ancient history.

Examination of the patient, apart from the pulse, played little part in diagnosis. Indeed, high-class ladies would not be examined at all by the practitioner. A small wax or ivory model was employed on which the patient could point out the site of her pain and discomfort to her physician.

Dissection was frowned upon since ancestor worship forbade the mutilation of the body of a dead person, so that knowledge of anatomy was primitive and restricted to accidental glances at dead or wounded persons or butchered animals. Surgery, apart presumably from the treatment of wounds and other injuries, was almost non-existent in contrast to the flourishing art in neighbouring India. Indeed, there appears to have been only one ancient Chinese surgeon of note, Hua Tuo (?AD 190–265), who is pictured operating on the upper arm of the war lord general Kuan Yun (Figure 2.9) for what was probably an infected wound of the arm. He offered trephination of the skull to Prince Sao, who was suffering from severe headaches. Unfortunately the Prince suspected that the surgeon wished to murder him and ordered his execution. Hua Tuo indeed might well have been a

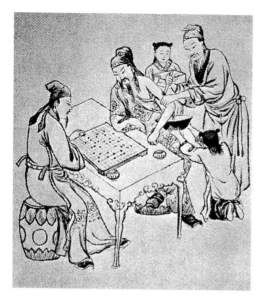

Figure 2.9 Hua Tuo drains an abscess on the arm of General Kuan Yun who shows his indifference to pain by playing a board game with his aide-de-camp.

foreigner who entered China from India who was therefore acquainted with the Indian art of surgery.

The single operation that was carried out in ancient China was not as a treatment of disease. Many court employees and officials were eunuchs. The operation of castration would have been dangerous, since probably all the external genitalia were removed – an operation that persisted into the 20th century. According to tradition, when the surgeon Hua Tuo was imprisoned by order of the emperor, he entrusted his manuscripts to his jailer who burned them all except his improved castration method.

India

As with the other ancient civilisations, there is much controversy concerning the early dating of Indian culture in general and the development of surgery in particular. In about 1500 BC, the Aryans invaded the Indian subcontinent from Central Asia and brought with them the Sanskrit language. The earliest writings on Indian medicine are to be found in the Vedas, the books of knowledge which were believed to be of divine origin. Here we can read of sages who would carry bags of healing herbs and who would care for the injured, remove arrows and spears from the wounded, and who would employ a plant named after the god Soma, which would relieve pain. In addition, they would cauterise wounds and snake bites and might even have developed a catheter in order to relieve retention of urine and which would 'open the flow of urine again like a dam before a lake'.

The earliest Indian surgical author was Susruta. It will probably never be ascertained whether he was an actual historical personage or a name to which collected works of surgical literature are attributed. The time of his existence is also vague, but it was some time after Christ. His works were translated into Arabic around AD 800 and are often quoted in the writings of Rhazes.

Susruta stressed the requirements for students who wished to study medicine and surgery. They should be of tender years, born of a good family, possessing the desire to learn, strength, energy of action, contentment, character, self-control, a good retentive memory, intellect, courage, purity of mind and body, have clear comprehension, command a clear insight into the things studied and should have thin lips, thin teeth, a thin tongue and be possessed of a straight nose, large, honest, intelligent eyes, with a benign contour of mouth and a contented frame of mind, be pleasant in speech and dealings and painstaking in their efforts. Even today, it would be difficult to find medical students who are such paragons of virtue!

Today, much emphasis is placed on surgical training using models in order to improve technique. The writings of Susruta include advice on how surgeons should practise the art of suturing on animal skins or strips of cotton, improve their bandaging on life-sized dolls, practise surgical incisions on water melons or cucumbers, cauterise a piece of meat before trying this method on their patients, and practise the ligature of blood vessels

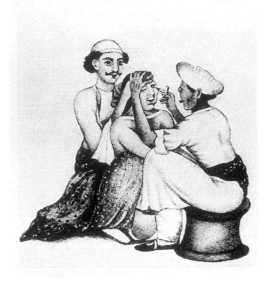

Figure 2.10 Couching for cataract. This early 19th century drawing shows the procedure as described by Susruta.

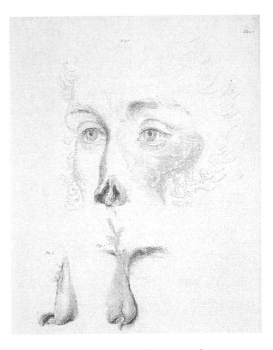

Figure 2.11 Joseph Carpue's illustration of reconstruction of the nose in 1814 using the Indian technique. ('An account of two successful operations for restoring a lost nose from the integuments of the forehead' London, 1816)

and of blood letting on lotus stems and the veins of dead animals. A disciple was expected to study for a period of at least six years.

It is quite evident that Hindu surgery at this time had reached a high state of excellence. For example, there is a detailed description of the operation for removal of a cataract, in which the opaque lens of the eye is mobilised and then pushed downwards into the lower part of the globe in order to allow restoration of vision:

In the morning in a bright place, the temperature being moderate, let the surgeon sit on a bench as high as his knee opposite the patient. The latter, having washed and eaten and been tied, sits on the ground. After he has warmed the patient's eye with the breath of his mouth, rubbed it with his thumb and detected the uncleanness which has formed in the pupil, he orders the patient to look down at his nose. Then, while the patient's head is held firmly, he takes the lancet between his forefinger and middle finger and thumb and introduces it into the eye towards the pupil, on the side, half a finger's breadth from the black of the eye (the pupil) and a quarter of a finger's breadth from the outer corner of the eye. He moves it back

and forth and upwards. Let him operate on the left eye with the right hand or on the right side with the left. If he has probed correctly, there is a sound and a drop of water comes out painlessly. Speaking words of courage to the patient, let him moisten the eye with women's milk, then scratch the pupil with the tip of a lancet without hurting. If the patient can see objects, the doctor should draw the lancet out slowly, lay cotton soaked in fat over the wound and let the patient lie still with bandaged eyes. (Figure 2.10)

Susruta also describes what must have been the earliest plastic surgical procedure, the restoration of an amputated nose by means of a skin graft turned down upon the forehead. Removal of the nose was a punishment for adultery in those days, so there was no shortage of patients for this procedure. Interestingly, it evidently remained in practice in India among itinerant surgeons for hundreds of years. A newspaper account of this in 1814 prompted

Joseph Carpue of London to perform a very similar operation, using the forehead skin flap, with success in two army officers (Figure 2.11).

The first patient had lost his nose from syphilis. A forehead flap was fashioned and stitched around the defect. The viability of the flap gave some initial anxiety but it fortunately recovered and the cosmetic result was good. The second patient, another officer, was a hero of the battle of Albuera, in the Peninsular War in 1810. In saving the regimental colours, the poor fellow lost an arm and sustained five other wounds, one taking off part of the cheek and the nose. Again, the operation was a success.

Carpue was born in 1764 in Hammersmith. He was a catholic, who first considered entering the Church, but instead studied at St.George's hospital under Sir Everard Home, becoming a member of the Company of Surgeons in 1798. The following year he was appointed to the surgical staff at the Duke of York's Hospital, Chelsea. He died in 1846.

3

Surgery in Ancient Greece and Rome

Ancient Greece

It can be truly said that 'modern' rational medicine, divorced from the supernatural forces of possession by the devil or by evil spirits, was founded in Ancient Greece.

An important concept that influenced not only medical but also lay concepts of disease was the humoral theory of Empedocles (?500–430 BC), developed by later Greek philosophers, in particular Aristotle (384–322 BC). This theory stated that everything derives from four elements – water, air, earth and fire – with their associated qualities respectively of wetness, coldness, dryness and heat. With this theory, later writers combined the somewhat similar doctrine of Hippocrates, which held that the body was composed of the four humors or fluids, black bile, yellow bile, blood and phlegm, with their associated temperaments – melancholic, choleric, sanguine and phlegmatic. A balance of these humors determined the health of the individual and the subject's temperament also resulted from his prevailing humor, thus the sanguine, phlegmatic, choleric or melancholic temperament. To this day, we still talk of an 'aerial spirit' or of a 'fiery nature' and indeed this doctrine of the four elements persisted into the 17th century. Much of our modern medical traditions and many of today's medical terms derive from Ancient Greece.

The Greek culture absorbed knowledge from Mesopotamia via Asia Minor and also from Egypt. By the 6th century BC, medical schools were flourishing on the island of Cos and on the adjacent peninsula of Cnidos, which is now in modern Turkey.

The most famous medical teacher of Cos was the man who is commonly regarded as the 'Father of Medicine', Hippocrates (470–400 BC). He was born on Cos, the son of a physician (Figure 3.1). Such a person undoubtedly existed and he is mentioned by his younger contemporary, Plato. However, the collection of Hippocratic writings, comprising some 70 works, probably represents the teachings of a number of authors associated with Hippocrates during and after his lifetime and often expresses contradictory views. Their titles include Fractures, Aphorisms, Epidemics, Prognostics, Ulcers, Surgery, Fistulae, and Haemorrhoids.

The Hippocratic writings are characterised by being factual; they contain descriptions of careful observations of actual patients, they resist elaborate theories of disease and emphasise the power of nature to heal, encouraged by suitable diet, rest and exercise. In severe cases, further aid may be given by blood letting, purging or sweating, and occasionally radical surgical intervention is required.

Modern doctors find it a fascinating exercise to interpret some of the clinical descriptions in these writings. For example, case nine of The Epidemics states:

The woman who lodged at the house of Tisamenas had a troublesome attack of Iliac passion (acute abdominal pain and distension), much vomiting; could not keep her drink; pain about the hypochondria, and pains also in the lower part of the belly; not thirsty; became hot; extremities cold throughout with nausea and insomnolency; urine scanty and thin; dejections undigested, thin, scanty. Nothing could do her any good. She died.

16

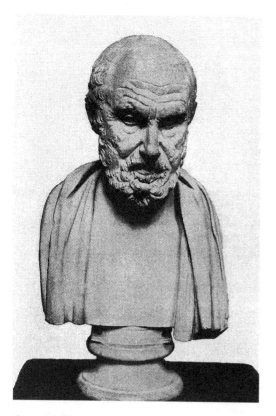

Figure 3.1 Hippocrates: a conventional bust, since no one knows what he really looked like!
From William Osler: *Evolution of Modern Medicine.* New Haven, Yale University Press, 1921.

This sounds to me like an attack of appendicitis with rupture and peritonitis. Perhaps the best known of his clinical descriptions is that of the patient dying of infection, which we still term the Hippocratic Facies:

Nose sharp, eyes hollow, temples sunk, ears cold and contracted and their lobes turned out, the skin about the face dry, tense and parched, the colour of the face as a whole being yellow or black, livid or lead coloured.

From the surgical point of view, Hippocratic writings give us descriptions of how to carry out treatment of wounds, fractures and dislocations; there are also descriptions of elective operations for a number of surgical conditions. Careful advice

is given to the surgeon on how to conduct himself. He is told that:

The nails should be neither longer nor shorter than the points of the fingers and the surgeon should practise with the extremities of the fingers, the index finger being usually turned to the thumb; when using the entire hand it should be prone; when both hands, they should be opposed to one another. Greatly promote a dexterous use of the fingers when the space between them is large and when the thumb is opposed to the index. One should practice all sorts of work with either hand and with both together, endeavouring to do them well, elegantly, quickly, without trouble, neatly and promptly.

Detailed advice is given about how to apply a bandage:

It should be done quickly, without pain, with ease and with elegance; quickly by despatching the work; without pain by being readily done; with ease, by being prepared for everything; with elegance, so that it may be agreeable to the sight.

In Articulations we find a description of the method of reducing a dislocation of the shoulder which is still used today and which, indeed, is termed the Hippocratic method (Figure 3.2):

The patient must lie on the ground on his back while the person who is to effect the reduction is sitted on the ground upon the side of the dislocation; then the operator seizing with his hand the affected arm, is to pull it while with his heel in the armpit he pushes in the contrary direction. A round ball of a suitable size must be placed in the hollow of the armpit, for without something of the kind the heel cannot reach to the head of the humerus.

In Wounds of the Head there is a detailed description of trephination of the skull. The surgeon is advised:

While trephining, often remove the instrument and dip it in cold water, if you do not do this, the trephine becomes heated by the circular motion and heating and drying the bone may burn it and cause an unduly large piece of the bone around the sawing to come away.

The trephine was held either between the palms of the hands and rotated by the action of rubbing them together, or was rotated by a cross-piece and thong.

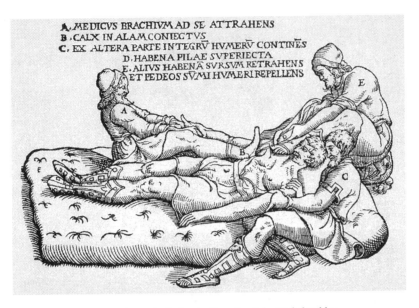

A. MEDICVS BRACHIVM AD SE ATTRAHENS
B. CALX IN ALAM CONIECTVS
C. EX ALTERA PARTE INTEGRV HVMERV CONTINĒS
D. HABENA PILAE SVPERIECTA
E. ALIVS HABENĀ SVRSVM RETRAHENS
ET PEDEOS SVMI HVMERI REPELLENS

Figure 3.2 The Hippocratic method of reduction of a dislocated shoulder.
From an edition of Galen's works published in Basel in 1562.

In the book On Haemorrhoids there is a rather horrifying description of the surgical treatment of piles and one can only stand amazed at the courage of the patient submitting himself to this treatment:

Having laid him on his back, and placing a pillow beneath the breach, force out the anus as much as possible with the fingers and make the irons red hot and burn the pile until it be dried up and so that no part may be left behind.

Another method of curing haemorrhoids is as follows:

You must prepare a cautery and an iron that exactly fits to be adapted to it, then the tube being introduced into the anus, the iron, red hot is to be passed down it, and frequently drawn out so that the part may bear the more heat and no sore may result from the heating, and the dried veins may heal up.

However, should the patient decide against operative treatment, various local applications are described containing alum, honey, the shell of the cuttlefish and various other ingredients.

Malaria was very common and often fatal in Ancient Greece. A particularly serious variant is 'blackwater fever'; here the red cells are broken down by the malaria parasite in large numbers and the released haemoglobin pigment is excreted in the urine. The following case report seems to be a classical example of this condition:

Philliscus lived by the wall. He took to his bed with acute fever on the first day and sweating; night uncomfortable. Third day, until midday, he appeared to have lost the fever, but towards evening acute fever, sweating, thirst, dry tongue, black urine. Sleepless; completely out of his mind. Fifth day, distressing night, irrational talk, black urine, cold sweat. About midday on the sixth day he died. The breathing throughout as though he were recollecting to do it, was rare and large.

The irregular breathing of a dying patient, described in the last sentence, is termed Cheyne–Stokes respiration in commemoration of two Irish physicians in the 19th century who brought it to the attention of the medical profession. Here it is, described quite clearly in the Hippocratic writings.

Not only did Hippocrates and his followers lay down a rational approach to medicine but they also emphasised the importance of the doctor–patient relationship. Nothing better reflects the spirit of the Hippocratic physicians than the oath which was obviously designed for a young man to swear on entering his apprenticeship to his physician master. This lays down the regard he must owe to his teachers, and emphasises the overall importance of the patient and the sacredness of the patient's confidence:

I swear by Apollo the healer, invoking all the gods and goddesses to be my witnesses, that I will fulfil this oath and this written covenant to the best of my ability and judgement.

I will look upon him who should have taught me this Art even as one of my own parents. I will share my substance with him and I will supply his necessities, if he be in need. I will regard his offspring even as my own brethren, I will teach them this Art, if they would learn it, without fee or covenant. I will impart this Art by presence, by lecture and by every mode of teaching not only to my own son but to the sons of him who has taught me, and to disciples bound by covenant of oath, according to the law of medicine.

The regimen I adopt shall be for the benefit of the patients according to my ability and judgement, and not for their hurt or for any wrong. I will give no deadly drug to any, though it be asked of me, nor will I council such, and especially I will not aid a woman to procure abortion. I will not cut persons labouring under the stone, but will leave this to be done by men who are practitioners of this work. Whatsoever house I enter, there will I go for the benefit of the sick, refraining from all wrong-doing or corruption, and especially for any act of seduction of male or female, of bond or free. In my attendance on the sick, or even apart therefrom, whatsoever things I see or hear concerning the life of men, which ought not to be noised abroad, I will keep silence thereon, counting such things to be as sacred secrets. Pure and holy will I keep my life and my Art. While I continue to keep this oath unviolated, may it be granted to me to enjoy life and the practice of the Art, respected by all men in all times. But should I trespass and violate this oath, may the reverse be my lot.

Of relevance to today's debates on medical ethics, note the Hippocratic proscriptions against euthanasia and abortion.

Aristotle (384–322 BC) followed closely after Hippocrates and, although not himself a physician, had a profound effect on medical thought and practice for succeeding centuries. Indeed he can be regarded as one of the greatest scientific geniuses

the world has ever seen. Aristotle was the son of a physician and a pupil of Plato; later he became tutor to the young Alexander the Great. Although Aristotle never dissected a human being, he carried out anatomical studies of a wide range of animals, laid the foundation of embryology by studying the developing chick, and gave an accurate account of the life of bees. He laid the basis of the doctrine of evolution, describing a ladder of nature ascending through lower plants, higher plants, insects, fish, mammals to man.

Soon after the deaths of Hippocrates and Aristotle, the great days of Athens drew to an end. The Macedonian, Alexander the Great, the pupil of Aristotle, conquered Greece, Asia Minor and Egypt, marched through Persia and reached India. In his progress he founded a string of at least 17 Alexandrias but it was Alexandria of Egypt that was by far the most important. After the death of Alexander, one of his generals, Ptolemy, declared himself Pharaoh, took up residence in Alexandria and there founded a great medical school and library at about 300 BC; into these institutions were imported scientists, mainly from Greece. Unfortunately the vast library, said to have contained some 700 000 manuscripts, was burned by a mob of fanatics intent on destroying the past, a phenomenon not unknown in later periods of history! We have to rely, therefore, on the writings of Galen and other authors to learn something of the Alexandrian school of medicine. Of particular fame were two surgeons, Herophilos and Erasistratos, both of whom flourished around 300 BC. Their most important contribution was systematic dissection of human bodies; indeed, Celsus states that they actually performed vivisections on condemned criminals. Herophilos (flourished c. 300 BC) named the duodenum and prostate and established the brain as the centre of consciousness; his name survives in one of the venous sinuses of the brain. Erasistratos (? 330–250 BC) is regarded by some as the founder of physiology; he distinguished the cerebrum from the cerebellum, noted the difference between sensory and motor nerves, and gave a good description of the heart valves.

With the absorption of Egypt into the Roman Empire in 50 BC and with the death of Cleopatra in 30 BC, marking the end of the Ptolemaic dynasty, Alexandria ceased to have great medical influence and Rome became of central importance.

Ancient Rome

According to tradition, Rome was founded in 753 BC by Romulus and Remus. Be that as it may, a tribe called the Latins lived on the site of Rome at around this time and by 509 BC the Romans had driven out the Etruscans and established Rome as a republic. By 201 BC, Rome had defeated Hannibal, annexed Carthage on the coast of North Africa and dominated the Mediterranean.

Roman surgery was strongly influenced by Greece. Upper class Romans considered medicine in general, and surgery in particular, as being beneath the notice of a cultured individual, and most practitioners were imported from Greece. However, it was a Roman nobleman, Celsus (25 BC–AD 50), who wrote a great encyclopaedia dealing with philosophy, law, medicine and probably other subjects around AD 30. The only parts of this to have survived are the eight books entitled De Re Medicina. Celsus was almost forgotten for some centuries, but he was the first classical medical writer to appear in print (AD 1478) and his writings were highly valued during the Renaissance. The last two books deal with surgery. Celsus describes the surgery of injuries, fractures and dislocations, diseases of the nose, ear and eye, of hernia, bladder stone and varicose veins. He gives an account of the surgery for cataract; this is performed with a needle which is 'inserted through the two coats of the eye until it meets resistance, and then the cataract is pressed down so that it may settle in the lower part'. He describes how diseased tonsils can be removed: 'tonsils that are indurated after an inflammation, since they are enclosed in the thin tunic, should be disengaged all round by the finger and pulled out'.

Among the many Greek immigrant surgeons must be mentioned Soranus of Ephesus (AD 90–138),

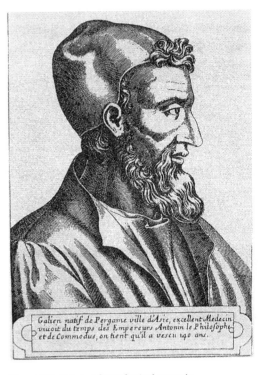

Galien natif de Pergame ville d'Asie, excellent Medecin vivoit du temps des Empereurs Antonin le Philosophe et de Commodus, on tient qu'il a vescu 140 ans.

Figure 3.3 Galen; a hypothetical portrait.

who studied in Alexandria and flourished under the Roman emperor Hadrian. As well as writing on fractures and skull injuries, Soranus can be regarded as one of the founders of obstetrics. He introduced the birth stool, which had supports for the back and arms and a crescent-shaped aperture. He also described the necessity of emptying the bladder before delivery of the baby.

Undoubtedly the most famous of the physicians of this period, and indeed perhaps of all time, was Galen (? AD 131–201) (Figure 3.3). He was born at Pergamon, in what is now Turkey, devoted himself to the study of medicine at an early age, and at 21 was a student of anatomy at Smyrna. He studied extensively in Asia Minor and Alexandria; here he had the opportunity of examining a human skeleton. In AD 158 he returned to Pergamon as surgeon to the gladiators and in the next five years developed an extensive practice in traumatic surgery. He then moved to Rome, where he became physician to the

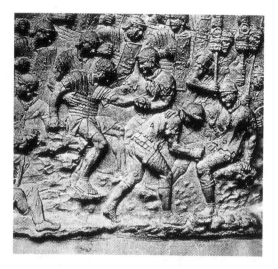

Figure 3.4 Detail of Trajan's column in Rome. Surgeons attending to wounded Roman legionnaires. Author's photograph.

emperor Marcus Aurelius. He dissected and experimented extensively on animals, since human dissection was not permitted, and wrote vast numbers of books on anatomy, physiology, pathology, therapeutics and, indeed, on every branch of medicine known at the time. He produced no specific surgical textbook, but his writings on surgery are scattered throughout his books. He describes operations for varicose veins, repair of a cleft lip, removal of polyps from the nose and suture of the intestine after penetrating injuries of the abdomen.

There was much that was good in Galen's didactic writings; for example, he gave excellent descriptions of the skeleton and the muscular system, worked out the physiology of the spinal cord by injuring it at various levels, and gave a description of the cranial nerves. However, he had no real knowledge of the circulation of the blood. He thought that blood passed from the heart to the tissues both in the arteries and the veins. New blood was manufactured in the liver and was burnt up in the tissues like fuel consumed by fire. He taught that there were invisible pores between the right and left sides of the heart chambers, which allowed blood to cross this barrier.

The whole corpus of Galen's knowledge was regarded as sacred by later generations. Galen's teachings remained almost unchallenged for the next 1500 years, until the 16th century, when men learned once more to observe nature. The dissections of Vesalius (1514–1564) swept away many of Galen's false anatomical concepts, and William Harvey (1578–1657), using experimental observations, proved the true nature of the circulation of the blood.

Before leaving Ancient Rome, mention must be made of the highly efficient and well planned hospitals that were established throughout the Empire to deal with wounded and sick soldiers. An inspection of Trajan's column in Rome (Figure 3.4) reveals reliefs of surgeons hard at work binding up the wounds of injured legionnaires.

4

The Dark Ages and the Renaissance

Alaric the Goth and his hordes entered Rome in AD 410, and this date marks the fall of the Roman Empire in the West. Following this, little progress was made in the art and science of medicine in general, and surgery in particular, until the beginning of the Renaissance after some 1000 years of the Dark, or the Middle, Ages. Much that had been learned by the Greeks and Romans was forgotten. The practice of tying blood vessels to control bleeding, for example, was abandoned and was replaced by the barbarous practice of using boiling oil or the red-hot cautery. Medical schools did not exist, dissection was forbidden by Church edict, and the practice of surgery was usually left in the hands of itinerant quacks. After all, knowledge other than that which made a man 'wise unto salvation' was useless; all that was necessary for this was either contained in the Bible or taught by the Church. Science was simply disregarded. Disease was the result of divine displeasure. When sinning became bad enough it would be punished by hell-fire and eternal damnation. A plague would be visited on a sinful community. Conversely, recovery from illness could be brought about by the faith of the sick subject or through the medium of prayer to God the merciful. This was the period of the healing saints, such as the twin brothers St Cosmas and St Damian, who became the patron saints of medicine and who will be encountered again in the chapter on transplantation (Chapter 15).

Illness might be caused by sin, but it also gave opportunity for redemption among the sick and an opportunity of service by the clergy, so that the Dark Ages saw the establishment by monks of hostels for the poor wanderers and infirmaries for the ill and dying (Figure 4.1). Some of these establishments, founded in the Middle Ages, still exist, for example the Hôtel Dieu in Lyon, which dates back to the 6th century, and the first in London, St Bartholomew's, which was founded in 1123 by Rahere, a canon of St. Paul's Cathedral, in the reign of Henry I.

The stream of scientific medicine, which dried up in most of the known civilised world, survived in three locations: Southern Italy, the Byzantine Empire and among the Arabs.

Southern Italy

Greek was the language of Southern Italy – a meeting ground of Latins, Greeks and Saracens. During the Dark Ages, the lamp of old learning was kept alight in the university in the town of Salernum (Salerno) 30 miles south-east of Naples, which was established about the 9th century AD. At the medical school dissection of animals, especially the pig, and occasionally of a human, was carried out. Medical and surgical clinics existed with both male and female professors and there were apothecaries and sisters of charity (Figure 4.2).

The medical school at Salerno reached its height of fame in the 11th and 12th centuries and perpetuated the authority of Hippocrates and Galen. Its most prominent teacher was Constantinus Africanus (1010–1087), a native of Carthage in North Africa (as shown by his name) and a Christian monk.

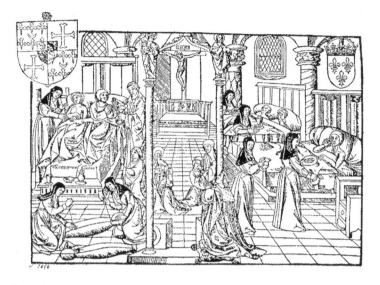

Figure 4.1 A hospital ward in the 1500s; the Hôtel Dieu, Paris. Note two patients to a bed, being ministered to by nuns and a priest, and bodies being sewn into their shrouds.
From Singer C, Ashworth Underwood E: *A Short History of Medicine.* Oxford, Oxford University Press, 2nd edition, 1962.

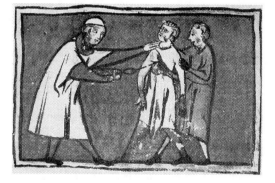

Figure 4.2 Extraction of an arrow from the arm.
From a 14th century manuscript of Roger of Salerno.

He was familiar with the writings of both the Greeks and Arabs, and his translations of the works of the Arab physicians Rhazes and Avicenna were responsible for their being introduced into the West.

One work among all others spread the fame of the School of Salerno. This was the Regimen Sanitatis, a poem on popular medicine, diet and household remedies. It was originally written as a work of medical advice for Robert, Duke of Normandy, the eldest son of William the Conqueror. It spread throughout the civilised world in numerous manuscript copies and remained popular for centuries. Indeed, the first English translation was published in 1607 by Sir John Harington, an Elizabethan courtier, and it is well worth reading today:

Another piece of medical wisdom might not be so socially acceptable today:

Great harmes have grown, and maladies exceeding
By keeping in a little blast of wind.
So crampes and dropies and colickies have their breeding –
For want of vent behind.
Drink not much wine, sup light and soon arise,
when meat is gone, long sitting breedeth smart:
and afternoon still waking keep your eyes.
When moved you find yourself to nature's needs,
forbeare them not, for that much danger breeds,
use three physicians still; first Dr Quiet,
next Dr Merry man and Dr Diet.

By the 15th century, the School of Salerno was declining in relation to other universities in Italy and was finally suppressed in 1811 by Napoleon Bonaparte.

Byzantium

Between the 3rd century and the fall of Constantinople to the Turks in 1453, a series of Byzantine physicians kept alive the Greco-Roman traditions of medicine. These included Oribasius, Aetius of Amida and Paul of Aegina. Oribasius (325–403) of Pergamum, the birthplace of Galen, wrote the Encyclopaedia of Medicine which included descriptions of screw traction and elaborate pulleys for the reduction of fractures. Aetius of Amida (502–575), physician to Justinian I, also produced extensive compilations with emphasis on the Greek medical authors. However, he is also credited with the first description of ligation of the brachial artery for aneurysm:

An aneurysm located at the end of the elbow is thus treated. First we carefully trace the artery leading to it from the armpit to the elbow along the inside of the arm. Then we make an incision on the inside of the arm, three or four finger breadths below the armpit, where the artery is easily felt. We expose the blood vessel, and when it can be lifted free with the hook, we tie it with two ligatures and divide it between them. We fill the wound with incense and a lint dressing and then apply a bandage. Next we open the aneurysm itself and no longer fear bleeding. We remove the blood clot present and seek the artery which brought the blood. Once found, it is lifted free with the hook and tied as before. By again filling the wound with incense we stimulate good suppuration.

Aetius gave descriptions of other surgical operations, including tonsillectomy and excision of haemorrhoids, but whether he actually carried out the procedures remains somewhat doubtful.

Paul of Aegina (625–690) studied and practised in Alexandria. He too produced a massive compendium of Greek and Roman medicine in Greek in seven volumes. His writings were translated into Arabic and then back into Latin in the Renaissance. His sixth volume is entirely devoted to surgery. He advises removal of the testis in hernia repair, describes removal of the breast for cancer and trephination of the skull, and gives this account of tracheostomy:

In inflammation about the mouth and palate and in cases of indurated tonsils which obstruct the mouth of the windpipe, as the trachea is unaffected it would be proper to have recourse to pharyngotomy in order to avoid the risk of suffocation. When we engage in the operation we slit open a part of the trachea below the top of the windpipe, about the third or fourth ring, for this is a convenient situation, being free of flesh and because the vessels are at a distance from the part which is divided. Therefore, bending the patient's head backwards so as to bring the windpipe better into view, we make a transverse incision between two of the rings so that it may not be the cartilage which is divided but the membrane connecting the cartilages . . . we judge that the windpipe has been opened from the air rushing through it with a hissing noise and with the voice being lost. After the urgency of the suffocation has passed over, we pare the lips of the incision so as to make them raw surfaces and then have recourse to sutures, but sew the skin only without the cartilage.

This description would well serve a modern textbook.

Paul's accounts of bleeding, cupping and the extensive use of the cauterising iron for all sorts of conditions were going to dominate surgical treatment when the fall of Constantinople dispersed many Greek scholars and medical manuscripts to Western Europe.

Arabian Medicine

The third and by far the most important preservers of Greek culture were the Arabians.

From the beginning of the 7th century to the beginning of the 8th, in a period of less than 100 years, an empire spread from the Arabian Peninsula along North Africa, across the Straits of Gibraltar to Spain, and through the Middle East, Egypt and Palestine to the Caspian Sea. Shortly after the conquest of Egypt, Greek works were translated into Arabic and these, of course, included the writings of Hippocrates, Aristotle and Galen. The writings of the physicians of India and Persia were also translated and, by the end of the 9th century, this influx of culture produced notable scientists and physicians, of which the most famous were Rhazes, Avicenna and Albucasis.

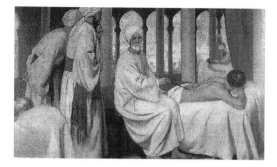

Figure 4.3 Albucasis applying the cautery to the back of a patient.

Rhazes (854–925), a native of Ray, near modern Tehran, became the Caliph's personal physician in Baghdad. He wrote extensively, gave a careful account of smallpox, which he differentiated from measles, and produced the largest and heaviest medical book printed before 1500! The Persian Avicenna (980–1037) was a child prodigy. By the age of 10 he could recite the Koran by heart. He trained in medicine, practised in Baghdad and published The Canon, a codification of Greek and Arabic medicine. Translations of this work were appearing until the 17th century, the last edition being printed in 1663.

Schools of medicine were founded in Spain in Cordoba, Seville and Toledo, as well as in the important cultural centres in Cairo, Baghdad and Damascus in the East. The most famous professor in Cordoba was Albucasis (926–1013) (Figure 4.3), who wrote the only textbook in Arabic that treated surgery as a separate subject. This was the last of his 13 volumes, termed The Collection. In his introduction, Albucasis complained that surgery had almost completely disappeared as a specialty in Spain. Proficient surgeons could no longer be found as a result of the absence of anatomical knowledge; dissection indeed was prohibited. It gives several examples of surgical incompetence:

I have seen an ignorant physician incise of a scrofulous tumour of the neck in a woman, open the cervical arteries and provoke such haemorrhage that the patient died in his hands. I have seen another doctor undertake the extraction of a stone in a very old man. The stone was huge; in performing the extraction he removed a portion of the bladder wall. The patient died in three days.

Albucasis' textbook included many illustrations of surgical instruments, among which can be found a guillotine for removal of the tonsils, a trocar for draining off ascitic fluid from the abdominal cavity, and a concealed knife for drainage of an abscess. Surgery is to be avoided wherever possible and the cautery preferred to the knife. Bleeding, cupping and the use of leeches are important means of treatment. An interesting finding in his chapters on the treatment of fractures is a good description of a fracture of the penis. He recommends splinting it by means of the skin of a goose neck, which is pushed over the member.

In the 12th century, a translation institute was founded in Toledo and vast numbers of works on philosophy, mathematics, astronomy and medicine, representing much Greek, Roman, Persian and Indian culture, as well as Arabic, were translated into Latin and so became available in Western Europe.

The Renaissance

The Renaissance ('rebirth') in the arts, science, medicine and, of particular interest in this book, surgery in Europe after the long centuries of the Dark Ages was not a sudden phenomenon; indeed, it spread over a long period from its first glimmerings in the 12th century to its full flourishing in the 15th through to the end of the 16th century. Moreover, this awakening occurred at very different times in different parts of Europe, as it steadily spread from the South. Its causes were multiple: the development of new universities; the introduction of printing, which is attributed to Johannes Gutenberg (1400–1468) of Mainz and which allowed more rapid dissemination of knowledge; the conquest of Constantinople by the Turks in 1453, which saw an influx of Byzantine scholars into the West, especially Italy; the development, or rather the

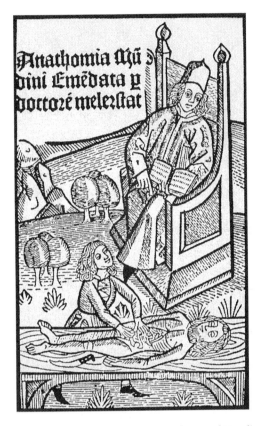

Figure 4.4 A dissection from the Anathomia of Mundinus, 1316. The professor sits in his professorial chair while an assistant dissects under his instruction. Compare this with Figure 4.13.

rediscovery, of the concept of learning by direct observation than by rigid adherence to ancient authority; and, finally, the papal ban on human dissection became less and less strict and was eventually lifted in the early 16th century, thus allowing an enormous expansion in anatomical, physiological and pathological knowledge.

Certainly the new universities, which were established in the 12th and subsequent centuries, played an important part in the awakening of medicine, even though medical teaching at first was entirely theoretical, based on the ancient Greek and Roman writings, and with no element

of instruction at the patient's bedside or in the autopsy room.

An important landmark in medical teaching took place in Bologna, in Northern Italy where, under the influence of the School of Salerno, a medical faculty was established in the 12th century by Hugh of Lucca (1160–1257). Here, public dissection of the human body was first performed in the 14th century. However, these post-mortem examinations were for forensic rather than scientific purposes, in an attempt to establish the cause of death of the victim. The anatomical dissections were simply used as a teaching aid to verify the writings of Avicenna, themselves, of course, based on those of Galen. The classical illustrations of dissections at that time (Figure 4.4) show the dissection itself being carried out by a lowly servant, while the professor, seated aloft and aloof on his professorial chair, reads from a large tome and certainly keeps well clear of the bloody and smelly proceedings below.

Little is known directly of Hugh of Lucca, founder of the Bologna school, but his contributions have come down to us in the writings of his most distinguished disciple, the Dominican friar Theodoric (1205–1296) (Figure 4.5). The latter was one of a small group of clerics who were trained in surgery as well as medicine. In 1257 he published his Chirurgia, which disputed the currently held view, based on the teachings of Galen and the subsequent Arabic authors, that suppuration and the formation of pus were the necessary adjuncts of wound healing. If this failed to occur, it was promoted by the surgeon's use of packs and dressings of various rather foul and greasy ointments. Indeed this theory that pus was 'laudable' and should be encouraged, held sway until the teachings of Lister, and was only denied by a number of independent surgical thinkers, of whom Theodoric must count as the first. He wrote:

As all modern surgeons profess, pus should be generated in wounds. No error can be greater than this. Such a practice is indeed to hinder nature, to prolong the disease and to prevent the consolidation of the wound.

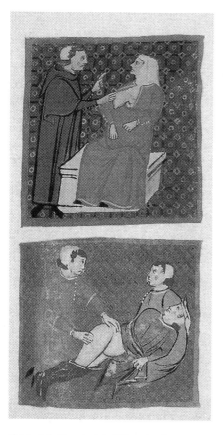

Figure 4.5 Theodoric's Chirurgia of 1257; examinations of the breast and rectum.

His advice on wound management has a modern ring to it:

In whatever part of the body a cut may have occurred, let everything be done in order. Indeed, above all else a wound must be made clean. Secondly, having brought the lips of the wound together, they should be replaced accurately in the position which they had in their natural state; if necessary they should be held there by stitches taken in accordance with the size of the wound. Let the size and depth of the wound determine the closeness and depth of the stitches . . . after the suturing has been properly done and the dressings have been carefully arranged, let the wound be bound up skilfully as the position and condition of the part require, that is to say so that neither the stitches nor the dressings can be disturbed at all. And, just as we have often said before, do not undo the dressing until the third or fourth or fifth day if no pain occurs. Afterwards let the dressings be changed every third day unless too much putridity should occur in the wound, in which case it should be changed every day. And always, whenever the dressing is changed, by pressing gently upon the wound with a little wine-soaked tow you may express any retained bloody matter. Afterwards let it be bound up according to the aforesaid method and let it be kept thus until the patient has completely recovered.

An important contemporary of Theodoric was William of Salacet (1210–1277), who taught surgery at Bologna and later at Verona. At the end of his career, in 1275, he published his major work Cyrurgia, which was the first systematic treatise on surgery to emerge after the Middle Ages. One of its five volumes was devoted to surgical anatomy. William advocated the use of the knife rather than the cautery and initiated the practice of quoting patients he had treated personally rather than quoting from the classical authors. His book was full of good advice to the young surgeon:

The wise physician does not commit any wickedness, he does not sow or excite discord among the relatives of the patient, he does not give any advice that is not asked for, he does not employ people who have a bad reputation or a vice which is displeasing to respectable persons. He should not have any quarrel with the inhabitant of the house, for all this spoils the operation and degrades the physician.

With regard to fees, he advises as follows:

Know just this; a remuneration worthy of your labours, that is to say, a very good fee, makes for the authority of the physician and increases the confidence which the patient has in him, even if the physician be of great ignorance (!).

The third of the great surgical teachers of Bologna was perhaps the most important of them all as regards historical significance. Mondino de Luzzi (?1275–1326), usually known by his Latin name of Mundinus, must be given the credit of reviving the study of the anatomy of the human body by systematic dissection, which had remained dormant for some 1500 years since the days of the great Alexandrian anatomists, Erasistratus and Herophilus (see Chapter 3). Mundinus was born in Bologna and

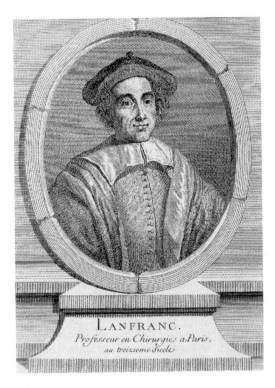

Figure 4.6 Lanfranc.
From Zimmerman L, Veith I: *Great Ideas in the History of Surgery*. Baltimore, Williams and Wilkins, 1967.

spent his life there, receiving his medical degree in 1290 and becoming Professor of both Anatomy and Surgery at the University, a joint chair which became traditional and which persisted for the next two centuries at this and at other Italian universities. It says much for Mundinus that he descended from the height of his professorial chair and performed dissections personally. We can presume that his subjects for dissection were mainly executed criminals for he writes 'Having the body of one that had died from decapitation or hanging on his back . . .' and then proceeds with his anatomical description.

The treatise on anatomy, Anathomia, by Mundinus was published in 1316 (see Figure 4.4) and was the first modern textbook on the subject. Many manuscript copies were circulated and it appeared in print in 1478. It remained as a standard text for

some 200 years until replaced by the great Fabrica of Vesalius that we shall describe later.

However, although Mundinus revolutionised the study of anatomy by performing human dissections personally and publicly, he himself was far from having a revolutionary outlook on the subject and remained firmly convinced that the writings of Galen were infallible. For example, the description of the liver in Galen's writings, which was based on dissection of lower animals, presented it as having five lobes. Mundinus, in spite of the fact that he could observe that this was not true in man, states 'the intrinsic and integral parts are five lobes. Yet in man these lobes are not always distinct'.

A bridge between Italian surgery and the renaissance of surgery in France was created by Guido Lanfranchi, known as Lanfranc (?–1315) (Figure 4.6), who may be regarded as one of the founders of the French School of Surgery. Trained in Milan, he left Italy as a result of the unrest in the feuds between the Guelphs (supporters of the Pope) and the Ghibellines, their aristocratic rivals, and moved to Paris in 1295. There he joined the Guild of Barber Surgeons, the College of Saints Cosmos and Damien (the patron saints of surgery), which had been founded in 1260. Lanfranc's teachings in Paris attracted surgeons from near and far and his book Chirurgia Magna appeared in many editions and translations. He describes at length the requirements of a good surgeon:

He must have a balanced temperament, his hands must be well shaped with long slender fingers and he should not tremble. He should be humble, of a strong mind but not over-confident. He should be versed in all the sciences not just medicine, should live a virtuous life without greed, adultery, jealousy or envy. In the home of the patient, he should not look at any woman nor quarrel with the patient's family. He should avoid dealing with hopeless cases but should give assistance to the poor.

Lanfranc deals with haemorrhage in great detail; he recognises arterial, venous and capillary bleeding. If the haemorrhage cannot be stopped with the application of a simple bandage soaked in the white of an egg, he advises compression of the bleeding vessel with the finger for well over an hour (during which time, of course, clotting will occur). If this does not succeed, the surgeon must pull out the end of the blood vessel in order to twist it or to tie it using a silk thread or otherwise to sear it with a cautery. He describes nerve injuries and notes that, when a nerve has been completely divided, the limb loses its feeling and mobility. For this, he advises applying sutures in order to approximate the nerve endings.

Here he describes his successful treatment of a patient with, as any surgeon today would recognise, Ludwig's angina:

I will set in this place a cure that befell a lady in the city of Milan of a lady that was fifty winters old and had a quinsy of phlegm that occupied all her neck in front within and without, except that most of the swelling was outward, and the woman could not speak or swallow. And this woman was under the cure of a young man that was my scholar, and he could not well fare therewith and so he was in despair of her life. I was sent after and found her in a wicked state, for she ate no meat for many days before, and she dared not sleep, lest she should be choked. Then I felt her pulse and it was remarkably feeble, and I felt the base of the abscess and I knew well that she would choke before the abscess broke externally or internally, for the matter was so great. And then I took a razor and looked where the matter was most collected to accomplish drainage and it was most able under the chin, and I felt the base with my hand and palpated it about that I might beware of nerves and arteries, and there I made a wound and drew out the matter that was corrupt, and all and it was foul stinking matter and all might I not avoid anon. And so the patient had bettered breathing, and her pulse was comforted that the lungs might take in air and herewith the heart was comforted, and then I gave her broth, and that escaped through the most part through the wound, so I studied how I might best do, and I had made a pipe of silver and put it in her mouth and passed it beyond the wound, that it might fulfil the place of the throat . . . and the woman began to be stronger and when the wound was made clean I dried it up and sewed it, and it is in this manner the patient was made well.

Another important link between Italian and French surgery took place at the end of the 13th century, when a Frenchman, Henri de Mondeville (1260–

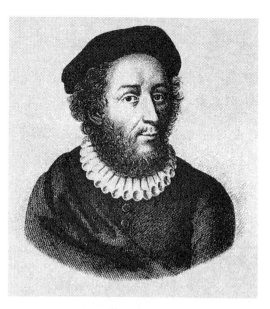

Figure 4.7 Guy de Chauliac.
From Zimmerman L, Veith I: *Great Ideas in the History of Surgery*. Baltimore, Williams and Wilkins, 1967.

1320), came to Bologna and studied under Theodoric. In 1301 he moved to the medical school at Montpellier in Southern France. Here, as in Paris, a guild of barber surgeons had been established in 1252 – indeed, rather earlier than in the capital city. Like his teacher, de Mondeville believed that primary healing of wounds was possible and desirable. His textbook, *Chirurgie*, was the first to be written by a Frenchman. It became popular and many manuscript editions have been preserved. It was soon translated into French from the original Latin and also appeared in a Dutch translation. Of the major operations, de Mondeville only describes amputation, which he performed in cases of gangrene. However, he recognised that once gangrene had progressed above the knee the patient was doomed. Unfortunately, de Mondeville died, probably of tuberculosis, before his great textbook could be finished.

An important contributor to the development of French surgery was Guy de Chauliac (1298–1368), a cleric who studied at Toulouse, Montpellier and Paris (Figure 4.7). Like Henri de Mondeville, he

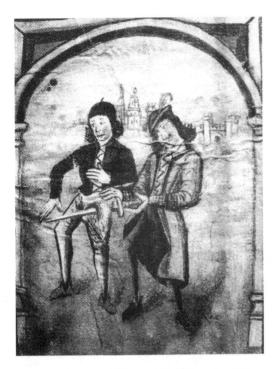

Figure 4.8 Extraction of a sword blade from the thigh. From Guy de Chauliac's *Chirurgia Magna.*

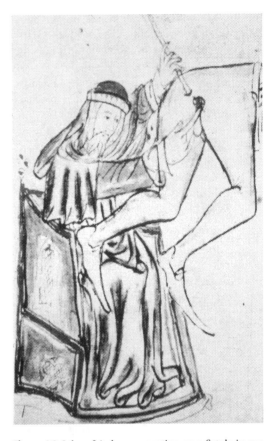

Figure 4.9 John of Arderne operating on a fistula in ano. From John of Arderne: *Treatises of Fistula in Ano, Haemorrhoids and Clysters* (edited by D'Arcy Power, London, Keegan Paul, 1910).

spent some time in Bologna. He became the personal doctor of three successive Popes in exile in Avignon. When in his sixties, he wrote his seven-volume *Chirurgia Magna*, one of the highlights in surgical history. It appeared in many manuscript editions and, after the invention of printing, in several languages and some 56 printed editions, one as late as 1683. As well as quoting extensively from the great authorities of the past, it is based also on a lifetime of practical experience (Figure 4.8). De Chauliac described a variety of operations for hernia, cataract extraction and amputation, a procedure he was reluctant to perform.

The first English surgeon of distinction, John of Arderne (1306–1390), flourished at about this period (Figure 4.9). We do not know where he trained, but he obtained considerable surgical experience during the Hundred Years' War as a surgeon first to the Duke of Lancaster and later to John of Gaunt.

His war service included the Battle of Crécy in 1346 and he would have seen some of the earliest examples of gunshot wounds. Leaving the army in 1349, John settled in Newark and moved to London 20 years later. He served as Serjeant surgeon to Edward III.

John of Arderne was particularly interested in rectal diseases and indeed is regarded as the father of proctology. He wrote the first book dealing with this topic, *Treatises of Fistula in Ano, Haemorrhoids and Clysters*. Fistula in ano was particularly common in those times and regarded usually as incurable. John realised that this condition was

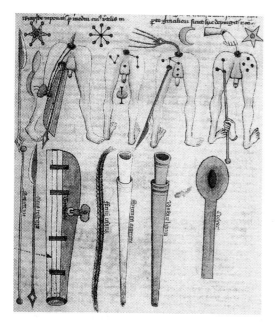

Figure 4.10 Illustrations of fistula in ano and the surgical instruments used in its surgery. Note the multiple external openings of these complex cases of anal fistulae.
From John of Arderne: *Treatises of Fistula in Ano, Haemorrhoids and Clysters* (edited by D'Arcy Power, London, Keegan Paul, 1910).

often the result of a perianal abscess and both these conditions were common among the nobility who spent many hours in the saddle in their suits of heavy armour, drenched in sweat, alternating in periods of cold and damp. Not surprisingly, therefore, many of John's patients came from the upper ranks of society. He realised that early treatment of abscesses around the anus was important and wrote:

And I have proved it for certain experience that an abscess breeding near the anus should not be left to burst by itself, but the leech should visually for to feel with his finger the place of the abscess, and whereso is found any softness, there, the patient not knowing, be it boldly opened with a very sharp lancet so that the pus and the corrupt blood may go out. Or else, forsooth, the gut or the bowel that is called rectum that leads to the anus will burst within the anus . . . if it bursts both within and without, then it can never be cured except by a surgeon full expert in his craft. For then may it from the first day be called a fistula. (Figure 4.10)

For the established fistula, John of Arderne's operation was similar to the technique employed today; a ligature was threaded through the track into the anus and then tied tightly to prevent bleeding. He then incised the tissue in the grasp of the ligature to lay open the entire track. If multiple sinuses were present, each of them had to be opened. He stressed the importance of after-care, which insisted upon cleanliness and the avoidance of irritating ointments and salves used by other practitioners.

Bold as a surgeon, John was also not hesitant in charging large fees:

Therefore for the cure of Fistula in Ano, when it is curable, ask he competently of a worthy man and a great a hundred mark or forty pounds with robes and fees of a hundred shillings term of life by year. Of lesser men forty pound or forty mark ask he without fees and take he naught less than a hundred shillings. For never in my life took I less than a hundred shilling for cure of that sickness.

During the long blossoming of the Renaissance, great advances were also being made, of course, in many branches of science and discovery. The sea voyagers of Spain, Portugal, England and the Low countries were enlarging the known world; Christopher Columbus reached the Americas in 1492. Nicholas Copernicus (1473–1543) published *On the Revolutions of the Celestial Spheres* and placed the Sun, not the Earth, at the centre of the Universe. Galileo Galilei (1564–1642) invented the telescope and the compound microscope and was one of the fathers of modern physics. Santorio Santorio (Sanctorius) (1561–1636), Professor of Medicine at Padua, measured the pulse of patients using the pendulum and studied the body temperature by means of a thermometer devised by Galileo – he may be regarded as the father of modern physiological measurements. William Harvey (1578–1657), who studied at Cambridge and Padua and was physician to Charles I, published *De Motu Cordis* (*The Motion of the Heart*) in 1628 and demonstrated, on the basis of detailed animal and human observations, the mechanism of the circulation of the blood. The final element in Harvey's argument, the actual passage of blood from the arteries to the veins via capillaries, as he postulated, was demonstrated by Marcello Malpighi (1628–1694) of Bologna in his microscopic study of the lung of the frog. Malpighi established microscopic anatomy as a subject; he demonstrated the fine anatomy of the spleen, liver and skin, and laid the basis of early embryology by his study under the microscope of the development of the chick embryo.

The renaissance of anatomy

In the history of surgery, the importance of the Renaissance was that it saw the birth of modern anatomy. For centuries, surgeons and anatomists 'saw what they believed' – the teachings of the ancient Greeks and Romans, often handed down to them in inaccurate translations. Now they were to learn to 'believe what they saw' and to trust their own observations.

Many of the great artists of the Renaissance, including Dürer, Michelangelo and Raphael, began to study anatomy closely, realising that a knowledge of the muscles and bones in particular was essential for accurate reproduction of the human form in their paintings and sculptures. Some, at least, actually engaged in dissection for this purpose; this was undoubtedly true of Leonardo da Vinci (1452–1519), who carried out detailed studies in some 100 dissections of the human body. He made meticulous drawings of the internal viscera, the pregnant uterus and the fetus, injected wax to study the ventricular cavities of the brain and introduced cross-sectional studies of the limbs. He never published his work although his superb illustrations (Figure 4.11) have come down to us today. There can be little doubt that he shared his detailed knowledge with others. Interestingly, he delineated the maxillary sinus, the cavity in the maxilla which so regularly gets infected as a complication of the common cold, a century before its 'official' description by Nathaniel Highmore (1613–1688), a physician at Sherborne ('the antrum of Highmore').

We have already noted the important contribution of Mundinus, Professor of Surgery and

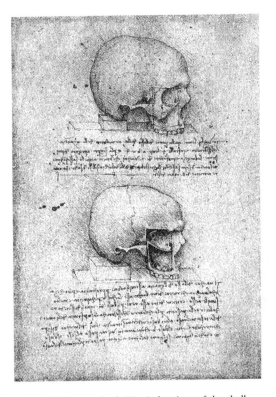

Figure 4.11 Leonardo da Vinci, drawings of the skull. The lower one demonstrates the maxillary antrum (for the first time).
From the Queen's Collection at Windsor Castle, reproduced with permission of The Royal Collection © 2008, Her Majesty Queen Elizabeth II.

Anatomy at Bologna until his death in 1326, who advocated and performed direct dissection of the human body. However, it was the surgeon-anatomist Andreas Vesalius (1514–1564), more than two centuries after Mundinus, who most significantly affected the evolution of the science of medicine at this period and must be regarded as the father of modern anatomy (Figure 4.12). Vesalius was born in Brussels the son, grandson and great-grandson of physicians and apothecaries, and studied first at Louvain and then Paris. Here his teacher was Jacobus Sylvius (1478–1555), who, although he introduced the injection technique for the study of blood vessels, was a confirmed Galenist who taught

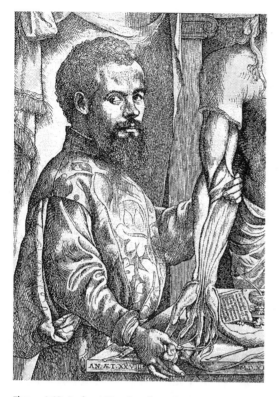

Figure 4.12 Andreas Vesalius, from De Humani Corporis Fabrica 1543.

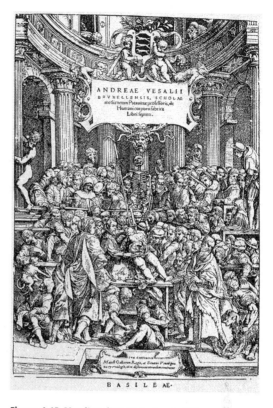

Figure 4.13 Vesalius dissects in front of his students at Padua. The frontispiece to De Humani Corporis Fabrica 1543.

from the textbook rather than from dissection, in the best medieval tradition. Vesalius moved back to Louvain and then to Padua, where he received his doctorate in medicine with highest distinction and was immediately appointed Professor of Surgery at the age of 23. In the footsteps of Mundinus, but unlike his immediate predecessors, he performed his own dissections. His masterly demonstrations attracted crowds of students from all over Europe.

In 1538 Vesalius published his *Tabulae anatomicae Sex*, six sheets of anatomical charts, three depicting the arterial, venous and caval vascular systems, which were probably drawn by Vesalius himself, and three drawings of the skeleton, drawn by the Flemish artist, John Stephen of Calcar (?1499 –?1546), who had trained under Titian. These were an immediate success, but were soon followed, in

1543, by the most famous anatomical atlas and text of all time, the *De Humani Corpora Fabrica*, (*The Structure of the Human Body*), in seven volumes, of a total of more than 700 pages, and with 250 illustrations. This was published in Basle when Versalius was a mere 28 years of age.

There is still something of a mystery, and some debate, as to the artist, (or artists?) of the *Fabrica*. John Stephen of Calcar is the most likely, but his name is nowhere mentioned in the text. He is believed to be the beardless man with the floppy hat immediately to the left and above the head of Vesalius in the frontispiece (Figure 4.13), but this head is 'brushed out' from the second edition, published in 1555, some nine years after Calcar's death.

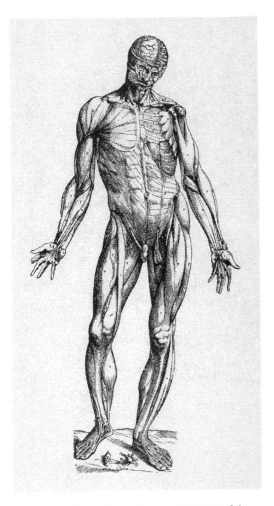

Figure 4.14 The muscles of the anterior aspect of the body. A woodcut from the Fabrica of 1543. Illustrations such as these are often better than those found in some modern texts!

The woodcut illustrations are highly accurate and obviously made directly from the dissected body; they are works of art that can be, and indeed frequently are, used to illustrate today's textbooks and lectures (Figure 4.14).

Although an instant success, the *Fabrica* (so well-known that its shortened title is often used) also aroused envy and attack. Vesalius had no hesitation in pointing out mistakes in classical writings, even those of the sacred Galen. For this he was attacked by a number of his teachers and colleagues, including Sylvius.

Vesalius realised that many of the mistakes in Galen arose from dissections having been made on animals and not on man. For example, the human liver does not possess five lobes, nor is the kidney lobulated as it is, for example, in the pig. Other classical errors were simply nonsense. For example, men do not have a rib missing ('Adam's rib') but have 12 on each side just as in the female! Galen had postulated that pores existed between the right and left chambers of the heart to enable blood to pass from one to the other. Vesalius pointed out in the *Fabrica* that this was not so:

Not long ago I would not have dared to diverge a hair's breadth from Galen's opinion. But the septum is as thick, dense and compact as the rest of the heart. I do not, therefore, see how even the smallest particle could be transferred from the right to the left ventricle through it.

Overall, Vesalius corrected 200 of Galen's anatomical mistakes.

A year after the publication of his masterpiece, Vesalius retired from academic life at the age of only 29 and entered the service of Charles IV and then Philip II of Spain as a practising surgeon. In 1563 he set off on a long pilgrimage to the Holy Land but on his return was shipwrecked on the islet of Zante in the Peloponnese and died of exposure and hunger.

To defy dogma was often dangerous in those days. The Spanish anatomist Michael Servetus (1511–1553) was burned at the stake by order of John Calvin for the heresy of writing that the blood, having been mixed with air in the lungs, passes back into the heart. He was a true martyr for anatomical truth.

5

The Age of the Surgeon-Anatomist: Part I – From the mid 16th century to the end of the 17th century

Following the renaissance in anatomy, and the publication of The *Structure of the Human Body* by Andreas Vesalius in 1543, there began a long period of surgical development – a period that will take us up to the discoveries of anaesthesia and antisepsis in the mid 19th century. These 300 or so years were characterised by the evolution of the surgeon-anatomists; these were men well acquainted with the anatomy of the human body, most of whom spent a considerable part of their training in the dissecting room, and who would push forward the frontiers of surgery as far as possible with the primitive means available to them. Remember their disadvantages: no means except alcohol or opium to assuage the agonies of their manipulations; no knowledge of bacteria and the causes of the wound inflammation that bedevilled their operations; primitive ideas of the body's physiology and of the underlying pathology of most of the diseases they encountered – cancer, tuberculosis, syphilis and so on. Yet, within these severe limitations, they devised methods of dealing with fractures, bladder stones, arterial injuries and diseases, hernias, cataracts and many superficial tumours. Of course, the patient would only submit to the surgery if the condition rendered life in peril, the deformity unbearable or the pain intolerable.

We can perhaps best illustrate this period by describing some of the surgical giants of these centuries; men who, by their example, their ingenuity, their teachings and their writings, alone or in combination, justify their inclusion in these pages.

The 16th century

One of the leading surgeons of the 16th century is acknowledged as the father of war surgery, and he will be encountered again in Chapter 9. Ambroise Paré (1510–1590) (Figure 5.1) was a barber-surgeon who trained at the Hôtel Dieu in Paris, stressed the importance of anatomy, and indeed kept with him for many years a dissected specimen. He writes:

I attest having a body given me after execution by the Criminal Lieutenant. I dissected it 25 years or more ago. I dissected nearly all the muscles of the right side so when I wanted to make some incision, seeing the parts afresh made me more sure in my work; the left side was left complete. To preserve it better, I punctured it in many places with a punch to let the liquor penetrate deeply into the muscles and upper parts. One can still see the entire lungs, heart, diaphragm, stomach, spleen and kidneys. Similarly one can see the hair of the beard, the head and other parts, the nails which I have noticed growing evidently after cutting them several times.

Here is an example from Paré's case reports that demonstrates the value of fundamental anatomical knowledge:

At this point I want to advise the young surgeons that sometimes the testes are not yet descended into the scrotum. They are retained in the groin and make a painful tumour, and since it is considered an intestinal hernia it is treated with astringent plasters, trusses and bandages to restrain it. This increases the pain and prevents descent of the testis. Not long ago I was called to such a case and after finding a single testis in the scrotum, the child not having been castrated, had the plaster and

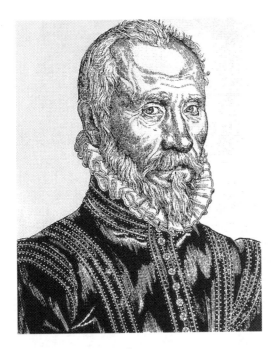

Figure 5.1 Ambroise Paré.
From Keynes G, ed.: *The Apologie and Treatise*. London,
Falcon Press, 1951.

the truss he wore removed. I told the father to let the child
run and jump to help the testis descend to its natural
place, which it did little by little without any complication.

One of Paré's most important contributions was
to teach the use of the ligature in preventing haemorrhage from blood vessels in trauma and in limb
amputation. He describes the following case:

A sergeant of the Châtelet got a sword thrust in the throat
in Pré-au-Clercs [the Pré-au-Clercs field outside the walls
of Paris which in Paré's day was much used for private
duels. Being convenient to his house, he treated many of
the casualties!]. It cut the external jugular vein completely
across. As soon as he was injured he put a handkerchief on
the wound and came to my house to find me. When he
removed the handkerchief blood flowed very freely.
I immediately tied the vein towards its root; thus it was
stanched and he recovered, thanks to God.

If you had followed your method of stanching the blood
with cauteries, I wonder if he would have recovered.
I believe he would have died in the hands of the operator.

Paré published his extensive writings, not in Latin
(which he never learned), but in his native French
so that the humblest surgeon apprentice could
learn from him. Reading the above pithy examples
of his style, one is not surprised at the popularity of
his numerous books, whose publications were
spread over his long life, from his first *The Method
of Treating Wounds Made by Firearms* in 1545, a
little work of 64 pages illustrated with 23 figures, to
his *Apologie and Treatise Containing the Trips
Made in Divers Places* in 1585.

A less well known French-born contemporary of
Paré, but one who well deserves our recognition as
a shining star of Renaissance surgery, was Pierre
Franco (?1500–1561). He was born in Provence of
humble parents and had little schooling, but was
early apprenticed to a barber-surgeon. As a Protestant, he was forced to flee from France and practised
his calling in Lausanne in Switzerland, although
he eventually returned to Orange in France and his
major work, *Treatise on Hernias*, was published in
Lyon in 1561, just before his death. He deplored the
fact that surgeons of his day rejected the use of open
operations. This was because of the risks involved
in such procedures, which they would often leave
in the hands of charlatans. Franco was obviously
a bold surgeon who carried out a wide range of
the operative procedures known at that time. He
describes in great detail his method of radical surgery for strangulated hernia, devising an incision at
the base of the scrotum which he claimed was less
dangerous than the higher incision. He also carried
out cataract surgery and plastic operations on the
face and described a new method for operating on
cleft lip. In the surgery for bladder stone he was
equally inventive; in Chapter 12 we shall encounter
him again as the first surgeon to remove a bladder
stone successfully via an abdominal approach.

In Italy, Gaspare Tagliacozzi (1545–1599) was
another example of a pioneer who did not fear to
attempt, with all its difficulties at that time, major
surgery. He can be regarded as the father of plastic
surgery and we shall meet him again in Chapter 15.
He was born, trained and practised in Bologna,
where he was appointed Professor of Surgery.

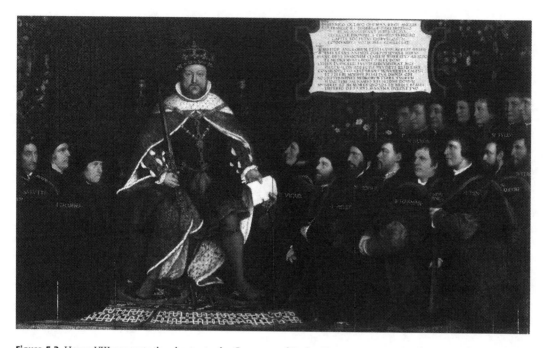

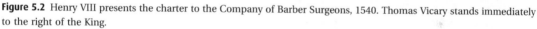

Figure 5.2 Henry VIII presents the charter to the Company of Barber Surgeons, 1540. Thomas Vicary stands immediately to the right of the King.
This painting is in the Hall of the Company of Barber-surgeons, London (reproduced by kind permission of the worshipful company). The cartoon is to be seen in the Edward Lumley Hall of the Royal College of Surgeons of England.

Two years before his death he published *On the Surgery of Mutilations by Grafting* which describes the operative methods evolved by him over many years of trial and error and which was illustrated with numerous clear drawings. He described reconstruction of the ears and lips, and his description of replacement of the nose lost either as a result of trauma or of syphilis by means of an arm flap pre-dated the pedicle flap of Harold Gillies in the First World War by some 300 years (see Chapter 9).

In England, a trivial event was to have important consequences in the evolution of surgery in this country. In 1525, King Henry VIII visited Maidstone in Kent. There he met a local surgeon, Thomas Vicary (?1495–1561), who treated his chronic varicose ulcer of the leg with some success. Vicary was promptly appointed Surgeon to the King and in 1530 became Master of the Company of Barbers as well as the Serjeant Surgeon. This appointment carried with it the requirement to accompany the sovereign into battle – a duty last called upon when John Ranby (1703–1773) was present at the battle of Dettingen with King George II. Vicary's genius lay in administration and organisation, so that in 1540 he no doubt used his royal influence to obtain a charter from Henry to incorporate the Company of Barbers and the Guild of Surgeons into the Company of Barber-surgeons. This event has been immortalised in the painting by Hans Holbein, the cartoon of which hangs in the Great Hall of the Royal College of Surgeons of England and the painting itself in the hall of the Company of Barbers. This is probably the best known medical group portrait in the United Kingdom (Figure 5.2).

Vicary became the first Master of the Barber-surgeons Company, which decreed that surgeons should no longer act as barbers and that barbers should restrict their surgery to dental extractions.

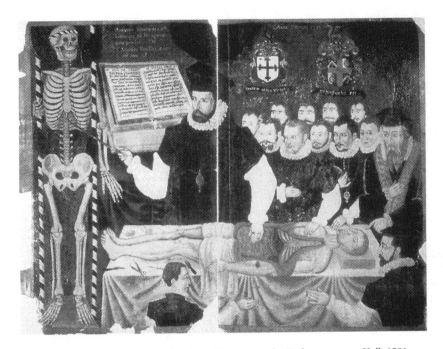

Figure 5.3 John Bannister giving the Visceral Lecture at the Barber-surgeons Hall, 1581. From a print at Barber's Hall. The original is in the Glasgow University Library.

The Company was entitled to fine unlicensed practitioners in London and also to have the bodies of four executed prisoners each year for the purpose of dissection (Figure 5.3). Apprentices were to serve for seven years and then to attend the Barbersurgeons Hall for examination. Even after qualification, members of the Company were obliged, under penalty of a fine, to attend the anatomical dissections and the lectures given in their Hall. They were allowed to treat 'all outward hurts and tokens of disease' but were not permitted to administer medicine for internal complaints. The Company existed until 1745 when the union was dissolved, the Surgeons and the Barbers reverting to their former independent states. The Worshipful Company of Barbers still exists as one of the ancient Livery Companies of the City of London. The Company of Surgeons was the forerunner of the Royal College of Surgeons of England.

Vicary himself was no pioneer surgeon. He appeared to ignore the discoveries of Vesalius even though a pirated version of the *Fabrica* had been published in English by Thomas Geminus in 1545. Three years later, Vicary's *A Treasure for the Englishman Containing the Anatomie of Man's Body* was published. This appears to be an abridgement of a 14th century manuscript and is nothing more than a medieval relic translated into English. However, it proved to be a popular work and reached its 11th edition in 1651. As a textbook on the subject it contributed nothing at all, indeed its influence was a retrograde one; its popularity seems to have rested on the useful recipes for medicaments which it included.

Vicary was appointed to the staff of St Bartholomew's Hospital in 1548. The cause of his death and his place of burial are unknown and there does not appear to be a monument erected in his memory.

The establishment of the Company of Barbersurgeons was typical of a move throughout Western Europe at about this time to organise surgeons

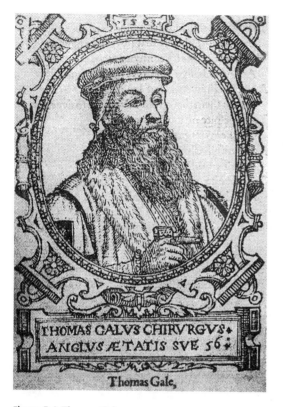

Figure 5.4 Thomas Gale.
Royal College of Surgeons of England.

into professional bodies and to distinguish them from the quacks, barbers, itinerant tooth-drawers and charlatans that provided much of the surgical care of former times. In Scotland, a decree by James IV established the Incorporation of Barber-surgeons in Edinburgh in 1505, and in 1599 the Faculty of Physicians and Surgeons received its charter in Glasgow. King Philip II of Spain, in his capacity as Count of Holland, in 1556 granted the Barber-surgeons Guild in Amsterdam, only recently detached from its association with the clog and patten makers, the status of an independent organisation with the annual privilege of dissecting a human cadaver. For this purpose, the judiciary had to place at the disposal of the Company the mortal remains of a criminal who had been executed.

In Paris, the Barber-surgeons had formed a guild in the mid 14th century. Since they carried out menial duties such as barbering and venesection, they were rather despised by the academic surgeons of the College of St Côme. Since the barber-surgeons were more accessible, greater in number and, perhaps, cheaper than their academic colleagues, they were certainly more popular, and undoubtedly the fame of Ambroise Paré contributed to this.

Three British surgeons of the 16th century are worthy of note.

Thomas Gale (1507–1587) (Figure 5.4) served as an army surgeon under Henry VIII and was Serjeant Surgeon to Elizabeth I. He succeeded Vicary as Master of the Company of Barber-surgeons. Gale wrote extensively – in English rather than Latin – and vigorously attacked quacks and charlatans who posed as surgeons. In 1563 he published his *Excellent Treatise of Wounds made with Gunshot* in which, like Paré, he denied that gunshot wounds were poisoned by gunpowder and needed to be treated by boiling oil.

Gale writes this vivid account of the maltreatment of the sick poor by quacks:

In the year 1562 I did see in the two hospitals in London called St Thomas' Hospital and St Bartholomew's Hospital to the number of 300 and odd poor people that were diseased of sore legs, sore arms, feet and hands, with other parts of the body, so sore infected that 120 of them could never be recovered without loss of a leg or of an arm, a foot or a hand, fingers or toes, or else their limbs crooked so that they were either maimed or else undone for ever. All these were brought to this mischief by witches, by women, by counterfeit rascals that take upon them to use the art, not only of robbing them of their money but of their limbs and perpetual health. And I, with certain other, diligently examining these poor people, how they came by their grievous hurts and who were their chirurgions that looked unto them and they confessed that they were either witches, which did promise by charms to make them whole, or else some women which would make them whole with herbs and such like things, or else some vagabond rascal which runneth from one country to another promising unto them health only to deceive them of their money.

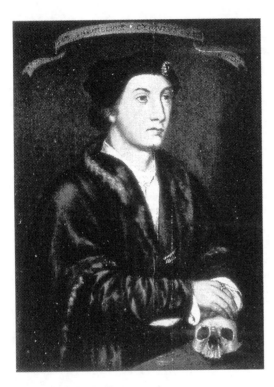

Figure 5.5 William Clowes.
Royal College of Surgeons of England.

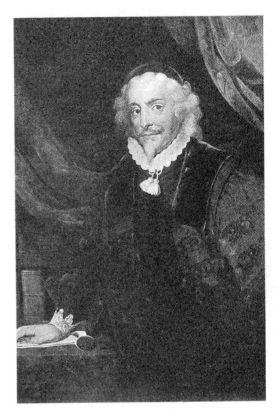

Figure 5.6 Peter Lowe.
Royal College of Surgeons of England.

William Clowes (1540–1604) (Figure 5.5) had an extensive experience of war surgery, both on land and at sea, and on the basis of this wide experience devised a surgical chest for the use of military surgeons with a carefully compiled list of the drugs and supplies it carried. Later he served on the surgical staff of St Bartholomew's Hospital, London. He published a book on syphilis, a disease which came under the care of the surgeon, entitled *A Brief and necessary Treatise, Touching the Cure of the Disease now usually called Lues Venera* as well as *A proved Practice for all Young Chirurgions, concerning Burnings with Gunpowder and Wounds made with Gunshot etc*. He indicated in his writings an earnest wish to pass on the benefits of his observations to younger surgeons and again wrote in English rather than Latin. He too did not believe that gunshot wounds were poisoned by gunpowder,

although he became convinced that it was possible for a bullet to be intentionally smeared with poison before firing.

Peter Lowe (1550–1612) (Figure 5.6) was one of the first, and certainly one of the most important of the early surgeons in Scotland. He left Scotland at about the time of the Reformation in that country and probably studied medicine in Orleans in France. After 30 years of practice on the continent of Europe, including six years of war surgery with the French army, he settled first in London in 1596, where he published a book on the 'Spanish sickness' (yet another euphemism for syphilis) before returning to Glasgow in 1598 as a salaried surgeon to the City. He must have been a man of considerable authority and persuasion because his efforts resulted in the foundation of the Faculty of Physicians and Surgeons of Glasgow with the powers to examine and license all practitioners of medicine and surgery in Glasgow and the surrounding countryside, which at that time embraced the entire western portion of Scotland. In 1597 Lowe published his *Chirurgerie*, which is the earliest systematic work on the whole of surgery to be published in Britain and is in part in the form of a dialogue between the teacher, Peter Lowe, and his son John. Much contains references to his own observations and experiences, as is shown in the following extracts on aneurysm, which I have transliterated into modern English:

Aneurisma is a tumour soft to touch, the which is engendered of blood and spirit under the skin and muscle which happens in diverse parts of the body, chiefly in the sides of the cragg (the neck). The cause is either dilatation, incision or rupture of the artery, which often chances to women in the time of their birth, to trumpeters, criers, watermen and others who use violent labour and great crying or other violence by the which some of the artery does dilate. The signs are tumour, in pressing on with the finger, great pulsation. The tumour is of the same colour as the rest of the skin, soft to touch, yielding to the finger, by reason of the blood and spirit retire unto the arteries and parts adjacent, having removed the finger it presently returns with a noise or bruit by reason of the blood and spirit that return. . . . those which are superficial in the exterior parts, as the head, legs and arms may be knit and are curable; those which are profound and interior, in the breast as often happens to those who sweat excessively of the venereal sickness and otherwise; also those in the neck under the arms and the roots of the thighs and when there is great dilatation of the arteries are not curable, but death ensues within a few days, or at the least are very perilous and if the tumour be opened, the patient dies presently. This happens often times by the unskilfulness of ignorant barbers and other abusers who meddle with this art . . . as I have often seen. Such ignorance do esteem all tumours that are soft should be opened as common apostumes (abscesses). I remember in Paris in 1590 there happened such a disease to a valiant captain on the right side of his cragg, which I as Surgeon Major to the regiment was sent for, and found it to be an aneurisme so not to be touched . . . we did ordaine remedies to let the increase of it, which receipt being sent to the Apothecary, who before

had seen the said captain, did think it no meat medicine for an apostume, as he termed it. So presently he sent for an ignorant barber like unto himself, who did swear unto the captain that they had salves and charms for all sores, so without further trial did open it, with a lancet to void the matter (as they thought) which being done, the spirit and blood came forth with such violence that the captain died a few hours after.

The 17th century

The 17th century was not marked by any great advances in surgery, which, once again, was mainly concerned with dealing with the injuries of peace and war and with superficial and readily accessible lesions.

The outstanding military surgeon of the century was an Englishman, Richard Wiseman (?1621–1676), of whom more will be heard in Chapter 9.

James Yonge (1646–1721), himself the son of a naval surgeon in Plymouth, served his apprenticeship as a naval surgeon and spent much of his time at sea. Captured by the Dutch, he was a prisoner in Amsterdam for a year. Yonge introduced the flap operation for limb amputation which allowed much more rapid healing than the classical guillotine procedure. Initially, a single flap was used but the operation underwent many modifications and usually a double flap replaced the single flap.

John Woodall (1569–1643) had extensive experience as a surgeon both at sea and on shore in the service of the East India Company and for some years acted as surgeon to a colony of English merchants in Poland. He wrote a number of books, including *The Surgeon's Mate* in 1617, which was one of the earliest books on medicine at sea. The East India Company decreed that every ship's surgeon in its employ was to own a copy. Woodall invented a new kind of trephine for use in cranial surgery, but a greater claim to fame was his remarkable advocacy of lemon juice as a cure for scurvy, some three centuries before the discovery of vitamin C. He wrote:

I find we have many good things that heal the scurvy well on land but the sea chirurgeon shall do little good at sea

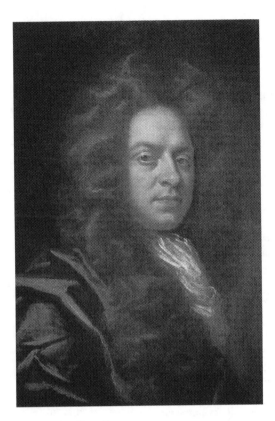

Figure 5.7 William Cowper.
Royal College of Surgeons of England.

with them, neither will they endure. The use of the juice of lemons is a precious medicine and well tried, being sound and good, let it have the chief place for it will deserve it . . . it is to be taken each morning two or three spoonfuls.

It was not until the publication of *A Treatise of the Scurvy* in 1753 by the naval surgeon James Lind (1716–1794) that a controlled trial showed that scurvy could be prevented by the adequate use of fresh fruit, the use of which became widespread in the English Navy.

On returning to England, Woodall was appointed Surgeon at St Bartholomew's Hospital and served on its staff for over 20 years. He also served as Master of the Company of Barber-surgeons.

William Cowper (1666–1709) (Figure 5.7) wrote a magnificent and beautifully illustrated book of

anatomy, much of which was 'lifted' without acknowledgement from the magnificently illustrated anatomical atlas by Govert Bidloo (1649–1713) of The Hague and later of Leyden. Cowper gave the first private lessons in anatomy in this country. He described the small glands at the base of the bladder which are still known as Cowper's glands. Perhaps his greatest contribution was to inspire William Cheselden – a man we shall meet as one of the important surgeons of the 18th century – with his love of anatomy and surgery. William Cowper should not be confused with Mr Cowper, a bone-setter in Leicester, who also had dealings with Cheselden and who may also have inspired him to undertake a career in surgery. It was the latter who, as Cheselden wrote many years later:

Set and cured a fracture of my own cubit (forearm) when I was a boy at school. His way was, after putting the limb in a proper posture, to wrap it up in rags dipped in the whites of eggs and a little wheat flour mixed; this drying, grew stiff, and kept the limb in a good posture. And I think there is no way better than this in fractures, for it preserves the position of the limb without strict bandage, which is the common cause of mischief in fractures.

Obviously a forerunner of plaster of Paris!

On the continent of Europe, perhaps the best known surgeon was Johannes Schultes (1595–1645), commonly called Scultetus. He was born in Ulm and at the age of 15 travelled to Padua to study medicine. He practised first in Padua, then in Vienna, but at the age of 30 returned to Ulm and served as City Physician until the time of his death. His fame rests on his *Armamentarium Chirurgicum*, published in Ulm after his death by his nephew who was also his namesake – Scultetus the Younger. The *Armamentarium Chirurgicum* was a remarkable book that contained a complete catalogue of all known surgical instruments, of all the methods of bandaging and splinting, and of a vast number of operative procedures, all of which are illustrated and cover the full range of operative procedures known in those days – operations on the mouth and ears, amputations (Figure 5.8), nasal reconstruction after the manner of Tagliacozzi, mastectomy

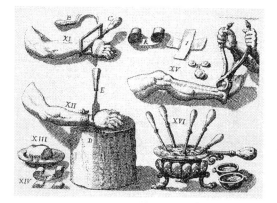

Figure 5.8 Amputations using a saw and a massive chisel, together with a selection of cauterising irons. From the *Armamentum Chirurgicum* of Scultetus.

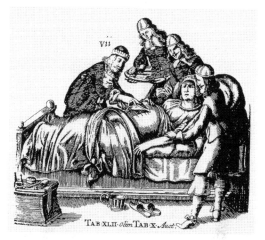

Figure 5.9 A caesarian section. From the *Armamentum Chirurgicum* of Scultetus.

for cancer of the breast and caesarean section (Figure 5.9). Although the original was in Latin, translations into French, English and German made the work available to surgeons throughout Europe who lacked the ability to read the original Latin. A sign of the importance and popularity of the book is that its illustrations were reproduced in many other publications throughout Europe over the next two centuries.

In France, Pierre Dionis (1643–1718) was appointed by Louis XIV in 1673 to carry out public anatomical dissections and operations in the Jardin du Roi in Paris for the benefit of students and without fee. This marked the beginning of the important French School of Surgery, whose influence we will see over the next two centuries. Dionis himself published important textbooks on anatomy and on surgical operations. The interest of Louis XIV in surgery was no doubt due to his own sufferings from a fistula in ano. His physicians sent several patients to various health resorts to try out the effects of conservative treatment: four of them spent a year taking the sulphur water of Barèges, four were sent to take the saline waters of Bourbonne-les-Bains; all failed to be cured. They then tried a salve invented by a Jesuit monk on further 'volunteers' with no effect. Charles François Félix (1650–1703), the court surgeon, was called into

consultation. He himself had never operated upon fistula in ano and promptly practised on patients with this disease collected from the charity hospitals of Paris. He then constructed a silver bistoury (a narrow-bladed knife) for the operation, which was carried out in the King's bedchamber in Versailles early in the morning of November 18th, 1686. Present were three other surgeons, four apothecaries, whose duty was to hold the patient still, a priest, the Minister of War and Madame de Maintenon (one of the King's favourites). Two incisions were made with the knife with a further eight cuts of scissors to lay the track widely open. Further operations were carried out on three occasions in December to prevent too rapid healing of the wound and, by January 11th, the King was well enough to walk in the Orangerie. Full recovery took place and Félix was elevated to the nobility, given a country estate and a magnificent fee of 300 000 livres. Surgery became fashionable and Félix, together with other popular surgeons, was bombarded with requests for similar operations from members of the Court even if they had nothing wrong with them!

If the 17th century was unremarkable in regard to significant surgical progress, it is important to note that major advances were made in knowledge

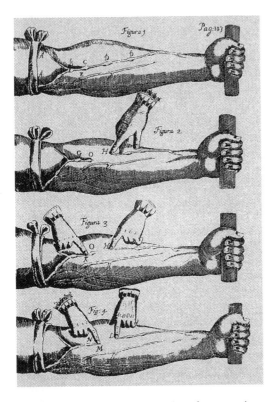

Figure 5.10 William Harvey's ingenious demonstration
of the function of the venous valves, using the
superficial veins of the arm.
From *De Motu Cordis*, 1628.

of the functions of the body. Indeed, whereas
the 16th century may be said to have heralded
the renaissance of anatomy, the 17th century saw the
beginnings of modern physiological knowledge.

Santorio Santorio (1561–1636), called Sanctorius,
studied medicine at Padua then practised medicine
in Poland and finally returned to Padua as Professor of Medicine. He was the first to study the pulse
rate in different individuals using a pendulum as
a timing instrument and the first to use a thermometer to measure body temperature in the study
of diseases in human patients. He fashioned a chair
suspended from a weighing machine which he
used to study himself under different conditions
of eating, resting and sleeping, and can be regarded
as the father of the modern study of metabolism.

William Harvey (1578–1657), after education at
Cambridge, studied in Padua and returned to
London to practise as a physician in 1602. After
many years of experimental and clinical studies
(Figure 5.10), he published *De Motu Cordis* (*The
Motion of the Heart*) in 1628, one of the most
important works published in the field of medicine.
In this, Harvey showed conclusively that the circulation of the blood was continuous and unidirec-
tional. Although he demonstrated the existence of
the circulation he did not see the capillary vessels
through which blood is conveyed from the terminal
branches of the arteries to the small tributaries of
the veins. This remained to be shown by Marcello
Malpighi (1628–1694) of Bologna, who demonstrated the capillaries in the almost transparent
lung of the frog. Using his microscope he also carried
out extensive investigations of the minute structure
of the skin, spleen and liver and made important
investigations in embryology. The lymphatics were
first described by Gaspare Aselli (1581–1626) of
Cremona, who noted fine ducts filled with creamy
fluid in the mesentery of the small intestine of the
dog. These were described in his book published
the year after his death, and his illustration of these
so-called 'lacteals' was the first time colour was used
in a medical textbook (Figure 5.11). Aselli himself
believed that the lacteals passed to the liver. The
means by which lymph returns to the circulation via
the great veins in the neck – the thoracic duct – was
discovered by Jean Pecquet (1622–1674) in 1647, and
the connection of the lymphatics of the gut with the
thoracic duct was demonstrated by Olaf Rudbeck
(1630–1702), a Scandinavian working at Padua.

The spirit of physiological enquiry is well demonstrated by the experiment of Timothy Clark,
who studied the effects of splenectomy in the dog;
he was particularly interested in the effect of this
procedure on the animal's sex life. He published
his findings in a volume entitled *Miscellanea Curiosa
Medico-physica*, first published in 1663:

In March 1663, with the assistance of Master Pearse, a
surgeon in ordinary to the Duke of York, I excised the
spleen from a stray dog of medium size and not well
nourished.

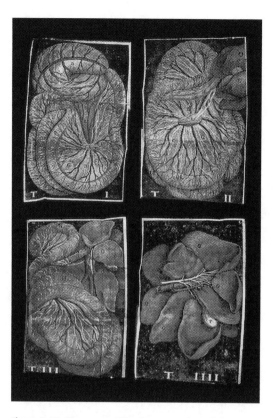

Figure 5.11 Gaspare Aselli's demonstration of the lymphatics in the mesentery of the small intestine of the dog (the lacteals). The first demonstration of this system and the first time colour was used in a medical illustration.
Royal College of Surgeons of England.

A transverse incision was made around the spleen, from which the enraged little creature extruded part of its bowel and intestines as well as the spleen itself, which we pulled out completely without any ligature but partly by section and partly by digital separation. Then, having replaced the other parts, we immediately closed the wound with stitches and entrusted the snarling animal to the care of an assistant who had to re-suture the wound shortly afterwards when the stitches were torn open by the enraged animal. From then on, however, the dog recovered its health, became tamer than before, and was subsequently enthusiastic in its pursuit of sexual activity.

In this manner the dog lived for a year a much happier life, and even put on flesh. In the following April, through what cause we do not know, at the front of the door it was found dead and rigid with a bruised head.

When we opened the cadaver we observed that the fleshy parts were redder and the fat everywhere whiter than in other animals. The mesentery was seen, in the spaces between the vessels, to be translucent, as one sees in the septum lucidum. The branches of the vessels were, however, covered over where the fat was whitest. All the other red parts were more florid than is usually seen in other animals, and the white parts much whiter, and this presented a not displeasing appearance. But where the spleen had been excised, part of the bowel and splenic artery were seen to be firmly adhered to the interior scar of the wound.

In 1676, in the same journal, Clark reported a remarkable clinical case of the effects of loss of the spleen in a suicide attempt:

A butcher named William Panier, living in the village of Wayford, near Crookhome in the County of Somerset, being greatly in debt, and fearing that lest he should be arrested, was constrained to go into hiding. The constables were about to capture him, and becoming desperate, and in order to avoid them, he drove a butcher's knife into his abdomen on the left side, thus causing a great wound through which part of the omentum, and of the intestine, and also the spleen protruded. The constables were horrified, and left the man for dead, as they believed. For three days the wound remained without a suture, but at last a surgeon was summoned. The surgeon replaced the intestines, and cut away part of the omentum, along with the spleen. The man rapidly recovered from the effects of the wound, and for the whole of the following year remained in good health and spirits. He soon afterward emigrated to New England, where not long ago he was so far living a healthy life. Doubeny Tuberville, M.D., a man renowned among our fellow-countrymen for his treatment of diseases of the eyes, has collaborated with me in communicating this observation.

Unfortunately, I can find no details of Timothy Clark, who was obviously a keen experimentalist and clinical observer.

6

The Age of the Surgeon-Anatomist: Part 2 – From the beginning of the 18th century to the mid 19th century

The 18th century

The 18th century has been termed the Age of Enlightenment. A wave of philanthropy and humanitarianism swept through Europe with the concept that Society is collectively responsible for its dependents, its mentally ill (in 1793 Phillipe Pinel, 1745–1826, freed from their chains the lunatics in the Bicêtre Hospital, Paris), its soldiers and sailors, the poor, women and children and the sick. In Britain, it saw the establishment of the great voluntary hospitals to complement the old religious foundations. For example, in London, the two original hospitals founded by the monks, St Thomas' (1173) and St Bartholomew's (1123), were added to by Westminster Hospital in 1716 (Figure 6.1), Guy's in 1726, St George's in 1733, the London in 1740 and the Middlesex in 1745. There was awakened concern with resuscitation of the drowned: in 1767 the Society for the Recovery of Drowned Persons was founded in Amsterdam; in 1771 a Humane Society was formed in Paris; and three years later the Humane Society (later to become the Royal Humane Society) was established in England in 1774 by Dr William Hawes (1736–1808), a London apothecary who obtained his MD at the age of 45. Hawes first had to overcome the dreadful superstition then current that it was unlucky to rescue, and especially to try to revive, the apparently drowned. One way in which he did this was to offer a reward of four guineas for any successful resuscitation.

The 18th century also saw steady growth in the technology and the stature of surgery, particularly in the schools of surgery in France and Britain, and the commencement of surgical training in the newly independent America. Still it was the case that the main endeavours of the surgeon were directed to the treatment of fractures and other injuries, the drainage of localised infections and removal of superficial lesions. Only when the patient could suffer his miseries no longer would he allow the surgeon to deal with his gangrenous leg by amputation, his strangulated hernia by relief from the knife or his bladder stone by lithotomy (see Chapter 12), by what was often a lethal operation.

France

We have already noted the improved status of surgery under the patronage of Louis XIV. This continued in the reign of Louis XV, whose personal surgeon, Georges Mareschal (1658–1736), successor to Félix and a surgeon at the Charité Hospital in Paris, persuaded the King to establish L'École de Chirurgie (the School of Surgery) in Paris in 1724 endowed by government grant. In 1775 this school was promoted to the title of Collège de Chirurgie and housed in a splendid new building. Mareschal, together with his successor at the Charité Hospital, François de La Peyronie (1678–1747), founded a scientific society in 1731 which became the Royal Academy of Surgery in 1748. This brought together the head surgeons under the chairmanship of the King's surgeon. Regular meetings and annual prize competitions were organised and regular

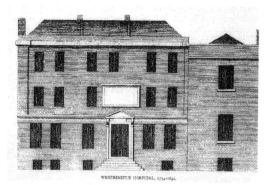

Figure 6.1 Westminster Hospital, first of the Voluntary Hospitals. Founded in 1716. This print shows the third building, erected in 1735, at the corner of James Street, now Buckingham Gate.

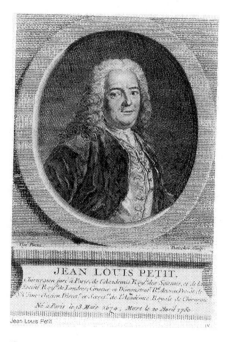

Figure 6.2 Jean-Louis Petit.
Royal College of Surgeons of England.

mémoires were published. Such measures ensured that surgery should have a scientific basis as well as being a practical art. Subjects taught at the Collège included physiology, pathology, chemistry and botany, as well as regular lectures on surgery and anatomy. In addition, the almost continuous continental wars of the century provided much practical experience for many young surgeons.

Another important step was that, in 1743, the surgeons at last became divorced from the barbers. A royal decree prohibited master surgeons from working, in addition, at the barbers' trade, with whom they had previously formed a single guild. In 1768, the apprenticeship system that dated back to the Middle Ages was abolished for the Master's examination in surgery and replaced by compulsory attendance at the Collège de Chirurgie.

Thus, during the century, Paris became one of the principal centres of surgery in Europe; among its leading teachers were Petit, Chopart, Desault and Bichat. Jean-Louis Petit (1674–1750) (Figure 6.2) was the outstanding surgeon in Paris in the first half of the 18th century. He was something of a precocious infant who even as a child preferred dissection to playing with his toys. By the age of 17 he was assisting his teacher, the anatomist and surgeon Alexis Littré (1658–1726), to teach anatomy. At the age of 18 he became an army surgeon before returning to Paris and establishing a private school of surgery. Petit was one of the founder members of the Académie de Chirurgie and eventually became its Director. He was the first to drain an infected mastoid (with success), invented a tourniquet with a screw to be placed directly over the artery, and improved the technique of limb amputation by incising the skin and muscles more distally to the bone, which allowed the 'flaps' to fall over the stump and thus speed the healing of the wound. In his *Treatise of the Diseases of Bones*, Petit describes in detail the mechanics and treatment of fractures by extension. He details the construction of a fracture bed that assisted traction by using an inclined plane. He also used overhead ropes to help the patient in moving about the bed. In a contribution to the Mémoires of the Royal Academy, he describes three patients in whom the inflamed gall bladder had been incised in the mistaken diagnosis of an abscess. One of the patients recovered and, from the post-mortem study of the two that died, Petit

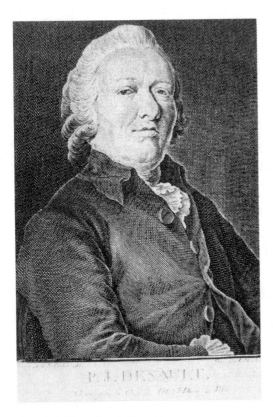

Figure 6.3 Pierre-Joseph Desault.
From Zimmerman L M, Veith L: *Great Ideas in the History of Surgery*. New York, Dover, 1961.

concluded that recovery was due to adhesions which had formed between the gall bladder and the abdominal wall. Although he probably had not done this operation himself, he advised opening the inflamed gall bladder and removing the stones; this was the operation of cholecystostomy, which was not, in fact, to be used until it was performed by John Bobbs in Indiana in 1867 (see page 92). Petit's contributions to the treatment of breast cancer will be described in Chapter 11.

François Chopart (1743–1795) published with Desault the influential *Traité des Maladies Chirurgicales et les Opérations qui leur Conviennent* in 1799 in two volumes. His name is perpetuated in the amputation through the forefoot at the mid tarsal joint using a long flap of the sole of the foot to cover the stump.

Pierre-Joseph Desault (1744–1795) (Figure 6.3) was the most influential surgeon and educator in France during the second half of the century, although his career was destroyed and his death hastened by the political disturbances of the French Revolution.

Desault was one of seven children of a poor peasant family but he soon proved to be a highly intelligent young man and became apprenticed to a local barber-surgeon. He moved to Paris and attended the lectures at the Collège de Chirurgie. At the age of 22 he began to give private lessons in anatomy and surgery and, although not a good lecturer, he attracted a large number of students by the clarity of his concepts. He insisted on the importance of practical dissection and emphasised that the functions of the parts under study and their pathological changes were more important than dry anatomical details. Eventually he became chief surgeon, first at the Charité and then at the Hôtel Dieu. Here he pioneered bedside teaching rather than formal lectures and case demonstrations in the newly constructed amphitheatre, which was packed with students both domestic and foreign. Among his many surgical trainees, the best known were Xavier, Bichat and Dominique-Jean Larrey, one of the most famous military surgeons (see Chapter 9).

Among Desault's surgical contributions were an ingenious bandaging technique for fractures of the clavicle (Figure 6.4) and ligation of the femoral artery for popliteal aneurysm in 1785, a few months before John Hunter performed this procedure, after whom it is named (see below). In 1791 he removed a large right-sided thyroid mass, five inches in diameter, in a female patient at the Hôtel Dieu. It was performed by meticulous dissection and ligation of the superior and inferior thyroid arteries – a remarkable procedure to perform without anaesthesia. The wound healed slowly and the patient left hospital completely cured on the 34th post-operative day.

At the height of his achievements, Desault's life, like that of so many others, was interrupted by the

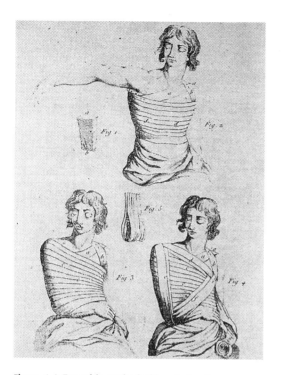

Figure 6.4 Desault's method of bandaging for fracture of the clavicle.
From Desault's *Oeuvres Chirurgicales*.

Revolution. He was actually arrested in 1793, but was released, by popular outcry, after a few days in prison. By now all institutes of higher education had been closed down, although he was appointed Professor of the new École de Santé in 1794; here, to his dismay, surgery and medicine were to be taught together. He was called to treat the 9-year-old Dauphin who was ill in prison and devoted lavish care to his young patient, but he himself became violently ill with what might have been some jail infection and died in 1795 at the age of only 51.

Xavier Bichat (1771–1802) had a brief but outstanding career. The son of a surgeon, he trained in Lyon; with the outbreak of war in 1793, he served as a military surgeon. The following year he joined Desault at the Hôtel Dieu, where his chief realised that he had an outstanding young student. Bichat was taken into Desault's home and became his private assistant at the age of 23. On the death of

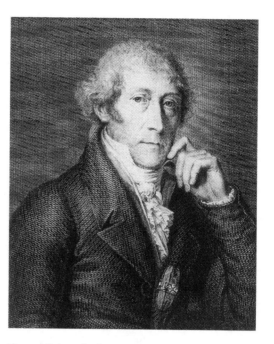

Figure 6.5 Antonio Scarpa.
Royal College of Surgeons of England.

his chief, Bichat established a private school and laboratory where he taught anatomy, physiology and operative surgery. He became completely engrossed in his scientific studies and abandoned surgery. His important contribution was to point out that organs were not homogeneous structures but were composed of different tissues. He died at the age of 31, probably of tuberculous meningitis, having suffered for years from pulmonary disease.

Italy

Italy, which had played such an important part in the development of surgery from the time of the Renaissance, lost much of its influence in the 18th century. The exception lay in one man, Antonio Scarpa (1752–1832) (Figure 6.5). He came from a humble background and was taught by his uncle, a priest. By the age of 15 he passed the entrance examination to the medical school at Padua and there came under the influence of Giovanni

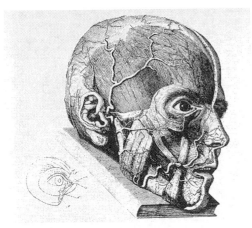

Figure 6.6 Anatomical illustration prepared by Scarpa. *Saggio di osservazioni e d'esperienze sulle principali mallattie degli occhi.* Venice, Giannantonio Pizzani, 1802.

Morgagni (1682–1771), the Professor of Anatomy. Morgagni laid down the principles of modern pathology and in his major textbook *On the Sites and Causes of Diseases* he carefully described each patient's case history, the events leading to the final illness and death, and then the detailed results of the post-mortem examination with an attempt to explain how the symptoms were the results of the pathology. Scarpa became Morgagni's assistant and personal secretary and from him developed his great interest in medical science, especially pathological anatomy, and his meticulous approach to investigations. Scarpa qualified at the age of 20 and two years later was appointed Professor of Anatomy and Clinical Surgery at the University of Modena, where he added to his duties that of teacher in obstetrics and chief surgeon to the military hospital. He visited Paris and London, where he befriended Percival Pott and the brothers John and William Hunter, and returned to Italy to the post of Professor of Anatomy at Padua in 1783.

Scarpa's talents were many; he was a brilliant anatomist, a surgeon with especial talents in ophthalmology and orthopaedics, an outstanding teacher and an excellent artist who illustrated his own numerous texts (Figure 6.6). His name is eponymously commemorated in Scarpa's fascia, the fibrous layer of connective tissue of the lower abdominal wall, Scarpa's triangle, the femoral triangle of the groin, and Scarpa's ganglion on the 8th cranial nerve. He studied the nerves of hearing and of smell, described the round window and the labyrinthine fluid of the ear and gave the first detailed description of the innervation of the heart. He gave an accurate description of sliding inguinal hernia, illustrated, of course, by his own drawings, and devised a shoe for club foot which is the basis of the one used today. Against all these achievements must be placed his ruthless character, promoting his favourites and destroying his enemies. He never married but had several illegitimate sons, whose careers he fostered. Soon after he died, at the age of 80, his reputation was attacked and the inscription on his memorial tablet was defaced. However, his head, preserved in spirit, remains to the present day in the medical museum in Padua!

Germany

Up until this period, Germany had lagged behind the other Western European countries in surgery; itinerant bone-setters, stone-cutters and charlatans vied with barber-surgeons for the practice of this art. One German surgeon, however, stood out as comparable in importance to any other in the 18th century, Lorenz Heister (1683–1758) (Figure 6.7). He was born in Frankfurt am Main and proved to be a gifted student. He studied first at the University of Giessen, then Leyden and then Amsterdam, where he sat at the feet of two outstanding surgeons and anatomists, Frederik Ruysch (1638–1731) and Johannes Rau (1668–1719). In 1707 he went as surgeon to the Dutch in their war against the French and then returned to Leyden for further study under Bernhard Albinus (1697–1770) and the great Herman Boerhaave (1668–1738); he obtained his Doctorate in 1708. That year he returned to his duties as an army surgeon. In 1710, Heister was appointed Professor of Anatomy and Surgery in the University of Altdorf in the Republic of Nürnberg, but before taking up his post he made a tour of surgical centres

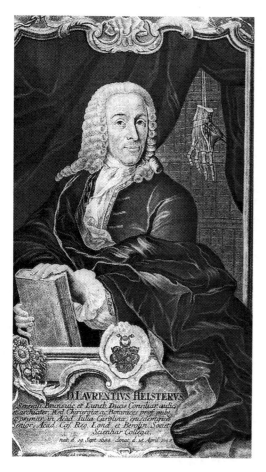

Figure 6.7 Lorenz Heister.
Royal College of Surgeons of England.

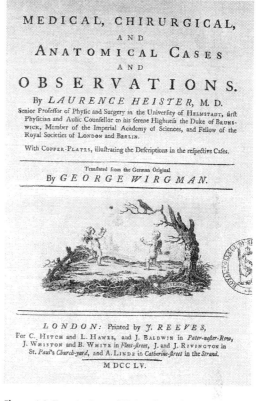

Figure 6.8 Frontispiece of Heister's Medical, Chirurgical and Anatomical Cases and Observations English edition, 1755.

in Great Britain. It was during his time at Altdorf that Heister published the first edition of his great *General System of Surgery* (Figure 6.8). Shortly after its publication, he was appointed to the Chair of Anatomy and Surgery at the University of Helmstadt, in the Duchy of Brunswick. Later the professorship of botany was added to his duties and he was responsible for the establishment of its famous botanical garden. Heister remained at Helmstadt for the next 38 years. Its school of surgery achieved a position of great importance due to his influence but its eminence disappeared rapidly after Heister's death in 1758.

Heister's great contribution to teaching was his surgical textbook, richly illustrated with 38 copper plates (Figure 6.9, and see Figure 11.3). It was originally written in German, in which it was published in seven editions, and was also translated into ten English and three Latin editions as well as being translated into Spanish, French, Italian and Dutch. I have a copy of the fifth English edition of 1755 at my side as I write this; its full title continues 'containing the doctrine and management of wounds, fractures, luxations, tumours and ulcers of all kinds. Of the several operations performed on all parts of the body. Of the several bandages applied in all operations and disorders to which is prefixed an introduction concerning the nature,

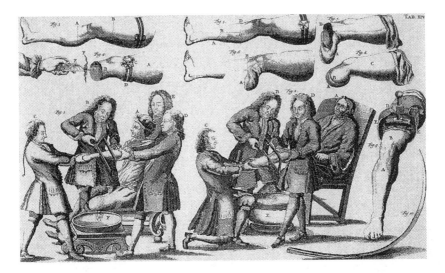

Figure 6.9 Copper plate illustration of amputations of arm and leg.
From Heister's *General System of Surgery*. London, English 5th edition, 1755.

origin, progress and improvements of surgery, with such other preliminaries as are necessary to be known by the younger surgeons. Being a work of 30 years experience.' It is a remarkable piece of work and does, indeed, cover the whole of surgery as known at that time and includes operative midwifery.

In dealing with strangulated inguinal hernia, Heister first of all gives a detailed account of attempting reduction of the hernia by manipulation. However:

When the surgeon perceives that it is impossible to return the intestine, and finds by the great inflammation, pain and vomiting, that the disorder will be fatal, he should acquaint his patient and his friends with the great necessity there is for him to undergo the operation, to prevent a mortification and consequent death . . . the integuments are next to be taken up on each side of the tumour by one hand of the surgeon and another of the assistant while he makes a longitudinal incision with the scalpel upon the middle of the tumour, after which he is to dilate or remove the sides of the wound from each other; but if the integuments cannot be thus elevated by reason of the violent inflammation, the surgeon should then grasp the tumour between the thumb and forefinger of his left

hand, making the incision downward in a right line and with a light hand but he may not divide deeper than the skin so as to injure the intestine. A director is then to be introduced between the tumour and divided skin and the wound is to be enlarged upward and downward by an incision knife or scissors, after which the sides of the wound are to be drawn asunder by hooks or the fingers and the remaining part of the membrana adiposa carefully divided 'til the intestine or its sacculus of the peritoneum appear to view . . . to avoid the intestine a small opening may be made in the peritoneum with the point of the scalpel to introduce the finger and if the surgeon should meet with a quantity of water or lymph discharging itself by the small apperture in that membrane, he should not be surprised, being no more than usual, but should proceed to divide that integument upwards with a pair of scissors or the scalpel 'til he comes to the rings of the abdomen; and if any large blood vessels should be by accident divided, which would obscure the work, it should either be taken up with a needle and thread or compressed by the fingers of an assistant who should also draw out the blood with lint or a sponge. If the intestine then appears to be found, it is to be returned by a gentle pressure through the ring of the abdominal muscles. But if any flatus or contained faeces prevents its return, they should be first gradually pressed out and if that also proves insufficient the ring of the abdominal muscles should be divided . . . when the ruptured part has been dilated and the intestine returned, the wound is to be dressed with linen compresses and retained by the bandage, though some scarify the ring of the abdomen to make a firmer cicatrix and prevent a return of the disorder.

No surgical condition known at that time was too major for Heister not to advise thereon nor too minor to be overlooked, thus he gives this advice for the treatment of an infected ingrowing toenail:

The great toenail sometimes turns too much in on one side so as to enter the flesh and cause violent pain and inflammation to such a degree that the patient cannot walk. The most general cause of this disorder is the wearing of too straight or narrow-toed shoes, which they will do well to avoid, who are desirous of being free from the complaint. But in order to set the nail at liberty from the tender flesh into which it has fixed itself the patient's foot is first to be held for an hour in hot water, to mollify the indurated nail and skin, and that the water may penetrate the farther, it may be proper to scrape off the outer surface every two or three minutes with a penknife or a piece of glass, after which the infected nail is to be gently elevated with the fingers or a probe and a piece of soft dry lint interposed betwixt it and the flesh, and so bound up with a compress dipped in warm spirit of wine, which operation is to be repeated again the next day 'til the pain and inflammation disappear. If the method before described proves insufficient to remove the disorder, we must then have recourse to the knife. In order to which, the foot being macerated in warm water, as before, is then to be placed and held in a convenient posture upon a chair by the hands of an assistant and the operator must insinuate the strong nail scissors gradually under the injurious part of the nail, to cut it off and then extract it, if it does not come away of itself with a pair of pliers; and though the operation itself may give the patient no small pain for a short time, yet he will quickly perceive the advantage by a more lasting ease.

In addition to this magnum opus, Heister wrote a textbook of anatomy which appeared in 25 editions in a variety of translations, books on eye surgery, botany and other subjects as well as a magnificent collection of case reports. One of these, describing the management of a massive tumour of the breast, will be described in Chapter 11.

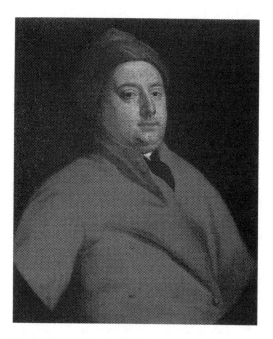

Figure 6.10 William Cheselden.
This portrait hangs in the Council Room of the Royal College of Surgeons of England.

Britain

It was, however, in the United Kingdom in particular that surgery flourished in the 18th century, especially London, where both the old and the newly founded teaching hospitals were attracting students from all over these islands and from abroad. A number of names towered above the rest and their influence can be felt even today; they include William Cheselden, Percivall Pott, John Hunter and Henry Cline.

William Cheselden (1688–1752) (Figure 6.10), the son of a Leicestershire farmer, came to London as a lad of 15 and was apprenticed to James Ferne (1672–1741), a young surgeon recently appointed to the staff of St Thomas' Hospital. He completed his apprenticeship in 1710, becoming a Freeman of the Barber-surgeons' Company. At that time no-one was giving regular lectures in anatomy in London so the following year, at the age of 23, he began private courses in this subject. In 1714 he was reprimanded by the Court of Assistants of the Barber-surgeons' Company, and we read in their minutes:

Our master acquainted the Court that Mr Wm Cheselden a member of the Company did frequently procure the dead bodies of malefactors from the place of execution and dissect the same at his own house as well during the Company's public lectures as at other times without the word of the Governors and contrary to the Company's By-law in that behalf by which means becomes more difficult for the beadles to bring away the Company's bodies and likewise drew away the members from the public dissections and lectures at the Hall. The said Mr Cheselden thereupon called in but having submitted himself to the pleasure of the Court with a promise never to dissect at the same time as the Company had the lectures at their Hall not without leave of the Governors for the time being the said Mr Cheselden was censured for what had passed with a reproof for the same pronounced by the Master at the desire of the Court.

This reprimand may well have biased Cheselden against the Barber-surgeons; later he was one of the instigators, in 1745, of the break-up of the Company, when the Company of Surgeons was formed as a separate body with John Ranby (1703–1773), Serjeant Surgeon to George II, as its first Master. Cheselden, in turn, became the second Master to the new Company. The Company, as such, had a short life since in 1800 it became the Royal College of Surgeons of London which, in turn, evolved into the Royal College of Surgeons of England in 1843.

In passing, we should note the difficulties in procuring bodies for dissection, usually executed criminals, and there was a brisk trade for the 'resurrectionists' in digging up recently buried corpses from the graveyards. Even the body of a beggar found dead from choking with bread outside St Thomas' Hospital was carried into the hospital by a passing stranger, who obtained a good price for 'his brother's body'.

A gruesome incident recorded in the minutes of the Barber-surgeons' Company in 1740 caused much consternation. The body of a youth aged 16 called Duell, hanged for rape, revived when laid out for dissection. He fully recovered within a couple of hours following blood letting and a glass of warm wine. Constantly glancing around the theatre in terror, he muttered repeatedly 'don't, don't, don't'. He was returned to Newgate Prison, but fortunately reprieved and transported. It was said that he later changed his name to Deverell, became a prosperous merchant and presented a gilded leather screen to the Company for saving his life.

Young Cheselden realised the need for a good, concise textbook of anatomy in the English language and published *The Anatomy of the Human Body* in 1713 when he was 25. This book maintained his popularity among students for more than a century, the 13th edition appearing in 1792. It was also published in America, where a second edition was published in 1806. The reason for its popularity was that it contained the essentials of gross anatomy mingled with physiological and clinical discussions. Thus, he illustrates the fact that an artery ruptured by traction goes into spasm and does not bleed with the following report:

The figure of Samuel Wood, a miller, whose arm with the scapula was torn off from his body by a rope winding round it, the other end being fastened to the cogs of a mill [Figure 6.11]. This happened in the year 1737. The vessels being thus stretched bled very little, the arteries and nerves were drawn out of the arm, the surgeon who was first called placed them within the wound and dressed it superficially. Next day he was put under Mr Ferne's care at St Thomas' Hospital, but he did not remove the dressings for some days. The patient had no severe symptoms, and the wound was cured by superficial dressings only, the natural skin being left almost sufficient to cover it.

Cheselden was undoubtedly the foremost surgeon of his day in London. He continued to insist on the importance of a sound knowledge of anatomy for the medical students and upon dissection to obtain this. He served on the staff of St Thomas', Westminster and St George's Hospitals and was a pioneer of ophthalmic surgery and a master of cutting for the bladder stone. We shall hear more of this in Chapter 12.

In his 50th year Cheselden gave up all his positions to devote himself entirely as surgeon to the Royal Hospital Chelsea, which had been founded by King Charles II for the care of old and disabled

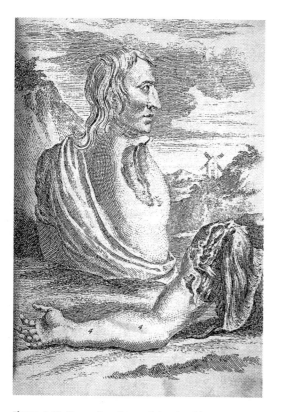

Figure 6.11 Case of avulsion of the shoulder. Cheselden's *The Anatomy of the Human Body* 1778, author's copy.

soldier pensioners. He died in 1752 on a visit to Bath, and this notice appeared in the *Gentleman's Magazine* in April of that year:

William Cheselden Esq.; an eminent anatomist, lithotomist and surgeon to the Royal Hospital Chelsea; at Bath; he had drunk ale after eating hot buns, upon which being very uneasy he sent for a physician who advised vomiting immediately, which advice, had he taken it might, it is thought, have saved his life.

The diagnosis of this catastrophe is subject for discussion.

Cheselden was buried in the grounds of the Royal Hospital and his tomb can be seen there to this day. It was my great privilege to serve for many years as surgeon to this hospital in very distant line of descent from William Cheselden.

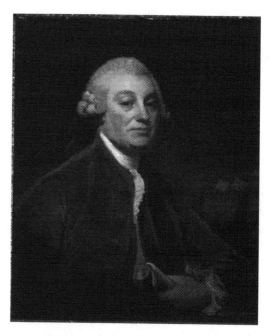

Figure 6.12 Percivall Pott. Royal College of Surgeons of England.

There remains one more incident of interest in the life of this great man. In 1748–1749 he had as one of his pupils John Hunter, at that time a youth of 20. It may well be that the veteran anatomist inspired the youth with some of his enthusiasm.

Percivall Pott (1714–1789) (Figure 6.12) was a cockney, born in Threadneedle Street in the City of London, the son of a greengrocer. He was apprenticed to William Nourse (1701–1761), one of the two surgeons at St Bartholomew's Hospital, at the age of 15 and obtained his Freedom of the Barber-surgeons Company in 1736 at the age of 22. Nine years later he was appointed Assistant Surgeon to Bart's and in 1749 became full surgeon. He was a highly intelligent person with a friendly personality and was a shrewd clinical observer. He advised gentleness in treatment, eschewing the use of the cautery, caustics and irritating medicaments.

At the age of 42, riding to hospital on a frosty morning, he was thrown from his horse and suffered a compound fracture of the tibia. He realised the seriousness of the situation, refused to be moved, and sent for two bearers. When they arrived with their poles, he purchased a door from a nearby shop, had this nailed to the poles and then had himself carried on this stretcher to his home. He was advised by his surgeons to have immediate amputation but as the instruments were being got ready, his old chief, William Nourse, arrived and advised conservative treatment. The fracture was reduced, the wound healed and his leg was saved. During his prolonged immobilisation, Pott used the time to commence his series of texts which are characterised by their high literary quality and wealth of clinical observation. His first treatise, *Ruptures*, was followed by others on congenital hernia, lachrymal fistula, head injuries, hydrocele, fractures and dislocations, palsy of the lower limbs and several other conditions.

Pott made numerous original observations. Thus, he first described 'chimney sweep's cancer', and can therefore be regarded as a pioneer of occupational disease. This is a cancer of the scrotum due to carcinogenic agents in soot. He wrote:

The fate of these people seems singularly hard; in their early infancy, they are most frequently treated brutally, and also starved with cold and hunger; they are thrust up narrow and sometimes hot chimneys, where they are bruised, burned and almost suffocated; when they get to puberty, they become peculiarly liable to a most noisome, painful, and fatal disease.

He described Pott's puffy tumour, the swelling of the scalp over an extradural abscess, and enumerated the signs by which it can be differentiated from an extradural haematoma. He also recognised the lucid period that can precede the coma of extradural haemorrhage and adds that the initial concussion causes a loss of consciousness which may blend into that of the brain compression without this period of lucidity. He advised the use of the trephine in head injuries and employed it much as modern neurosurgeons do when the presence of accumulation of blood beneath the skull cannot otherwise be excluded. He gave a classic description of tuberculous disease of the

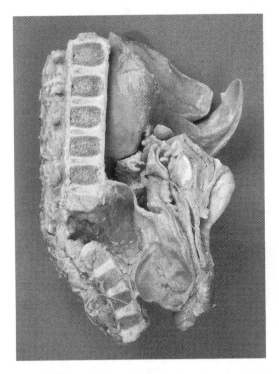

Figure 6.13 Pott's disease of the spine (tuberculosis). This specimen is in the Gordon Museum at Guy's Hospital. It demonstrates the bodies of the third, fourth and fifth thoracic vertebrae have been destroyed. In front of them is a thick-walled abscess cavity which is compressing the trachea. From a child aged three.

spine (Pott's disease of the spine) (Figure 6.13) and a detailed description of fracture dislocation of the ankle, again still to this day called Pott's fracture (Figure 6.14).

John Hunter (1728–1793) (Figure 6.15) was the first surgeon to apply the inductive system of observation and experimentation to the study of disease. He also realised that to understand the effects of the disease process on the body it is first necessary to study the form and function of the normal healthy individual. Indeed, he realised that pathological processes are 'the perversion of the natural actions of the animal economy'. He is rightfully regarded as the father of modern scientific surgery in the British Isles. His philosophy can

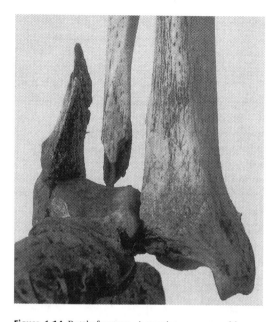

Figure 6.14 Pott's fracture. A specimen prepared by
Sir Astley Cooper and preserved in the Gordon Museum
at Guy's Hospital. It demonstates an oblique fracture of
the lower end of the fibula with gross lateral dislocation
of the ankle joint.

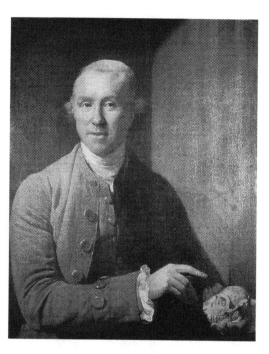

Figure 6.15 John Hunter (as a young man).
Royal College of Surgeons of England.

be summed up by a famous remark he made in a
letter to his friend and pupil Edward Jenner (1749–
1823), of smallpox vaccination fame, a copy of which
is carefully preserved in the Hunterian Museum
of the Royal College of Surgeons of England: 'Why
do you ask me a question, by the way of solving it.
I think your solution is just; but why think, why not
try the experiment?'

Indeed, an important part of Hunter's contribution to surgery was the way he inspired many of
his surgical students in the experimental method,
which they would take with them and pass on in
turn to their own students. Among his pupils we
must make mention of: Benjamin Bell (1749–1806),
Henry Cline (1750–1827), Everard Home (1756–1832),
who became Hunter's brother-in-law and later
Serjeant Surgeon and President of the Royal College
of Surgeons, John Abernethy (1764–1831), Anthony
Carlisle (1768–1840), who later served on the staff of

Westminster Hospital and also became a president
of the Royal College of Surgeons, and, most famous
of all, Astley Cooper (1768–1841). Several of these
we shall meet later in this chapter. Students from
America also came to Hunter; they included John
Morgan (1735–1789) and William Shippen (1736–
1808) who were co-founders of the first medical
school in North America, in Philadelphia, and also
Philip Syng Physick (1768–1837), who is often regarded as the father of American surgery.

John Hunter was born on a farm on the outskirts
of East Kilbride near Glasgow. He was the last of
ten children and his brother William, who was ten
years his senior, considerably influenced his early
career. John proved to be a boy who disliked his
school lessons but who was keen on natural history, which he studied in the woods and fields – a
story reminiscent of the early days of Astley Cooper
and of Charles Darwin.

At the age of 20, John joined his brother William who had established himself as a popular anatomy teacher in London, as well as being a highly successful obstetrician at the Middlesex Hospital; he was later to deliver Queen Charlotte of the future King George IV. John proved to have a brilliant flair for anatomy and became a skilled and energetic dissector. For the following 12 years he worked as assistant to William, while at the same time studying surgery under William Cheselden and Percivall Pott.

In 1760, Hunter joined the army; the following year, during the Seven Years' War, he saw active service, first in Belle Isle off the coast of France, and then in Portugal, gaining considerable experience in treating war wounds. He returned to London in 1763, set up a successful surgical practice and, in 1768, was appointed to the staff of St George's Hospital. His first episode of what was undoubtedly angina pectoris occurred in 1773. He died on October 16th, 1793 at the age of 65 of a heart attack while being particularly aggravated at a board meeting at his hospital. A post-mortem performed by Everard Home, his brother-in-law, demonstrated severe calcification of the arteries of the heart and of the brain. Originally Hunter was buried in the crypt of the church of St Martin-in-the-Fields, but the coffin was reinterred at Westminster Abbey in 1859.

Among the vast number of Hunter's experimental contributions may be listed his studies on descent of the testis, during which he described and named the gubernaculum testis, the demonstration of fat absorption by the lacteals, the lymphatics of the small intestine, the demonstration of the blood supply of the placenta, the proof that the seminal vesicles do not act as a sperm reservoir, and his interesting studies on grafting. These latter demonstrate what today we would term an autograft, in which Hunter transplanted the spur of a cock into its comb, and what would be termed today an allograft, in which he grafted the testis of a cock into the abdominal cavity of a hen and, finally, a xenograft in modern terms, the transplantation of a human tooth into a cock's comb. These specimens can still be seen in the Hunterian Museum.

Indeed, many would regard Hunter's greatest contribution to be his museum; which grew, in his lifetime, to 13 682 specimens. Before Hunter, museums of natural history were collections of curiosities, however Hunter arranged his museum into a dynamic teaching exercise. The specimens were grouped into three main categories; the first demonstrated the inter-relationship between structure and function, whether plant, animal or human. For example, the section on the nervous system demonstrated the evolutionary series from the primitive nerve chain of the earthworm to the highly developed central nervous system of man. The second group demonstrated the preservation of the race and comprised the reproductive organs and the development of the fetus. The third series demonstrated pathological changes.

After Hunter's death, the collection eventually passed into the custody of the Royal College of Surgeons of England. On the night of May 10th, 1941 the College was extensively damaged by both incendiary and high explosive bombs, and over half the specimens were destroyed. However, much of the collection remains to be inspected today and has been supplemented by many magnificent specimens.

Certainly the most famous specimen is the skeleton of Charles Byrne, 'Obrian the Irish Giant' (Figure 6.16). This young man earned his living being exhibited as 'the tallest man in the world'. His skeleton measures 7 feet 8 inches, so in life he was probably a couple of inches taller than this. He was a heavy gin drinker and died at the early age of 22. He greatly feared being 'anatomised' and arranged to be buried at sea in a leaden coffin. However, Hunter's associates bribed the pall bearers and carried the body off to Hunter's country house at Earl's Court, to be prepared as a skeleton. Harvey Cushing (see Figure 9.27) asked to open the back of Byrne's skull; this demonstrated a very large pituitary fossa (later confirmed on X-ray) which shows that the pathology was acromegaly due to a massive tumour of the anterior pituitary gland.

Hunter's most famous technical contribution to surgery was his operation of ligation of the femoral artery in the subsartorial canal of the thigh, often with consequent death from haemorrhage. After animal studies, in which he showed that there was an excellent collateral circulation after ligation of the artery in the thigh, Hunter carried out this procedure in 1785 with great success. This patient was described by Sir Everard Home in 1793:

> Mr Hunter, from having made these observations, was led to propose that in this operation the artery should be taken up in the anterior part of the thigh, some distance from the diseased part, so as to diminish the risk of haemorrhage, and admit of the artery being more readily secured, should any such accident happen. The force of the circulation being thus taken off from the aneurismal sac, the progress of the disease would be stopped; and he thought it probable, that if the parts were left to themselves, the sac, with its contents, might be absorbed, and the whole of the tumour removed, which would render any opening into the sac unnecessary.

A number of specimens of successful Hunterian ligations, in patients who survived for years after the operation, can be seen today in the Hunterian Museum.

In Scotland, the leading surgeon of his time was Benjamin Bell (1749–1806). He was born in Dumfries and studied in Edinburgh, Paris and London, here as a pupil of the Hunters, before returning to join the staff of the Edinburgh Royal Infirmary. He wrote a six volume *System of Surgery*, which was designed to become a comprehensive text in competition with Heister's book. It went through seven editions and was translated into German and French. Bell also wrote a book on venereal diseases in which he corrected one of the errors made by John Hunter, who, as the result of experimental inoculations of venereal matter, believed that syphilis and gonorrhoea were the same disease. The error probably arose because the scrapings of pus Hunter used were presumably taken from a patient with both diseases.

Benjamin Bell's two sons both became Edinburgh surgeons, as did two of his grandsons. One of these, Joseph Bell (1837–1911), a brilliant teacher of clinical observation, had as one of his pupils Arthur Conan Doyle, who used him as the model for the famous fictional detective Sherlock Holmes.

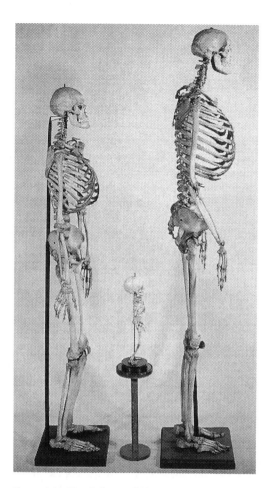

Figure 6.16 The skeleton of Obrian, the Irish giant, in the Hunterian Museum of the Royal College of Surgeons. To his left is the (much smaller!) skeleton of the American giant and between is seen the skeleton of the Sicilian dwarf. All in their life times had been side-show exhibits.

now called Hunter's canal, for aneurysm of the popliteal artery. This was common in those days in coachmen and horse-riders, probably as a result of repeated pressure from the upper edge of the high riding boot on the artery. Up to the time of Hunter, surgeons either refused to operate or tied the artery immediately above the aneurysm, where the vessel was frequently diseased and could easily rupture

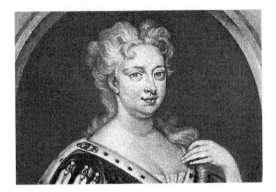

Figure 6.17 Caroline of Ansbach as a young woman.

What would it have been like, to have been a patient with some serious illness who had to undergo the agonising and dangerous emergency surgery of the 18th century? How better to illustrate this than to use the case history of the first lady of the land in the London of 1737.

Caroline of Ansbach (Figure 6.17) was born in 1683 and married George, Prince of Wales, in her early twenties. She possessed ample Germanic charms: flaxen hair, sky-blue eyes, fair skin, and a voluptuous figure. She was also highly intelligent and enjoyed theological speculation. Her husband, like his father George I, was, in contrast, rather stupid, although he had a passion for the genealogy of European nobility and an extensive knowledge of the uniforms of all the regiments of Europe.

On the death of George I in 1727, George and Caroline ascended the throne, but by now, seven children and innumerable banquets had converted Caroline to an obese middle age. Her sixth pregnancy, in 1723, had also left its mark – a large umbilical hernia – which she successfully disguised from her husband for many years.

The emergency began on Wednesday, November 9th, 1737. Caroline was seized with severe colicky pain and vomiting while at St James' Palace, London. Dr George Tesier, physician to the household, and Dr Noel Broxolme of St George's Hospital were summoned. The usual polypharmacy of the early 18th century was immediately put into operation; snake root and brandy, Daffy's elixir, and

Sir Walter Raleigh's cordial were prescribed and just as quickly vomited. The Queen was relieved of twelve ounces of blood and was given an enema, which, we read, 'came from her just as it went into her'. Much to the Queen's inconvenience, the King insisted on sharing her bed that night, where neither could he sleep nor could she roll about as readily as she would wish in her pain.

On the next morning, Thursday, another twelve ounces of blood were drawn from the Queen and two more enemas given, which returned 'immediately and pure'. Two additional physicians were called in, Sir Hans Sloane and Dr Hulse; they ordered blisters and aperients which, again, were vomited.

On Friday morning the poor woman was bled yet a third time. Early on Saturday morning, the Queen, no doubt by now weak from loss of blood, consented to the indignity of clinical examination; John Ranby, Surgeon to the King, was allowed to feel the royal abdomen. At once he realised the seriousness of the situation and more surgical consultants were immediately summoned. Ranby advised simple lancing of the hernia and opposed the suggestion of his colleagues that the neck of the navel should be divided wide enough to thrust the gut back into its place, saying that, at this stage, the strangulated bowel would prolapse out of the body into the bed. There is little doubt that, in those pre-anaesthetic days, and without the advantages of modern relaxant drugs, his advice was probably sound. At six o'clock that evening Ranby lanced the swelling at the umbilicus and let out some matter but not enough to abate the swelling to any degree or to give any hope of her recovery.

On Sunday, the lips of the wound were seen to have mortified, and the surgeons, indeed everyone in the royal household, realised that the prognosis was now hopeless. Caroline called George to her side and told him that on her death he should marry again. George was beside himself in misery and with tears streaming down his face, sobbing between every word, said 'No, I will never marry again, I will simply have mistresses'. This was no doubt a great compliment in the early 18th century,

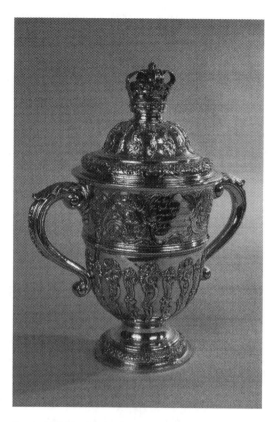

Figure 6.18 The Ranby Cup.
Royal College of Surgeons of England

when so many husbands expected to outlive one or more of their wives.

Day after day the poor woman's sufferings continued but she bore them, together with repeated painful dressings of the wound, with considerable courage and without complaint. On Thursday, the strangulated bowel burst and excrement gushed out of the wound in immense quantities, flooding the bed and flowing all over the floor. When her companions hoped the relief would do her good, the Queen replied, very calmly, that she hoped so too, for that was all the evacuations she should ever have.

Hour by hour the Queen weakened, and indeed the bystanders believed each hour would be her last, but peace did not come until ten o'clock on Sunday night, November 20th. Her last word was to her children; it was 'Pray'. Today, how often does a patient die of a strangulated umbilical hernia? Even the old and feeble can readily be rescued by the surgical house staff. Yet, in the 18th century, the first lady in the land, obese but otherwise fit, could not be given even the slightest relief by the most distinguished coterie of physicians and surgeons that London could muster.

John Ranby (1703–1773), who operated on the Queen, was an interesting man. He was a Londoner and was only 34 years of age at the time of this royal operation. He continued to serve the royal family for many years and was appointed Serjeant Surgeon in 1740. In 1745 he became the first Master of the Company of Surgeons at the break-up of the United Company of Barbers and Surgeons. This Company of Surgeons later became the Royal College of Surgeons of England. Visitors to the College, to this day, will be shown one of its most precious possessions, a magnificent silver cup (Figure 6.18) on which is inscribed in Latin, 'John Ranby dedicates this memorial, such as it is, to the very worshipful Company of Surgeons on the first day of July 1745, as a token of regard for his brethren'. Surprisingly, there is no known portrait of this distinguished man.

America

Surgery in America began to develop towards the end of the 18th century. The American colonies broke away from the mother country in the War of Independence (1775–1783). In the early days of the colonies, there were few doctors and still fewer surgeons; most patients depended on what help they could get from intelligent and interested laymen. Those surgeons who were to be found were either immigrants from Europe or Americans who would travel to Europe to study, especially to London and Edinburgh. Among these students, the most notable were William Shippen, John Morgan, Philip Syng Physick and John Collins Warren. William Shippen (1736–1808) came to London at the age of 22 and studied with John Hunter. He kept

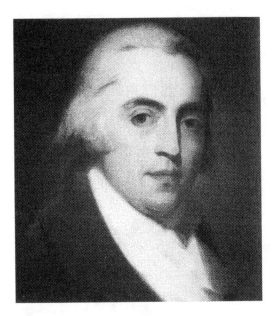

Figure 6.19 Philip Syng Physick.
Royal College of Surgeons of England.

a diary during his stay which gives a clear picture of a medical student's life in those days. A typical day is recorded as follows: 'Rose at six, operating 'til eight, breakfast at nine, dissected 'til two, dined 'til three, dissected 'til five, lectured 'til seven, operated 'til nine, supper 'til ten, then bed'.

Hospitals were visited daily and often on Sundays. Shippen's particular pleasure was to sit late into the night talking to John Hunter, who stimulated his students to observe, enquire and to try the experiment.

Shippen spent two years in London and a year in Edinburgh, where he obtained his MD for a thesis on *Attachment of the Placenta to the Uterus*, and six months in France. He then returned to Philadelphia and helped John Morgan in the foundation of the first medical school, part of the University of Pennsylvania, in 1765 and was appointed its first Professor of Anatomy and Surgery.

John Morgan (1735–1789) served as an apprentice to a Doctor Redmon in Philadelphia then studied with the Hunters in London in 1760, followed by two years in Edinburgh, where he obtained his MD for his thesis on *Suppuration and the Formation of Pus*. In this he pointed out that pus was formed only in inflamed blood vessels and was always preceded by evidence of inflammation. Morgan returned to Philadelphia in 1763, helped to found the School of Medicine and was appointed its first Professor of Medicine. During the American War of Independence both Shippen and Morgan held high rank in the medical services.

John Hunter's last American student and the man often called 'the father of American surgery' was Philip Syng Physick (1768–1837) (Figure 6.19). Like so many of the early American doctors, he hailed from Philadelphia and was one of the early students at the University of Pennsylvania. He completed his training in Edinburgh and London, where he served as Hunter's house pupil and helped him with his dissections. He was also appointed for a year as house surgeon at St George's Hospital. Physick returned to practise in Philadelphia, began giving private lectures on surgery in 1800, and in 1805 was appointed Professor of Surgery at the University. For the rest of his life he was the best known surgeon in that city and probably in the whole of the USA. Except for a few reports in medical journals, he wrote little, although he introduced a number of innovations.

John Collins Warren (1778–1856), a Bostonian, served as a dresser at Guy's Hospital in 1799, returned to Boston in 1802 and became one of the founders of the Massachusetts General Hospital. He served later as Professor of Surgery and Anatomy at the Harvard Medical School. We shall meet him again in the next chapter since he had the honour to perform the first operation under ether anaesthesia.

The first half of the 19th century

During the early part of the 19th century, pioneering surgeons took the art and science of their subject as far as, indeed I consider further than, one might imagine possible with the constraints they faced. They had to cope with the absence of means of relieving the pain of surgery, so that speed was of the essence, and the absence of knowledge of the bacterial nature of wounding sepsis, so that any operation they performed, no matter how skillfully, faced the strong possibility of being followed by suppuration, often with generalised spreading infection, and with consequent prolonged morbidity and often death.

Important advances were made during these decades. They saw the beginning of what is now popularly called 'key-hole surgery', when Jean Civiale (1792–1867) in Paris invented the lithotrite, which could be passed along the urethra into the bladder to crush a bladder stone without the necessity of open surgery. This remarkable advance will be detailed in the chapter devoted to bladder stones (Chapter 12). The first successes were reported for elective, that is to say non-emergency, operations within the abdominal cavity; these were performed for removal of massive ovarian cysts and tumours. Vascular surgery, with the exposure and ligation of the major arteries of the body for injury and aneurysm, was taken to its potential limits. Radical surgery for breast cancer, with removal even of invaded adjacent lymph nodes, was carried out (see Chapter 11) and amputations through the hip joint and shoulder joint for injury and disease were performed with survival of the patients.

An important factor that facilitated surgical progress at this time was the rapid dissemination of the news of important discoveries and of major advances in the well-established medical press in Europe and America. Thus, the oldest journal still published in the United Kingdom, the *Edinburgh Medical Journal* (originally the *Edinburgh Medical and Surgical Journal*), first appeared in 1805. *The Lancet*, edited by Thomas Wakley, a general practitioner turned journalist, commenced publication in 1823. This was soon followed by the *Glasgow Medical Journal* in 1828 and the *Dublin Medical Press* in 1839.

Let us now consider some of these advances in more detail and comment upon the surgical pioneers responsible for them and upon their remarkably courageous patients.

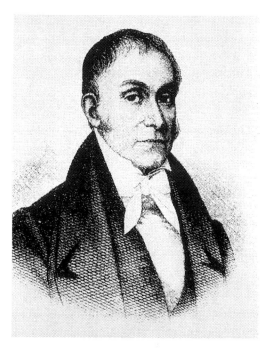

Figure 6.20 Ephraim McDowell.
Royal College of Obstetricians and Gynaecologists.

It is incredible that the first successful removal of an abdominal tumour was carried out, not in some great teaching hospital in Europe, by an eminent professor of surgery, but in 1809 in Danville, Kentucky. The surgeon was Ephraim McDowell (1771–1830) (Figure 6.20). McDowell was born in Virginia but moved to Kentucky as a schoolboy when his father was appointed a judge at Danville, the first capital of that state. Like so many American students, he went to Edinburgh; here he attended the sessions of 1793 and 1794 where he followed the anatomy lectures of Alexander Monro Secundus (1733–1817) and studied surgery under John Bell (1763–1820). The following year he returned to Danville as its only surgeon and built up an extensive practice covering hundreds of miles of frontier and where a call might mean a long ride on horseback, where Indians and wolves still posed a threat.

On December 13th, 1809, McDowell was called to see Mrs Jane Todd-Crawford, a lady of 44, who

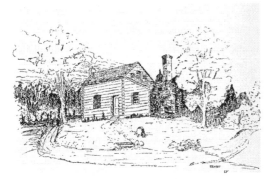

Figure 6.21 Mrs Crawford's house in Green County, Kentucky.
From Schachner A: *Ephraim McDowell*. Philadelphia, JB Lippincott, 1921.

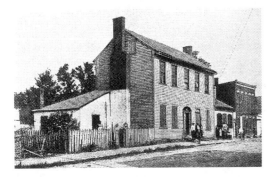

Figure 6.22 Ephraim McDowell's house. The first ovariotomy was performed in the front room. The building is carefully preserved and is now a museum. Royal College of Obstetricians and Gynaecologists.

lived with her family in a log cabin some 60 miles from Danville (Figure 6.21). She was thought to be in the last stages of pregnancy and he was asked to help in delivering her. When McDowell examined the patient he found that the abdomen was considerably enlarged and indeed had the appearance of pregnancy. However, the tumour was inclined to one side and was mobile, and vaginal examination showed nothing in the uterus and the cervix pushed to one side; all the indications were that the mass was 'an enlarged ovarium'. He promised that should

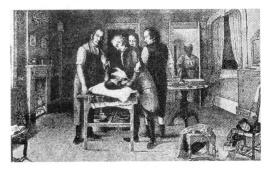

Figure 6.23 The first ovariotomy, painting by George Knapp. McDowell stands to the left of the patient.
From Schachner A: *Ephraim McDowell*. Philadelphia, JB Lippincott, 1921.

she be able to travel to Danville, he was prepared to perform an experiment on her. Mrs Crawford was a tough frontier woman and a few days later she appeared at his home in Danville, having made the long, difficult and dangerous journey by horseback. Interestingly enough, when McDowell operated upon her, he found that the abdominal wall was a good deal bruised and this he ascribed to 'the resting of the tumour on the horn of the saddle during her journey'.

At this time, McDowell's nephew Dr James McDowell, who had graduated a few months before from the new medical school at Philadelphia, joined the practice as a partner. The young man tried to dissuade his uncle from operating but McDowell and Mrs Crawford were determined on the experiment. The operation was performed in the front room of McDowell's home (Figure 6.22). Naturally the operation was performed without any anaesthetic on the classical 'operating table' of the time, brought in from the kitchen (Figure 6.23). During the operation, which took 25 minutes, Mrs Crawford recited psalms and hymns. McDowell describes the operation as follows:

Having placed her on a table of ordinary height, on her back, and removed all her dressing which might in any way impede the operation, I made an incision about three inches from the musculus rectus abdominis, on the left side, continuing the same nine inches in length, parallel with the fibres of the above-named muscle, extending into the cavity of the abdomen . . . The tumour then appeared full in view, but was so large that we could not take it away entire. We put a strong ligature around the Fallopian tube near the uterus, and then cut open the tumour, which was the ovarium and fimbrious part of the Fallopian tube very much enlarged. We took out 15 lbs of a dirty gelatinous-looking substance, after which we cut through the Fallopian tube and extracted the sack, which weighed 7 lbs and one-half. As soon as the external opening was made the intestines rushed out upon the table and so completely was the abdomen filled by the tumour that they could not be replaced during the operation, which was terminated in about 25 minutes. We then turned her upon her left side, so as to permit the blood to escape, after which we closed the external opening with the interrupted suture, leaving out at the lower end of the incision the ligature which surrounded the Fallopian tube.

Within five days Mrs Crawford was up and about making her own bed, and in 25 days she returned home in good health by the same means as she came.

McDowell did not immediately publish this triumphant result – the first elective laparotomy successfully carried out for an accurately diagnosed intra-abdominal pathology. Perhaps he was too diffident, or perhaps he did not realise the tremendous implications of the case; possibly his busy practice gave him little time for the niceties of writing, and he was certainly not a particularly literary man. Most likely he realised that a comparatively unknown country surgeon, publishing a single case report, might be ridiculed unless further 'experiments' were attempted. Whatever the reason, McDowell waited until he had performed two further successful operations, in 1813 and 1816, before publishing a report in 1817 of all three successes. His report appeared in the *Eclectic Repertory and Analytical Review*, published in Philadelphia. Two years later, McDowell's second contribution appeared in the same journal, reporting two further cases. One was successful, but the second patient died of peritoneal inflammation on the third post-operative day. Although McDowell published no more, he did continue with his experiments; between 1822 and 1826 he operated on three more women. In one, the ovarian mass was incised and drained,

and the patient lived for a considerable period of time. One operation involved complete excision, and the third had to be abandoned at laparotomy due to extensive adhesions. There is evidence from correspondence that McDowell performed at least 12 operations for ovarian pathology, but no details exist of the later cases.

It certainly took some time for McDowell's successes to be accepted by the establishment. A copy of the 1817 report was sent to his old teacher, John Bell of Edinburgh, who was then in Rome, where he died shortly thereafter; thus John Lizars (1783–1860), who later became Professor of Surgery at the Royal College of Surgeons of Edinburgh, received the report. Lizars did nothing about the paper until his own publication, *Observations on Extraction of Diseased Ovaria*, was published in 1825, in which he reported four cases, one of which was successful in February 1825. In his report, he quoted McDowell's paper, although by now two other American surgeons had performed successful ovariectomies – Nathan Smith (1762–1829) of Connecticut in 1821, and A G Smith, another Kentuckian, in 1823.

McDowell's first report received a cynical reception. Thus, an article in the *London Medical and Chirurgical Review* reads:

Three cases of ovarian extirpation occurred, it would seem, some years ago in the practice of Dr McDowell of Kentucky, which were transmitted to the late John Bell and fell into the hands of Mr Lizars. We candidly confess that we are rather sceptical respecting these things, and we are rather surprised that Mr Lizars himself should put implicit confidence in them.

However, the publication of McDowell's second report made even the unbelieving English repent and in 1826 we read in the same journal:

A back-settlement of America – Kentucky – has beaten the mother country, nay, Europe itself, with all the boasted surgeons thereof in the fearful and formidable operation of gastrotomy, with extraction of diseased ovaria . . . there was circumstances in the narrative of some of the first three cases that raised misgivings in our minds, for which uncharitableness we ask pardon of God and of Dr McDowell of

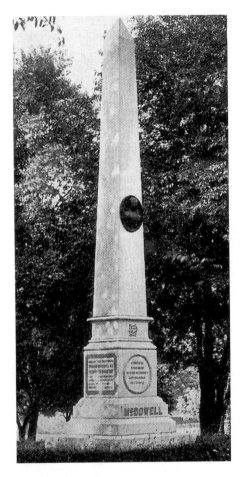

Figure 6.24 The memorial to McDowell in Danville.
From Schachner A: *Ephraim McDowell*. Philadelphia,
JB Lippincott, 1921.

Danville. Two additional cases now published . . . are equally
wonderful as those with which our readers are already
acquainted.

Ephraim McDowell is acknowledged as father not
only of ovariotomy but also of abdominal surgery.
His portrait was immortalised as a four cent stamp
by the United States Postal Service, and the most
senior gynaecological society in the USA is named
after him. Over his grave in Danville is a fine
memorial shaft in Virginia granite erected by the
Kentucky State Medical Society (Figure 6.24). The
inscription reads: 'Beneath this shaft rests Ephraim

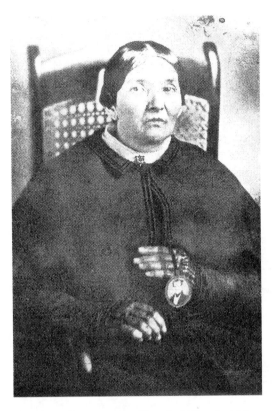

Figure 6.25 Daguerrotype of Jane Todd Crawford taken
in either 1840 or 1841 at the age of 78.
From Schachner A: *Ephraim McDowell*. Philadelphia,
JB Lippincott, 1921.

McDowell MD, the father of ovariotomy who by
originating a great surgical operation became a
benefactor of his race, known and honoured
throughout the civilised world'.

Mrs Crawford and her husband moved to Indiana,
where Mr Crawford was a substantial landowner
and a representative in the Indiana legislature. She
died in 1842 at the age of 78 (Figure 6.25).

The life of one surgeon can be used to illustrate
the heights achieved in the early 19th century.
Astley Cooper (1768–1841) (Figure 6.26), as well as
his other contributions, must be regarded as the
father of modern arterial surgery. If I spend a great
deal of space upon him it is because I freely admit
that he is my surgical hero.

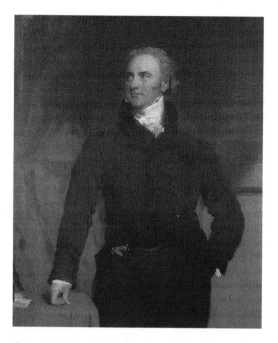

Figure 6.26 Sir Astley Paston Cooper.
Royal College of Surgeons of England.

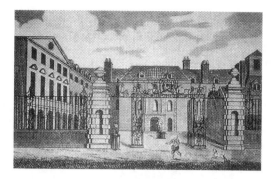

Figure 6.27 Guy's Hospital in 1734. The entrance is very much the same today.
Gordon Museum, Guy's Hospital.

Cooper was born in 1768, the son of a Norfolk country clergyman. At the age of 16 he became articled to his uncle, William Cooper (1724–c. 1800), who was the senior surgeon at Guy's Hospital. However, Astley lived with Henry Cline (1750–1827), surgeon at St Thomas'. In those days the two hospitals were opposite each other across St Thomas' Street and were known as the United Hospitals (Figure 6.27). Medical students were attached to both institutions, their lectures in medicine taking place at Guy's and those in surgery and anatomy at St Thomas'.

Cline encouraged young Cooper to attend the lectures of John Hunter and, six months after arriving in London, Astley transferred his apprenticeship to Cline. He now began his lifetime interest in anatomy. While still a pupil, he was appointed, first, demonstrator in anatomy and then, at the age of 23, helped Cline with his course of lectures. Cooper was appointed to the surgical staff at Guy's

Hospital in 1800 and there he spent the rest of his professional life.

He must have been one of the hardest working surgeons in history. At the height of his fame he would rise every morning by six, often by five and sometimes as early as four. He would go straight to his dissecting room, which was a shed at his own home, and there he would experiment until breakfast. From then until one o'clock he gave free consultations at his home. He then went to Guy's Hospital, where crowds of students would attend his ward rounds, clinical lectures and operating sessions. Visits to private patients and operations in their homes would follow. He would be home by seven, take a hurried meal, and then go out again to see more patients or to lecture, rarely arriving home before midnight. He used to say that a day spent without dissection was a day wasted.

His monograph on *Hernia*, published in 1804, gives an account of the anatomy of the groin which can be read with profit to this day. It contains the first description of the fascia transversalis, which he so named. His other monographs were *Fractures and Dislocations* (1822), *Illustrations of Diseases of the Breast* (1829), *Observations on the Structure and Diseases of the Testis* (1830), *Anatomy of the Thymus Gland* (1832) and *On the Anatomy of the Breast* (1840). The guiding principle in Cooper's teaching is stated in the preface to his treatise on *Hernia*, in which he writes: 'I have almost uniformly in this

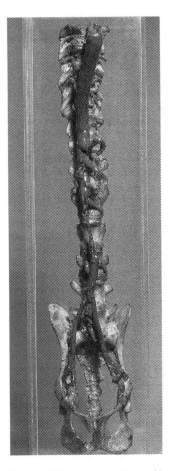

Figure 6.28 Injected specimen of ligated dog's aorta to show collateral channels, prepared by Astley Cooper. Gordon Museum, Guy's Hospital.

work avoided quoting the opinion of authors on this part of surgery . . . I have therefore related no case, and given no remark to the truth of which I cannot vouch'.

He lectured with remarkable clarity – no wonder his classes were always crowded – and his published lectures are well worth reading today, based as they were on careful clinical and experimental studies. He sought explanations for everything; in his monograph on the testis he notes that the reason that one testis is lower than the other is so that they do not become squashed when we stand with our thighs together – as good an anatomical reason as any other.

At the age of 57, Astley Cooper resigned as Senior Surgeon to Guy's Hospital but continued with his private practice and his dissections. In 1827 he was elected president of the Royal College of Surgeons and in 1836 was elected for a second term in office. He died in 1841, at the age of 72, from what was probably hypertensive cardiac failure.

We return now to Cooper's contributions to vascular surgery. He was not simply a bold surgeon, who ligated most of the major arteries of the body; his work was based on careful observation and experimental studies. While still a student, he investigated the collateral circulation in the dog following femoral and brachial artery ligation. He made extensive studies on ligation of the carotid and vertebral arteries and had one dog that actually survived serial ligation of all four of these vessels. In 1811 he reported successful ligation of the abdominal aorta in the dog and demonstrated specimens to show the collateral circulation which follows this. One of these specimens still survives in the Gordon Museum at Guy's and is well worth a close inspection (Figure 6.28).

Cooper was the first to ligate the common carotid artery for aneurysm. His first patient, in 1805, died of suppuration of the sac but his second case, a man aged 50, operated upon in 1808, was entirely successful, the patient surviving 13 years until dying of a left cerebral haemorrhage, on the operated side.

Cooper ligated the external iliac artery for femoral aneurysm on nine occasions. One of these was performed on the same day as the successful case of carotid ligation, a remarkable operating list even for today! This patient died 18 years later.

When, in 1817, a patient presented at Guy's Hospital with a rapidly expanding iliac aneurysm, which was obviously on the point of rupture, Cooper had the opportunity to put his earlier experimental observations to the test. At this point he went to the post-mortem room and attempted to expose the aorta through a lateral retroperitoneal incision, found this to be 'utterly impracticable' and practised the trans-abdominal approach. His operation of aortic ligation had therefore been completely studied, both from its physiological and anatomical aspects.

As the following case report describes, the collateral circulation was indeed sufficient on the normal side, but on the side of the aneurysm, where collateral channels were no doubt disrupted and thrombosed, the leg became ischaemic and the patient died.

The following is a somewhat shortened version of Cooper's description of the operation:

Charles Hutson, a porter, aet 38, was admitted into Guy's Hospital, on the 9th of April 1817, for an aneurysm in the left groin, situated partly above and partly below Poupart's ligament. The swelling was very much diffused, and pressure upon it gave considerable pain. On the third day after he had been in the Hospital, the swelling increased to double its former size, and extended from three to four inches above Poupart's ligament to an equal distance below it, and was of great magnitude. Just below the anterior and superior spinous process of the ilium, a distinct fluctuation could be felt in the aneurismal sac, so that the blood had not evidently yet coagulated; and the peritoneum was carried far from the lower part of the abdomen, in such a manner as to reach the common iliac artery, and to render an operation impracticable without opening the cavity of the peritoneum. I therefore was extremely averse to perform an operation, and determined to wait and see if any efforts would be towards a spontaneous cure.

He was occasionally bled, kept perfectly quiet, and pressure was applied on the tumour. June 19th, a slough was observed on the exterior part of the swelling below Poupart's ligament, which, in part, separated on the 20th, and he had some bleeding from the sac, but it was easily stopped by a compress of lint, confined on the part by adhesive plaster. On the 22nd, after some slight exertion, he bled again, but not profusely. 24th, the bleeding again recurred, but stopped spontaneously. 25th, about half-past two o'clock, in consequence of a sudden mental agitation, he bled profusely, and became so much exhausted that his faeces passed off involuntarily; but Mr Key, then my apprentice, succeeded in preventing immediate dissolution by pressure. At nine o'clock the same evening I saw him, and found him in so a reduced a state, that he could not survive another haemorrhage, with

which he was every moment threatened. Yet still anxious to avoid opening the abdomen, to secure the aorta near to its bifurcation, I made an incision into the aneurismal sac, above Poupart's ligament, to ascertain if it were practicable to pass a ligature around the artery from thence. On introducing my finger, I found that the artery entered the sac above and quitted it below, without there being an intervening portion of vessel; I, therefore, was obliged to abandon that mode of operating; and as the only chance which remained of preventing his immediate dissolution, by haemorrhage, was by tying the aorta, I determined on doing it. The operation was performed as follows:-

The patient's shoulders were slightly elevated by pillows, in order to relax, as much as possible, the abdominal muscles. I then made an incision, three inches long, into the linea alba, giving it a slight curve, to avoid the umbilicus: one inch and a half was above, and the remainder below the navel. Having divided the linea alba, I made a small aperture into the peritoneum, and introduced my finger into the abdomen; and then with a probe-pointed bistoury enlarged the opening into the peritoneum to nearly the same extent as that of the external wound. During the progress of the operation, only one small convolution of intestine projected beyond the wound.

Having made a sufficient opening to admit my finger into the abdomen, I passed it between the intestines to the spine, and felt the aorta greatly enlarged, and beating with excessive force. By means of my finger nail, I scratched through the peritoneum on the left side of the aorta, and then gradually passed my finger between the aorta and spine, and again penetrated the peritoneum, on the right side of the aorta.

I had now my finger under the artery, and by its side I conveyed the blunt aneurismal needle, armed with a single ligature behind it; and Mr Key drew the ligature from the eye of the needle to the external wound, when the needle was withdrawn.

The next circumstance, which required considerable care, was the exclusion of the intestine from the ligature, the ends of which were brought together at the wound, and the finger was carried down between them, so as to remove every portion of the intestine from between the threads: the ligature was then tied, and its ends were left hanging out of the wound.

The omentum was drawn behind the opening as far as the ligature would admit, so as to facilitate adhesion; and the edges of the wound were brought together by means of a quilled suture and adhesive plaster.

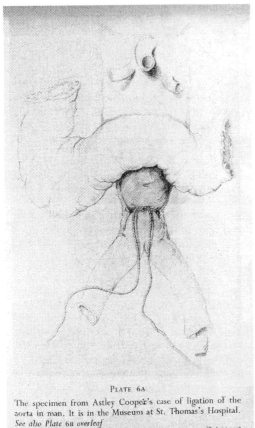

PLATE 6A

The specimen from Astley Cooper's case of ligation of the aorta in man. It is in the Museum at St. Thomas's Hospital. *See also Plate 6B overleaf*

[*To face page 58*]

Figure 6.29 Drawing of the autopsy specimen of Cooper's ligation of the abdominal aorta.
Guy's Hospital Reports 1940–41. The original specimen can be seen in the Gordon Museum at Guy's.

He remained very comfortable until the following evening, when he vomited, and his faeces passed off involuntarily. 27th, Seven o'clock am, had passed a restless night, and had vomited at intervals, pulse 104, weak and small; pain in head; great anxiety of countenance; very restless, and his urine dribbled from him. He gradually sunk, and died at eighteen minutes after one o'clock, having survived the operation forty hours.

Dissection

No peritoneal inflammation, but at the edges of the wound, which were glued together by adhesive matter, excepting at the part at which the ligature protruded. The thread had been passed around the aorta, about three quarters of an inch above its bifurcation, and rather more than an inch below the part at which the duodenum crosses the artery; it had not included any portion of omentum, or intestine. The aneurismal sac, which was of a most enormous size, reached from the common iliac artery to below Poupart's ligament, and extended to the outer part of the thigh. The artery was deficient from the upper to the lower part of the sac, which was filled with an immense quantity of coagulum.

The specimen can be seen today, carefully preserved, in the Gordon Museum at Guy's (Figure 6.29).

It was not until over a century later, in 1925, that Rudolph Matas (1860–1957) of New Orleans was able to report the first successful ligation of the abdominal aorta (see Chapter 14).

In addition to his work on arterial ligation, Cooper was one of the first to carry out a successful disarticulation at the hip joint. This was performed on January 15th, 1824, on a soldier who had had his leg amputated at the battle of Waterloo in 1815. He was now suffering from chronic osteomyelitis of the stump of the femur and was obviously sinking under the effects of the disease. Cooper first tied the femoral artery at the groin, then made an elliptical incision from below the groin to about one third down the back of the thigh. The head of the femur was disarticulated without difficulty. Four blood vessels were tied and a total of about 12 ounces of blood lost. The skin flaps were brought together with a stitch and strips of adhesive. The operation took a total of 35 minutes, the patient being given wine during the course of the procedure. The patient bore the operation with extreme fortitude. Recovery was retarded by infection of the stump, which was relieved by loosening the dressings and strapping and by incision of an abscess. By March 19th he was gaining strength and had been wheeled around the squares of the Hospital. By August the patient was perfectly recovered and was living in the country residence of his surgeon; it is an interesting light on Cooper's character that his interest in his welfare of his patient extended so far as to provide convalescence for him in his own country house (Figure 6.30).

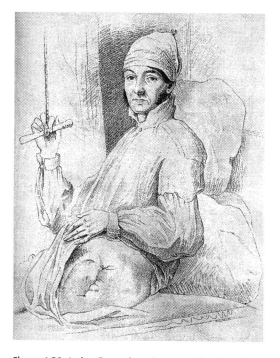

Figure 6.30 Astley Cooper's patient convalescing after disarticulation at the hip joint in 1824. Guy's Hospital Reports 1940–41.

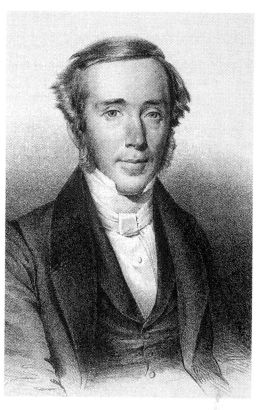

Figure 6.31 James Syme.
Royal College of Surgeons of England.

The following year, in September 1825, James Syme (1799–1870) (Figure 6.31), assisted by Robert Liston (1794–1847), performed an amputation at the hip joint for a tumour in Edinburgh. Unlike Cooper's operation, this was done at great speed, the actual removal of the limb taking no more than a minute. Syme paid no attention to bleeding until the limb was removed except that his assistant, Liston, 'covered the numerous cut arteries with his left hand and compressed the femoral in the groin by means of his right'. As soon as the femoral artery was secured, Liston released his hands and Syme writes:

And then had it not been for thorough seasoning in scenes of dreadful haemorrhage, I certainly should have been startled. It seemed, indeed, at first sight, as if the vessels which supplied so many large and crossing jets of arterial blood could never all be closed. It may be imagined that we did not spend much time in admiring this alarming spectacle. A single instant was sufficient to convince us that the patient's safety required all our expedition; and, in the course of a few minutes, haemorrhage was effectually restrained by the application of ten or twelve ligatures.

Syme's patient sank and died from exhaustion seven weeks after the operation.

A report of the operation, in the *Edinburgh Medical and Surgical Journal* sarcastically compared the time occupied by Syme to that by Cooper. The *Lancet*, in London, vigorously championed Cooper's technique, basing its criticism on the comparison between Cooper's meticulous care to secure the main vessels at first step in the operation in contrast to Syme's bloody procedure. The fact that Cooper's patient survived and Syme's patient died was also not overlooked!

Syme and Liston were leading surgeons in Edinburgh at this time. James Syme was born and trained in Edinburgh, opened a school of anatomy with Liston, and in 1833 became Professor of Surgery in the University of Edinburgh. He made numerous important contributions, including excision of the lower jaw for tumour in 1828, the introduction of his technique of amputation of the foot using a long heel flap which still bears his name, and advocating, in a monograph he published in 1839, the operation of excision of the joint for chronic conditions such as tuberculosis in preference to amputation. He was also a pioneer in the use of chloroform as an anaesthetic.

Joseph Lister, the father of antiseptic surgery (see Chapter 7), was his house surgeon and later married Syme's daughter Agnes.

Robert Liston was appointed Professor of Surgery at the University College Hospital, London in 1835 and will be encountered again as the first surgeon to use ether anaesthesia in Europe (Chapter 7).

7

The advent of anaesthesia and antisepsis

In the middle years of the 19th century, over a short period of only two decades, the two most important advances in the history of surgery took place. The first was the discovery of the effects of anaesthetic agents, which abolished the agonies of surgical procedures. The second was the realisation that wound suppuration was caused by bacteria and thus that the greatest hazard of open wounds produced by injury or by the surgeon's knife could be largely obviated by the introduction first of antiseptic and, soon after, aseptic surgical techniques.

Anaesthesia

From earliest times, attempts have been made to dull the pain of injuries and of surgery. Large doses of alcohol, of opium or of laudanum (tincture of opium and alcohol) taken by mouth, or mandragora (obtained from the mandrake plant, *Mandragora officinarum*, which contains hyoscine and other alkaloid drugs), were used. Much effort was expended on the psychological preparation of the patient before surgery and some good effects could be obtained by hypnotism, since its introduction as 'mesmerism' by Anton Mesmer (1734–1815).

However, it was the study of the effects of inhalation of various gases and vapours that initiated a truly effective method of anaesthesia.

Humphrey Davy (1778–1829), who later became Director of the Laboratory of the Royal Institution, described the analgesic effect of inhaling nitrous oxide while still a lad of 19. Davy himself gave it the name 'laughing gas' and wrote, in 1800: 'It appears capable of destroying physical pain, it may probably be used with advantage during surgical operations in which no great effusion of blood takes place'.

This appears to be the first suggestion that pain relief in surgery might be achieved by inhalation of some suitable vapour or gas. Nitrous oxide was widely used for its euphoric effects in so-called 'frolics' but no-one appears to have taken Davy's advice until Horace Wells (1815–1848), a dentist in Hartford, Connecticut, carried out dental extractions painlessly using nitrous oxide administered through a wooden tube placed in the mouth from an animal bladder distended with the gas. Wells, in order to popularise his discovery, went to Boston in 1845 and was introduced by his former partner, William Morton, to the surgeons at the Massachusetts General Hospital. A demonstration of dental extraction under nitrous oxide failed and Wells was booed out of the room. He continued to use the gas in his own practice but this was soon replaced by ether. It was some time before nitrous oxide returned as a popular method of anaesthesia for dental extractions and other relatively minor procedures.

Ether (or, to give it its full chemical name, diethyl ether) was first prepared in 1540. Like nitrous oxide, it was widely used in Europe and America as a party amusement, so there is nothing new in the behaviour of our modern youngsters in their experiments with mood-changing substances. Crawford Long (1815–1878), who was a general practitioner

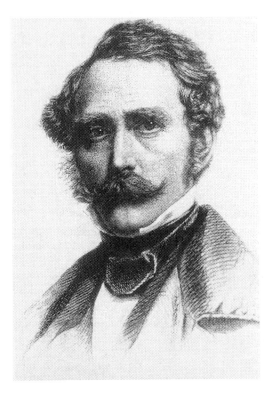

Figure 7.1 William Morton.
MacQuitty B: *Battle for Oblivion*. London, Harrap, 1969.

in Jefferson, Georgia, had himself inhaled ether and noticed that he might fall and bruise himself under the influence of the vapour without feeling any pain. He therefore tried out inhalation of the substance in 1842 in order to remove a couple of cysts from the back of a patient's neck and indeed carried out a number of minor operations over the next years. However, he did not publish his experiences until 1849, by which time the use of ether was well established. It is not sufficient to make a discovery, it is also necessary to let the world know about it.

William Thomas Green Morton (1819–1868) (Figure 7.1) can be regarded as the father of modern anaesthetics. He studied at the Baltimore College of Dental Surgery and became a pupil and then a partner of Horace Wells at Hartford. He then moved to Boston and was present when Wells gave his unsatisfactory demonstration of nitrous oxide. Ether was an obvious alternative, since Morton had observed its effects on his patients when they breathed the vapour after applying liquid ether to deaden painful tooth sockets. Morton tried the effects of ether on himself, on a dog and on his assistants and then, on September 30th, 1846, on his first patient, Eben Frost, who had a tooth pulled out under the influence of ether saturated into a handkerchief. The patient testified as follows:

This is to certify that I applied to Doctor Morton at nine o'clock this evening suffering under the most violent toothache; Doctor Morton took out his pocket handkerchief, saturated with a preparation of his, from which I breathed for about half a minute, and then was lost in sleep. In an instant more I awoke and saw my tooth lying upon the floor. I did not experience the slightest pain whatever. I remained 20 minutes in his office afterward, and felt no unpleasant effects from the operation.

Dr Henry Bigelow (1818–1890), who had recently been appointed to the staff of the Massachusetts General Hospital, having read the newspaper reports of Morton's work, went to see him and was impressed by what he saw. He introduced Morton to John Collins Warren (1778–1856) (Figure 7.2), the Professor of Surgery at the MGH, and a few days later Morton received the following letter: 'I write at the request of Dr John Collins Warren to invite you to be present Friday morning October 16, at 10 o'clock at the hospital to administer to a patient who is then to be operated upon, the preparation you have invented to diminish the sensibility to pain'. The letter was signed by the house surgeon, Dr C F Heywood.

It was now only two weeks since ether had been administered to Frost, but already Morton had progressed from a soaked handkerchief to a simple anaesthetic machine. This consisted of a two-necked glass globe, one neck allowing the inflow of air, the other fitted with a wooden mouthpiece through which the patient inhaled air across the surface of an ether – soaked sponge in the bottom of the jar (Figure 7.3).

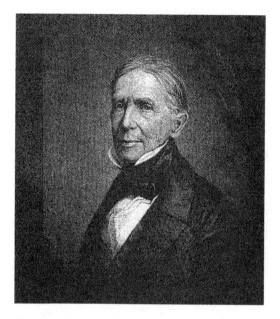

Figure 7.2 John C. Warren.
From MacQuitty B: *Battle for Oblivion*. London, Harrap, 1969.

All the anxieties of a great clinical trial are summed up by Morton's young wife, who wrote:

The night before the operation my husband worked until 1 or 2 o'clock in the morning upon his inhaler. I assisted him nearly beside myself with anxiety, for the strongest influences had been brought to bear upon me to dissuade him from making this attempt. I had been told that one of two things was sure to happen; either the test would fail and my husband would be ruined by the world's ridicule, or he would kill the patient and be tried for manslaughter. Thus I was drawn in two ways; for while I had unbounded confidence in my husband, it did not seem possible that so young a man could be wiser than the learned and scientific men before whom he proposed to make his demonstration.

The operating theatre at the Massachusetts General Hospital was situated just below the central dome of the old building (Figure 7.4). It is preserved to this day.

I have had the privilege of lecturing in what is now called the 'Ether Dome', a great thrill for anyone interested in surgical history.

On the morning of October 16th, it was crowded with surgeons and medical students. The audience included both Jacob Bigelow and his son, Henry. The patient was Gilbert Abbott, 20 years of age, who had a benign vascular tumour of the neck. Petrified at the thought of the pain of his operation, he had readily agreed to the experiment. Professor Warren explained to the audience how much he had always wished to free his patients from the pain of operation and for that reason had agreed to the experiment. The time of the operation arrived and passed. By ten minutes past ten Professor Warren picked up his knife and said 'As Dr Morton has not arrived, I presume he is otherwise engaged'.

Just as Abbott was being strapped down on the operating chair, a breathless and flustered Morton arrived; he had been modifying his apparatus up to the very last moment. Warren said, 'Well, sir, your patient is ready'.

'Are you afraid?' Morton asked the patient. 'No, I feel confident that I will do precisely what you tell me.' Morton applied his ether, its smell disguised by orange essence to prevent bystanders recognising its nature. Turning to Warren, Morton was now able to say, '*Your* patient is ready, doctor.' Many years later Mrs Morton described the scene:

Then in all parts of the ampitheatre there came a quick catching of breath, followed by a silence almost deathlike, as Dr. Warren stepped forward and prepared to operate . . . The patient lay silent, with eyes closed as if in sleep; but everyone present fully expected to hear a shriek of agony ring out as the knife struck down into the sensitive nerves, but the stroke came with no accompanying cry. Then another and another, and still the patient lay silent, sleeping while the blood from the severed artery spurted forth. The surgeon was doing his work, and the patient was free from pain. (Figure 7.5)

The operation took 30 minutes, and at the end Abbott agreed that the whole affair had been free from pain. Warren turned to the audience and said, 'Gentlemen, this is no humbug'. It took a few moments before the sensational importance of what they had seen struck the audience, who then rushed forward to congratulate Morton, to examine

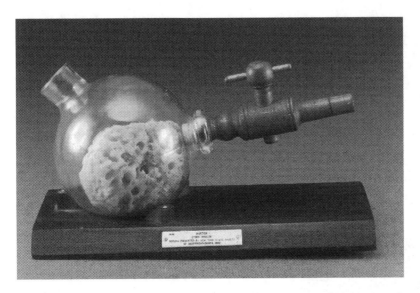

Figure 7.3 A model of Morton's ether inhaler. (The original is preserved in the Massachusetts General Hospital, Boston.)

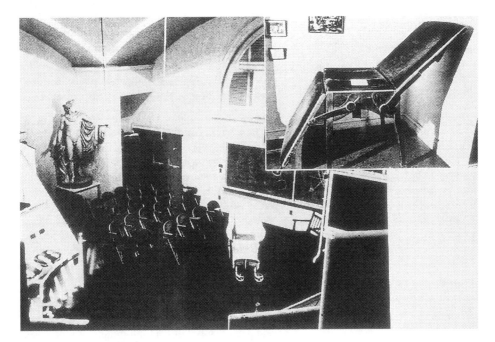

Figure 7.4 The 'Ether Dome' still carefully preserved and used today as a lecture theatre. Inset is the table on which the operation was performed.
Photograph provided by the General Director of the Massachusetts General Hospital, Boston.

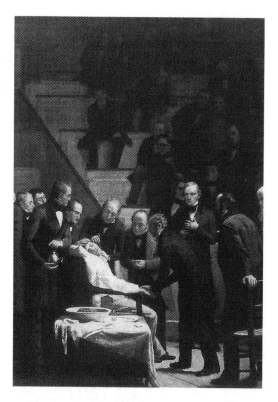

Figure 7.5 Painting of the first operation under ether. Morton holds his anaesthetic apparatus at the head of the table; Warren operates.
Photograph provided by the General Director of the Massachusetts General Hospital, Boston.

the patient and to ask him over and over again if the operation had really been painless. Everyone in that room must have realised that they had witnessed an historic occasion.

It was now necessary to proceed to the crucial experiment. The new agent might be effective in the removal of a subcutaneous lump from the neck, but would it work in a capital operation, an amputation? A case was duly scheduled, therefore, for November 7th. Before this could be put to the test, a burning ethical issue arose. Should Morton be allowed to administer a secret agent, beneficial though it might be, or should its use be prohibited until its nature was revealed to the medical profession? Warren was prepared to go ahead,

his only concern being relief of pain, but the Massachusetts Medical Society resolved unanimously – no formula, no patients. Even though Morton offered to supply the preparation free for use in the Boston hospitals, the doctors remained adamant.

On the very day of the operation the argument continued, with the patient waiting in the anteroom and the theatre packed to the ceiling with expectant doctors and students. Unable to bear the thought of the patient's suffering, Morton quietly announced that his liquid was indeed sulphuric ether.

The patient was a 21-year-old servant girl, Alice Mohan, who had been in the hospital since the previous March with tuberculosis of the knee joint. Dr George Hayward was to perform the amputation, with Warren and Bigelow in attendance. Morton administered the ether, and after some coughing, the patient fell into a deep sleep. Hayward stuck a pin into her arm and, when there was no reaction, rapidly amputated the leg. As he finished, Alice began to groan and move. Hayward bent over her and said, 'I guess you've been asleep Alice'. 'I think I have, sir', she replied. 'Well, you know why we brought you here; are you ready?' 'Yes sir, I am ready.' Hayward then reached down, picked up the amputated limb from the sawdust, showed it to her and said, 'It's all done, Alice'. (What Alice said when she saw her leg has not been recorded.)

Scenes of intense excitement then took place, with the medical audience clapping and shouting with amazement. Morton described the affair modestly: 'I administered the ether with perfect success. This was the first case of amputation'. The patient did well and was discharged from the hospital in time for Christmas.

The news of Morton's discovery spread with amazing speed through the civilised world. In December, Francis Boott (1792–1863), a medical practitioner in Gower Street, London, who had trained in America, received a letter written on November 28th by Bigelow giving a full account of the momentous events in Boston. Boott immediately encouraged a dental surgeon, James Robinson

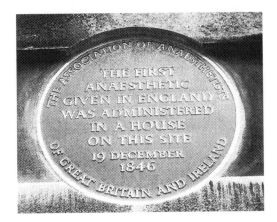

Figure 7.6 Plaque to commemorate the first operation under ether in Great Britain – a dental extraction in a house in Gower Street, London, along the road from University College Hospital.
Photograph by the author.

(1813–1862), who had studied at Guy's and was in practice in Gower Street, to give ether to a young woman for extraction of a molar tooth. The site of this first operation under anaesthesia in the British Isles is today commemorated by a plaque (Figure 7.6). Robinson went on to write the world's first textbook of anaesthesia *A Treatise of the Inhalation of the Vapour of Ether* the following year.

So successful was this experiment that Boott persuaded Robert Liston (1794–1847), Professor of Surgery of the nearby University College Hospital, to try the effects of ether for major surgery. The apparatus was made by Peter Squire, a nearby pharmacist, and the anaesthetist was his nephew, William Squire, a medical student at UCH aged 21. The operation was carried out just two days after the dental extraction, on December 21st.

The patient was Frederick Churchill, a butler who had been admitted a month previously with chronic osteomyelitis of the tibia. At two o'clock the operating theatre at the University College Hospital was packed to capacity. Squire called for a volunteer among the doctors and medical students present, saying that he had only tried the apparatus once before and would like one more rehearsal

before submitting a patient to its influence for a capital operation. No-one moved. The theatre porter, Shelldrake, was therefore asked to submit to the test. He was not a good choice to try out an anaesthetic as he was fat, plethoric, and with a liver no doubt very used to strong liquor. After a few deep breaths of ether, Shelldrake leaped off the table and ran out of the room, cursing Squire and everybody else at the top of his voice.

Fifteen minutes later, Liston arrived, and Churchill was brought into the theatre by the now sober and recovered Shelldrake. Squire took the precaution of choosing two hefty students to stand by in case the patient repeated the porter's performance. What happened next has been brilliantly described by a member of the audience, Dr F W Cock, and is illustrated in Figure 7.7:

A firm step is heard, and Robert Liston enters – that magnificent figure of a man, six foot two inches in height, with a most commanding expression of countenance. He nods quietly to Squire and, turning round to the packed crowd of onlookers, students, colleagues, old students and many of the neighbouring practitioners, says somewhat dryly, 'We are going to try a Yankee dodge, to-day gentlemen, for making men insensible.' He then takes from a long narrow case one of the straight amputating knives of his own invention. It is evidently a favourite instrument, for on the handle are little notches showing the number of times he had used it before . . . The patient is carried in on the stretcher and laid on the table. The tube is put into the mouth, William Squire holds it at the patient's nostrils. A couple of dressers stand by, to hold the patient if necessary, but he never moves and blows and gurgles away quite quietly. William Squire looks at Liston and says, 'I think he will do, sir.' 'Take the artery, Mr. Cadge,' cries Liston. Ransome, the House Surgeon, holds the limb. 'Now gentlemen, time me,' he says to the students. A score of watches are pulled out in reply. A huge left hand grasps the thigh, a thrust of the long, straight knife, two or three rapid sawing movements, and the upper flap is made; under go his fingers, and the flap is held back; another thrust, and the point of the knife comes out in the angle of the upper flap; two or three more lightning-like movements and the lower flap is cut, under goes the great thumb and holds it back also; the dresser, holding the saw by its end, yields it to the surgeon and takes the knife in return – half a dozen strokes, and

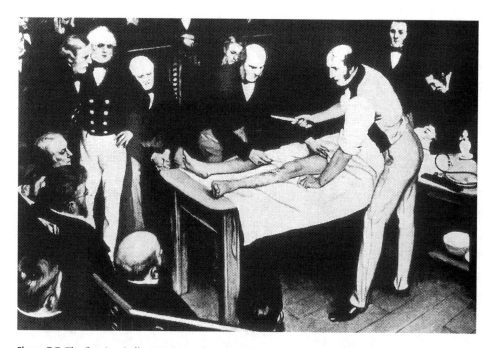

Figure 7.7 The first 'capital' operation under ether at University College Hospital. Professor Robert Liston operates in his shirt sleeves. The ether apparatus is placed on a small table; William Squire bends over the patient. The original painting is in UCH, courtesy of University College, London.

Ransome places the limb in the sawdust. 'Twenty-eight seconds,' says William Squire. The femoral artery is taken upon a tenaculum and tied with two stout ligatures, and five or six more vessels with the bow forceps and single thread, a strip of wet lint put between the flaps, and the stump dressed. The patient, trying to raise himself, says, 'When are you going to begin? Take me back, I can't have it done.' He is shown the elevated stump, drops back and weeps a little, then the porters come in and he is taken back to bed. Five minutes have elapsed since he left it. As he goes out, Liston turns again to his audience, so excited that he almost stammers and hesitates, and exclaims, 'This Yankee dodge, gentlemen, beats mesmerism hollow.'

Liston could hardly have realised at that moment that the need for rapid surgery, which his skill had brought to such a pitch of perfection, was now to be replaced by the new era, when anaesthesia would allow calm and unhurried operations.

As for Morton, the rest of his short life was not a happy one, although he had the compensation of using ether with great success during the American Civil War (see Chapter 9). He died in 1868 at only 48 years of age. The citizens of Boston erected a monument over his grave (Figure 7.8), the inscription of which was composed by Dr Jacob Bigelow:

> Inventor and revealer of anaesthetic inhalation
> By whom pain in surgery was averted and annulled
> Before whom in all time surgery was agony
> Since whom has controlled the pain.

The word 'anaesthesia' was suggested by Oliver Wendell Holmes (1809–1894), Professor of Anatomy and Physiology at the Harvard Medical School. He did so in November 1846, a few weeks after the first use of ether, in a letter to Morton, although the word anaesthesia had appeared in *Bailey's English Dictionary* in 1721 to mean loss of sensation. The word anaesthesia passed into the English language, although the term 'etherization' was widely used in the early years.

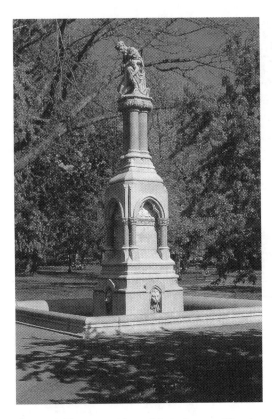

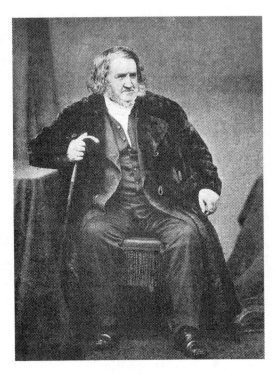

Figure 7.9 James Young Simpson.
Royal College of Surgeons of England.

Figure 7.8 The memorial over Morton's grave, Mount Auburn cemetery, Boston.
Photograph by the author.

Ether was probably given in Scotland on December 19th, 1846, the same day as the dental extraction by Robinson in London. This was at the Dumfries and Galloway Royal Infirmary. The news of Morton's success was taken there by William Fraser (1819–1863), a ship's surgeon who arrived in Liverpool from Boston. The surgeon was William Scott (1820–1887). Joseph Malgaigne (1806–1865) was able to report his first five cases of ether anaesthesia at the Académie de Médecine in Paris on January 12th, 1847. The first anaesthetic in the southern hemisphere was given by a general practitioner, Dr William Russ Pugh (1805–1897) in Launceston, Tasmania, on June 7th, 1847. The first major war in which anaesthetics were employed was the Crimean War of 1854–1855.

James Young Simpson (1811–1870) (Figure 7.9), Professor of Midwifery in Edinburgh, used ether in his obstetrical practice on January 19th, 1847 but the agent had the disadvantage of slow induction and associated vomiting. He and his two young assistants experimented by inhaling various drugs in Simpson's house and were impressed by the speed of action and pleasantness of chloroform in producing unconsciousness. It was easy to use, simply by pouring a drop of the agent on a piece of gauze or handkerchief held near the face of the patient each time the subject breathed (Figure 7.10). By November 10th, 1847, Simpson was able to report the use of chloroform in obstetric practice in a paper read to the Edinburgh Medical and Chirurgical Society. Simpson was attacked for using pain relief for women in labour but the cause of obstetrical anaesthesia was greatly strengthened

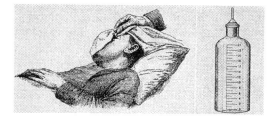

Figure 7.10 The simple 'rag and bottle' method of administration of chloroform used by Simpson.

when Queen Victoria had chloroform administered to her by John Snow (1813–1858) at the birth of her eighth child in 1853.

It is hardly surprising that the means of relieving the pain of surgery was so quickly adopted throughout the world. The story of the spread of knowledge of the cause of wound infection and its prevention was a much slower process.

Of course, the early anaesthetic agents had their disadvantages, even though their use was widespread well into the second half of the twentieth century. The author, for example, as a young doctor, became quite expert in the administration of both nitrous oxide and ether. Nitrous oxide is only suitable for a short anaesthetic, for example, dental extraction. Ether requires a long time to induce the patient, produces a good deal of nausea and is highly inflammable when mixed with oxygen. Chloroform, although easy to use, is associated with very occasional incidents of sudden death from cardiac irregularity. Numerous inhalation agents, used alone or in combination, were developed in the 20th century: cyclopropane and halothane, for example, were safer and more pleasant for the patient. Intravenous anaesthetic drugs, such as pentothal and ketamine, make the induction of anaesthesia rapid and reasonably pleasant.

Local anaesthesia was a relatively late development. It began when Carl Koller (1857–1944), a young ophthalmologist in Vienna, on the suggestion of his friend, Sigmund Freud, used cocaine applied as eye drops as a local anaesthetic for operations on the eye in 1884. It was soon taken up by surgeons in London, Paris and Berlin as a local

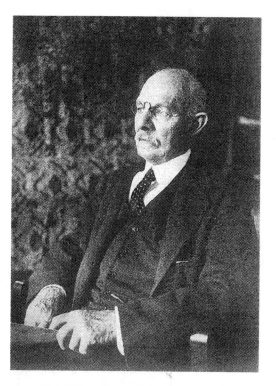

Figure 7.11 William Stewart Halsted. From MacCullum WG: *William Stewart Halsted, Surgeon.* Baltimore, Johns Hopkins Press, 1930.

infiltration for surgical procedures. In the same year as Koller's pioneering work, William Stewart Halsted (1852–1922) (Figure 7.11), a surgeon at the Roosevelt Hospital New York, began to experiment on himself and three of his young colleagues with cocaine for nerve blockade, infiltrating nerves of the face, jaws and limbs to produce regional anaesthesia. He did not realise that cocaine is a dangerously addictive drug; his three colleagues all died and Halsted himself, by 1886, required hospital admission for psychiatric care. The treatment appeared to be to wean him from cocaine on to morphine and it is probable that Halsted never overcame his morphine addiction. We shall meet Halsted again in Chapter 11 as he played an important part in the development of surgery for cancer of the breast, but he was now a changed person. From being a bold, rather flamboyant personality, he became, as Foundation Professor of Surgery at the Johns Hopkins Hospital in Baltimore, a slow, meticulous introvert; an unwitting martyr in the development of anaesthesia.

Fortunately, substitutes for the dangerous agent cocaine were soon developed, in particular novocaine, or procaine, in 1905. More recently a whole series of agents such as lignocaine (1943) have been synthesised and are in use today. Not only are these agents used to infiltrate skin or to block peripheral nerves, but they may be injected into the dural sac to block the spinal nerves (spinal analgesia) or infiltrated around the spinal nerves outside the dura within the vertebral canal (epidural or extradural analgesia) in modern surgical and obstetrical practice.

The development of antiseptic surgery

Few, if any, discoveries in science are sudden affairs; there is so often a series of steps, a slow realisation, leading to the important brilliant success. There are numerous examples of this throughout this book: the evolution of effective surgery for missile wounds, for bladder stone and for breast surgery for example. Nowhere is this better illustrated than the evolution of the control of surgical wound infection.

We have seen (Chapter 4) that Theodoric (1205–1298) denied that suppuration was an essential part of wound healing and wrote: 'It is not necessary that pus should be generated in wounds. No error can be greater than this. Such a practice is indeed to hinder nature, to prolong the disease and to prevent the consolidation of the wound'.

Most surgeons, however, both before and after him, considered suppuration and pus formation to be a normal accompaniment of wounding.

Bacteria were first observed by a remarkable man who had no medical or scientific training whatsoever. This was Antoni van Leeuwenhoek (1632–1723), a draper in Leyden, Holland, who can be regarded as the father of microscopy. He ground the lenses of his own microscopes, which were really no more than sophisticated magnifying glasses, and illustrated bacteria from his own mouth in 1683. It was to be nearly two centuries before their significance in the causation of diseases was established.

Many observers postulated a role for hypothetical 'effluvia' or 'miasmas' in the spread of infectious diseases. The very word 'malaria' comes from the Italian *mal aria* ('bad air') although now we know that it is the malaria protozoal parasite, carried by the Anopheles mosquito, which causes the illness and not the 'bad air' of the marshlands which are home to this insect.

Early important observations were made by obstetricians on the contagiousness of puerperal or childbed fever. This was the dreaded and often fatal infection of the birth canal and peritoneal cavity, usually associated with generalised sepsis and pyaemia (infection of the bloodstream) in women after childbirth. Alexander Gordon (1752–1799) in Aberdeen published a book in 1795 indicating that puerperal fever was carried from one patient to the other by the attending midwife or doctor; he considered that it was putrid matter from the uterus which caused the infection and advised cleanliness on the part of the attending doctor. Charles White (1728–1813) of Manchester emphasised the importance of cleanliness in obstetrical practice while Oliver Wendell Holmes (1809–1894) of Boston, in a paper *On the Contagiousness of Puerperal Fever* in 1843, argued that women in labour should not be treated by a doctor who had recently conducted an autopsy or who had treated a patient with puerperal fever. He quoted that a colleague had been able to halt an epidemic of puerperal fever in his practice simply by washing his hands in a solution of calcium chloride after attending any patient infected by this disease.

Important observations were made by Ignaz Semmelweiss (1818–1865) (Figure 7.12), a Hungarian who was appointed first assistant to the professor of obstetrics at the Allgemeines Krankenhaus in Vienna in 1846. The obstetrical clinic was divided into two divisions: the first was devoted to teaching post-graduate doctors and medical students, and

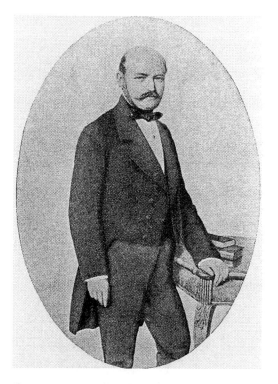

Figure 7.12 Ignaz Semmelweiss.
Royal College of Surgeons of England.

Semmelweiss found that this had an appalling maternal mortality, which could be as high as 18% of the patients. In contrast, the second division, which was staffed by midwives, had a maternal death rate of around 2%. Moreover, he noted that while childbed fever raged in the wards, no such epidemic existed in women delivered in their homes or even those who self-delivered in the streets of Vienna.

The following year, his colleague, the pathologist Jacob Kolletschka, died after performing a post-mortem examination during which he had pricked his finger. Semmelweiss noted that the post-mortem changes seen at the autopsy on his colleague were similar to those of the women dying of childbed fever. The cause of the difference in mortality between the two divisions of the hospital was now clear. The doctors and students in Division

One would perform post-mortems and practise obstetrical operations in the autopsy room, then go straight to the delivery ward bearing with them invisible 'cadaver particles', recognisable only by their characteristic and unpleasant smell, from the dead women to the birth canal of the women in labour. The midwives, who had nothing to do with post-mortems, were protected from this contagion. Semmelweiss immediately instituted a ritual of hand-washing, which comprised scrubbing with soap and hot water followed by a wash in chlorinated water until the smell of the post-mortem room had been completely eliminated. At the same time, instruments, basins, linen and dressings were also cleaned. The results were soon apparent, with maternal mortality falling to the region of 1%.

Semmelweiss returned to Budapest in 1850 and became Professor of Obstetrics there, achieving a maternal mortality rate of 0.85% at the Rochus Hospital.

Unfortunately, Semmelweiss did not publish his work until 1860. His *Aetiology, Concept and Prevention of Puerperal Fever* was difficult to follow, wordy and repetitious; it was not translated into English until 1941. In it he states:

The carrier of the decomposed animal-organic material is the examining finger, the operating hand, instruments, bed linen, atmospheric air, sponges, the hands of the midwives and ward attendants that come into contact with the discharges of other ill parturients . . . in a word the carrier is anything contaminated with decomposed animal organic-material that comes into contact with the vaginal tract.

By 1862 Semmelweiss was showing obvious features of mental deterioration and in 1865 he was admitted to a private asylum in Vienna, where he died. There is some poignancy in the date of his death, since this was the year in which Joseph Lister carried out his first operations using the antiseptic technique.

The important link in the chain, the proof that micro-organisms are the cause of wound infection, remained to be demonstrated. This vital evidence was produced, not by a medical researcher, but by an organic chemist. Louis Pasteur (1822–1895)

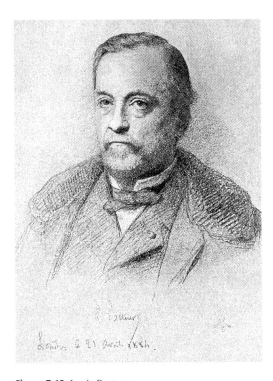

Figure 7.13 Louis Pasteur.
From William Osler: *Evolution of Modern Medicine.* New Haven,
Yale University Press, 1921.

249

air but the solids which cause the decomposition. Take any fermenting liquid, say
wine, and place it in a flask with an extended neck so that the heat may be carried up to 212°, and then apply a spirit lamp
below the flask so as to expell the air and
destroy any thing that may be alive in it.
Take away the spirit lamp
and the air will reenter,
but any germs which may
happen to pass up the tube
will be killed by the heat.
What will be the result?
You have let the air reenter
but this air has been de-
prived of its germs and
the wine in the flask will remain for any
length of time, 20 years or more perfectly
sweet because the air that is now in the
flask deprived of its power of decomposition by being heated in a way calculated
to kill any thing that may be alive in it.

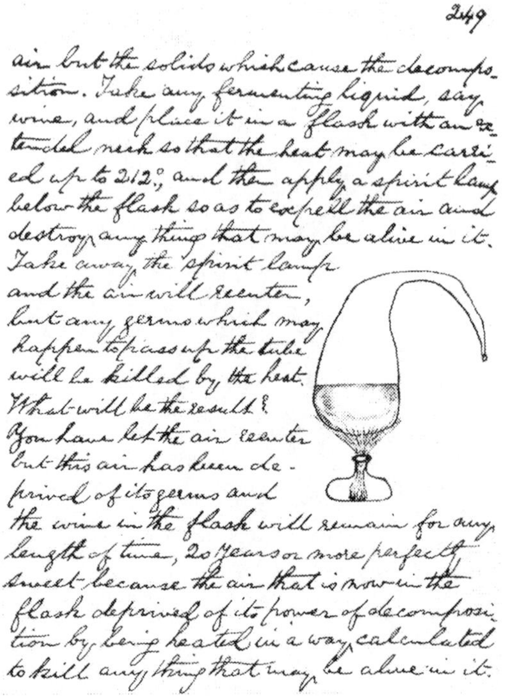

Figure 7.14 Pasteur's experiment with broth, illustrated in the lecture notes of WS Anderson, a medical student attending Lister's surgical lectures in Glasgow.
From Guthrie D: *Lord Lister, his Life and Doctrine.* Edinburgh, Livingstone, 1949.

(Figure 7.13) studied at the École Normale in Paris, worked at the University of Lille and was later appointed Professor of Chemistry at the Sorbonne, Paris. His studies on fermentation of wine and putrefaction of milk, butter and broth demonstrated that this putrefaction process was produced by what he called 'ferments', micro-organisms which he could demonstrate under the microscope.

In a series of brilliant, but simple, experiments, Pasteur was able to show that broth sterilised by boiling would remain so if placed in a flask plugged by sterilised cotton wool, which would allow access to the atmospheric air but not to organisms in the air, which would be filtered by the wool. Remove the plug, and the broth would become putrid after a couple of days. A broth infusion, sterilised by boiling, could be left open to the air indefinitely if the neck of the flask was drawn out into a curve whose convexity pointed upwards. This enabled the broth to be in contact with the outside air, but bacteria were prevented by gravity from doing so and were deposited in the double bend of the neck. Breaking off the neck close to the top of the flask, so that air and its contained organisms now had direct access, produced rapid infection of the broth (Figure 7.14).

Pasteur's studies on fermentation proved to be the catalyst to the work of Joseph Lister on the causes and prevention of surgical wound infection.

Few could deny that Joseph Lister (1827–1912) (Figure 7.15) was the greatest surgical benefactor to mankind. He was born in Upton, Essex. His father Joseph Jackson Lister, a devout Quaker, was a wine merchant and also a distinguished microscopist.

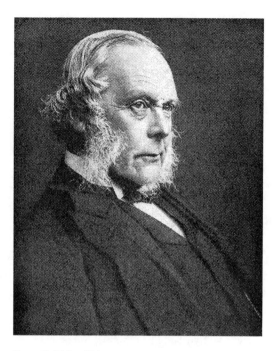

Figure 7.15 Lord Lister.
Royal College of Surgeons of England.

Lister commenced his medical studies at the age of 17 at University College, London, and was said to have been present at Liston's historic amputation of a leg while the patient was anaesthetised with ether (see above). In 1853, Lister became house surgeon and then assistant to James Syme (1799–1870) in Edinburgh, married his daughter Agnes and was appointed assistant surgeon at the Edinburgh Royal Infirmary. In 1860 he was appointed Regius Professor of Surgery at Glasgow and it was here that he laid the foundations of his life's work. Lister was interested in inflammation and in wound healing; he had already carried out important studies on the inflammatory process by observing the vascular changes that take place in the blood vessels of the frog's foot web under the microscope. Like so many surgeons before him, Lister was puzzled by the observation that a closed fracture, no matter how severe, would heal without infection. In contrast, a compound fracture, complicated by perhaps only a minor puncture wound, could suppurate and the victim would be lucky to get away with his life, let alone his limb. In some way, the exposure of the fracture to air could be lethal and many surgeons advised urgent packing of the wound to prevent such contamination.

In 1865, Thomas Anderson, the Professor of Chemistry in Glasgow University, told Lister of Louis Pasteur's publications between 1857 and 1860 which proved conclusively that putrefaction was due to bacteria and not merely to exposure to air. At once it became obvious to Lister that it was not the air but the organisms contained in it and carried into the wound which resulted in the suppuration, the pus and the gangrene that plagued the surgical wards of his days. It was obviously impossible to kill microbes by means of heat, as Pasteur had done in his experiments; some chemical substance must be used. He wrote:

When it had been shown by the researches of Pasteur that the septic property of the atmosphere depended, not upon the oxygen or any gaseous constituent, but on minute organisms suspended in it, which owed their energy to their vitality, it occurred to me that decomposition of the injured part might be avoided without excluding the air, by applying as a dressing some material capable of destroying the life of the floating particles.

Lister tried a number of different substances such as zinc chloride and sulphite of potash with little success. He then heard or read about the application of carbolic acid in the effective treatment of sewage in Carlisle and obtained a sample of the crude acid from his colleague, Professor Anderson. In 1865 his first two experiments with carbolic acid were failures: the first an excision of the wrist for tuberculosis and the second on a patient aged 22 with a compound fracture of the leg. In both cases suppuration occurred. The first successful use took place on August 12th, 1865, an operation that might be regarded as the watershed between two eras of surgery, the primitive and the modern. Of this patient Lister wrote:

On the 12th of August 1865, a boy named James Greenlees, aged 11 years, was admitted to the Glasgow Royal

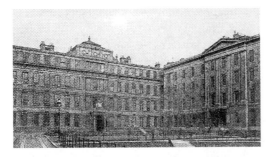

Figure 7.16 The Royal Infirmary, Glasgow, in 1865. From Guthrie D: *Lord Lister, his Life and Doctrine.* Edinburgh, Livingstone, 1949.

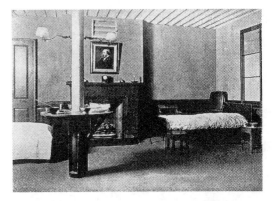

Figure 7.17 The room in the Glasgow Royal Infirmary where the first compound fracture was treated by the antiseptic method. Photograph taken before this part of the hospital was pulled down for rebuilding. From Guthrie D: *Lord Lister, his Life and Doctrine.* Edinburgh, Livingstone, 1949.

Infirmary (Figures 7.16 and 7.17) with compound fracture of the left leg, caused by the wheel of an empty cart passing over the limb a little below its middle. The wound, which was about an inch and a half long and three quarters of an inch broad, was close to, but not exactly over, the line of fracture of the tibia. A probe, however, could be passed beneath the skin over the seat of the fracture and for some inches beyond it.

The treatment consisted of careful application of undiluted carbolic acid to all parts of the wound, which was then dressed with lint soaked in the same fluid. The lint was covered with a sheet of tinfoil to prevent evaporation, and the leg was then carefully splinted. Under the dressing, the blood and carbolic acid formed a protective crust, beneath which, miracle of miracles, the wound began to heal soundly.

After four days, the first dressing was removed. Although the wound was sore, no doubt from the crude carbolic, there was none of the usual horrible smell of hospital infection or the other familiar signs of putrefaction, which would have been expected in the normal course of events within three to four days. Lister dressed the wound again in the same way and left it untouched for another five days. The patient remained comfortable. The skin around the wound had been burned by the carbolic acid, so Lister changed the dressing to gauze soaked in a solution of carbolic acid in olive oil. Six weeks after his accident, James Greenlees walked out of the hospital.

The outcome of the second case was less happy. This was a 32-year-old labourer, whose compound fracture of the tibia produced only a small external wound. He was admitted to the hospital under Lister's care on September 11th and identical treatment was employed. After 11 days, progress seemed to be excellent and Lister went for a short holiday, leaving the house surgeon in charge. Unfortunately, gangrene developed and the leg had to be amputated.

There was now a dearth of compound fractures on Lister's unit, but he spent the time experimenting with carbolic acid in the treatment of leg ulcers and in the use of the antiseptic technique in removing diseased bones from the wrist of a young girl named Janet Forgie. At last, a third patient with a compound fracture was admitted on May 19th, 1866, a 21-year-old man whose leg had been smashed by a heavy iron box at work. Treatment was successful, as was that of a fourth case, a nasty compound fracture of the forearm in a 10-year-old boy.

Lister delayed publishing his results until a total of 11 patients had been managed by the antiseptic technique. *On a new method of treating compound fracture, abscesses, etc., with observations on the conditions of suppuration* was published in

Table 7.1 Lister – the first eleven cases of compound fracture treated by the antiseptic method

No.	Sex	Age	Site and Injury	Result
1	M	11	Tibia – cart wheel	Recovery
2	M	32	Tibia – horse kick	Hospital gangrene amputation
3	M	21	Tibia – heavy box	Recovery
4	M	10	Radius and ulna – machine strap	Recovery
5	M	7	Tibia – omnibus wheel	Recovery
6	M	57	Femur – quarry	Death – haemorrhage
7	F	62	Radius and ulna – fall	Recovery
8	M	13	Femur – engine governor	Recovery
9	M	33	Tibia – omnibus wheel	Recovery
10	M	52	Tibia – waggon wheel	Recovery
11	M	55	Tibia – jump from window	Recovery

The Lancet in five successive issues from March 16th to July 27th, 1867 (Table 7.1). Of the 11 cases of compound fracture, Lister reported only one death, the sixth in the series. John Campbell was a 57-year-old quarryman with a compound fracture of the thigh resulting from a large falling rock. There was a six-hour delay and considerable loss of blood before he was admitted to the hospital. After making good progress for several weeks, he died from haemorrhage following the perforation of the femoral artery by a sharp fragment of the fracture.

It must be remembered that, at this time, many compound fractures required amputation, and this procedure was often fatal. The improvement in the statistics on Lister's own service, after the adoption of his antiseptic method, is demonstrated by his published figures. Between 1864 and 1866 there were 35 amputations with 16 deaths, a 46% mortality. Between 1867 and 1870, when amputations were carried out using the antiseptic technique, 40 operations were performed with only 6 deaths, a 15% mortality. Such results were quite extraordinary in those days.

Before Lister, surgeons hesitated to inflict an incision through the intact skin because of the extreme risk of wound infection, which was often fatal. Even the simplest procedure, such as removal of a sebaceous cyst, might be followed by a lethal erysipelas. However, by December 12th, 1870, Lister was sufficiently confident to operate on a man whose gross malunion of the ulna had left the limb more or less useless. Under antiseptic precautions and with the addition of a carbolic spray, Lister performed an open osteotomy on the malaligned bone, which of course involved transforming the situation into what amounted to a compound fracture. In those days, this could almost be considered malpractice. The wound healed by something rarely seen before Lister – healing by first intention!

Enormous new vistas of surgery now lay open. Lister performed an open reduction of a fractured patella, daring to open the intact knee joint and wire the two fragments together; the wound healed. He wired together a displaced fracture of the olecranon, with safe fracture union (see Figure 10.5). Success followed success as the new antiseptic method became firmly established.

While these experiments were going on, Lister was also deeply involved in the problems of arterial ligation. The standard practice for centuries had been to ligate major blood vessels, usually with silk, and then to leave the ends of the ligature long and dangling out of the wound. As the wound suppurated, the ligatures would gradually come away, often helped by a tug from the surgeon and often accompanied by secondary haemorrhage. It is interesting that Sir Astley Cooper (see Chapter 6) in a case of popliteal aneurysm tied the femoral artery using catgut and cut the ends short; the wound healed by first intention. This was back in 1817.

Lister believed that bacteria-free ligatures might be left safely within the wound, and in 1867 he tied the carotid artery of a horse with a piece of silk soaked in carbolic acid. The ends of the ligature were cut short and the wound closed. First intention healing took place, and at autopsy the silk was found to be unchanged and embedded in fibrous tissue. Following this, Lister ligated the external iliac artery in a 51-year-old woman with an aneurysm of the femoral artery. Again, he used silk soaked in carbolic acid, and the operation was successful. He still worried that, even without suppuration, the unabsorbed silk might cause irritation later, and so he turned to catgut prepared from sheep's intestines as a more suitable agent. Over Christmas 1886 he carried out his classical experiment on a calf, tying the carotid artery with catgut sterilised in carbolic acid. The operation was a complete success; when the wound was explored a month later, the original catgut had been entirely replaced. For the rest of his life, Lister remained interested in the best means of sterilising catgut, and some of his original tubes can be seen to this day in the Hunterian Museum at the Royal College of Surgeons of England in London.

Douglas Guthrie gives a vivid account of Lister at work:

The technique of an operation by Lister . . . was very simple. He never wore a white gown and frequently did not even remove his coat, but simply rolled back his sleeves and turned up his coat collar to protect his starched collar from the cloud of carbolic spray in which he operated. Sometimes he would pin an ordinary towel around his neck. The skin of the patient and the hands of the operator and his assistants were treated with carbolic solution (1 in 20). Towels soaked in the solution were placed around the wound. Instruments and sponges were steeped in the same fluid. Neither the operating theatre nor its furnishing were specially adapted for the purpose. The rough wooden floor bore the marks of previous operations,

the table was a plain deal board padded with leather, while gas or candles supplied artificial light when required. One advantage of so simple a method was that the student who saw it practised in hospital could reproduce it when he commenced practice and had occasion to operate in the homes of his patients. It has been alleged that he was a poor operator, but that is not true. He may have been slow; he had none of the dramatic dash and haste of the surgeon of previous times. But there was now no need for rapid operating. The introduction of anaesthetics allowed the surgeon to proceed with his work calmly, deliberately and carefully. On the occasion when rapid action was demanded, Lister showed that his dexterity was equal to that of other surgeons. As he told his students, 'anaesthetics have abolished the need for operative speed and they allow time for careful procedure', and he would often add a favourite maxim, 'success depends upon attention to detail'.

One might have expected that Lister's results of what we can call the antiseptic technique of surgery would have spoken for themselves and that his methods would have been accepted rapidly throughout the civilised world. Those surgeons who visited him and learned his meticulous ritual of wound care were impressed and reproduced his results in their own practices. This applied particularly to continental visitors, so early supporters included Saxtorph of Copenhagen (1870), Volkmann of Halle (1874) and Nussbaum of Munich and Thiersch of Leipzig, both in 1875. However, many others, especially in Britain, simply regarded carbolic acid as just another of the many substances that had been advised as wound applications, and indeed surgeons had experimented with this very compound in the past. Without all the other adjuncts of the method, it is not surprising that Lister's results under these circumstances would not have been repeated. Still other surgeons could not believe that invisible microbes could produce wound infection. Lawson Tait (1845–1899), one of the fathers of modern abdominal surgery, for example, derided Lister's ideas. It is interesting that Tait's own excellent results were due to his meticulous cleanliness; he was, in fact, practising an early form of *aseptic* surgery. A full two decades

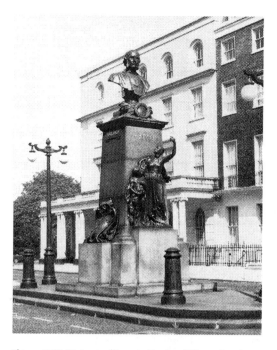

Figure 7.18 Statue to Lister in Portland Place, London. Photograph by the author.

of patient experiment, demonstrations, lectures and learned articles in the journals were required before surgeons were entirely won over to Lister's ideas.

In 1869 Lister transferred from Glasgow to become Professor of Clinical Surgery in Edinburgh, and in 1877 he accepted an invitation to the Chair of Surgery at King's College, London. It was probably the very resistance of the London surgeons that persuaded Lister to leave Edinburgh. He wrote to a friend that his new appointment would: 'Enable me to carry out the two objects which I should in reality have in view, viz, the thorough working of the antiseptic system with a view to its diffusion in the metropolis and the introduction of a more efficient method of clinical surgical teaching than has hitherto prevailed in London'.

Lister died in 1912, having been created a baronet in 1883 and being the first surgeon to obtain a peerage, in 1897. He served on the Council of the Royal College of Surgeons and was one of the first

recipients of the Order of Merit. He shares the honour of being one of the two surgeons in the United Kingdom who have a public monument. It stands for all to see in Portland Place in London, just south of Park Crescent, where he lived for many years when he was Professor of Surgery at King's and where a plaque commemorates his residence. His monument bears but two words; on one side 'Surgery' and on the other 'Lister' (Figure 7.18).

The other statue, by the way, is to John Hunter and this is to be found in Leicester Square.

The development of aseptic surgery

Lister constantly worked at perfecting his surgical technique, chiefly in the direction of using milder antiseptics and adapting heat for the sterilisation of his instruments and dressings. He abandoned the use of carbolic spray (Figure 7.19) when he realised that the risk of wound infection was greatest from the surgeon's hands, instruments and swabs rather than from bacteria in the air. This came as a great relief to the surgeon and his assistants who had had to work for some years under the discomfort of an aerosol of irritating carbolic acid.

The use of steam sterilisation of instruments, dressings and gowns, the wearing of masks, caps and gloves, air filtration and the other rituals of the operating theatre today were introduced over the next couple of decades. Among the pioneers must be mentioned Gustav von Neuber (1850–1923) of Kiel, Kurt Schimmelbusch (1860–1895) of Berlin and Ernst von Bergman (1836–1907) of the same city. William Macewen (1848–1924) a student of Lister at Glasgow, who became Professor of Surgery at that university, did much to popularise aseptic surgery. His technique included scrupulous preparation of the patient's skin, of his own hands and arms and those of his assistants and nurses. It was he who introduced the sterilisable surgeon's gown and his specially designed all-steel instruments sterilised by boiling. It was Macewen who carried out the first successful removal of an intracranial tumour in 1879. With his other contributions,

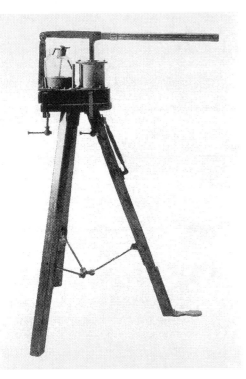

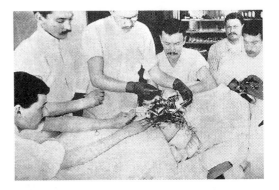

Figure 7.20 An operation in 1893. Only the surgeon is wearing rubber gloves. His assistants are bare-handed.

Figure 7.19 Lister's carbolic spray; nick-named 'the donkey', it produced an aerosol of carbolic in the room, much to the discomfort of the surgeon and his assistants. (This is preserved in the Hunterian Museum at the Royal College of Surgeons of England.)

including the treatment of intracranial and intra-spinal abscess and intracranial haematoma, he can be regarded as one of the father figures of neuro-surgery (see Chapters 8 and 10 and Figure 10.16).

In recent times, Sir John Charnley (1911–1982) (Figure 10.18), one of the pioneers of joint replace-ment surgery, who well knew the disaster of wound infection in this type of procedure, introduced what might be thought of as 'super asepsis'. In addition to the standard precautions, the surgeon and his team operate in a laminar flow tent in a stream of filtered air and wear what look like space suits to ensure that their exhaled breath is shunted away from the patient.

It is interesting that sterile rubber gloves, now regarded as an essential part of the operating theatre ritual, were introduced initially not to protect the patient from the surgeon's bacteria, but to guard the surgeon and his staff from the irritat-ing effects of antiseptics.

Indeed, even before the era of antiseptic surgery, gloves made from cotton, silk, leather and, finally, rubber were employed to protect the hands from injury during operations and autopsies – when a trivial cut in a septic case might prove lethal to the operator. Rubber became the material of choice following the invention of the vulcanisation pro-cess by Charles Goodyear in 1844 to stabilise the rubber.

William Halsted (1852–1922), Professor of Sur-gery at the Johns Hopkins Hospital Baltimore (see Figure 7.11) was most disturbed when, in 1889, his theatre sister, Miss Caroline Hampton, announced that she was going to have to retire because she could no longer tolerate the intense irritation of her hands produced by constantly dipping them into the antiseptic solution then used, corrosive sub-limate. Halsted arranged for rubber gloves to be made by the Goodyear Rubber Company and brought them back for Miss Hampton to use; the skin irritation disappeared. It was only subsequent to this that the use of gloves slowly became routine, but now as an antibacterial barrier between the surgeon's hands and the patient (Figure 7.20). The ending of the Halsted–Hampton story is a romantic one; the following year they married!

Although Halsted never publicised the use of gloves, his trainees no doubt spread the idea. Johann Mikulicz of Breslau, (see page 97), observed Halsted at work and helped to popularise the use of gloves in Germany. The first publication on the use of boiled sterilised rubber gloves in surgery appears to have been by Werner von Manteufel in 1897, Professor of Surgery at Tartu, Estonia. 'To wear boiled gloves is as if to operate with boiled hands,' he wrote!

8

The birth of modern surgery – from Lister to the 20th century

The years from the 1860s to the outbreak of the Great War in 1914 saw an extraordinary burgeoning of surgery. At last surgeons were able to operate untroubled by the need for speed, undisturbed by the screams of their patients and without the high risks of often fatal post-operative infection. The great bulk of the standard operative procedures of today was laid down; for example, the routine surgery of the abdominal organs, of the urinary tract, the endocrine glands, bones and joints, the nervous system, hernia repair and ear, nose and throat surgery. The first attempts were made into the field of chest surgery. Only the surgery of the heart, the reconstructive surgery of arteries, the transplantation of organs and joint-replacement procedures were to remain as major fields of surgical development, and these will be considered in later chapters.

This remarkable era will be illustrated by picking out some of the great men and some of the important developments that still shine out of that remarkable half century of rapid change.

Gall stone surgery

Gall stones have been found in ancient Egyptian mummies and have presumably troubled the human race since the earliest days. Certainly 'inflammation of the liver' was recognised by the Greeks and described by Paulus Aeginata, who flourished in the 7th century. Giovanni Morgagni (1682–1771) reported 20 post-mortem examinations in which he found gall stones. Jean-Louis Petit (1674–1750) (see Figure 6.2) in Paris in 1743 described a lady who had her distended gall bladder drained under the impression that it was an abscess. Several months later he was able to extract a stone the size of a pigeon's egg from the depths of the persistent fistula. However, it was a physician who encouraged surgeons to carry out a deliberate operation for gall stones. John Thudichum (1829–1901) of St Thomas' Hospital, London, published a treatise on the chemical composition of gall stones and in 1859 he advised that the surgeon could fix the gall bladder to the abdominal wall through a small incision and then, having allowed adhesions to form, could open the gall bladder, extract the stones and then allow the resultant fistula to heal spontaneously. It was not until 1867 that John Stough Bobbs (1809–1870), Professor of Surgery in Indianapolis (Figure 8.1) who was apparently unaware of Thudichum's paper, performed the procedure and published it the following year. The operation was carried out under chloroform in a third-floor room above a drug store where Bobbs had rented the room for his operation. The procedure was performed, of course, without antiseptic precautions – Lister's paper on antisepsis was published in this same year (see Chapter 7). The patient was a lady aged 30 who presented with a large abdominal mass which was thought probably to be an ovarian cyst. When the mass was opened, limpid fluid escaped under considerable force, together with a number of gall stones. Apart from wound infection, the patient made a good recovery and outlived not only her

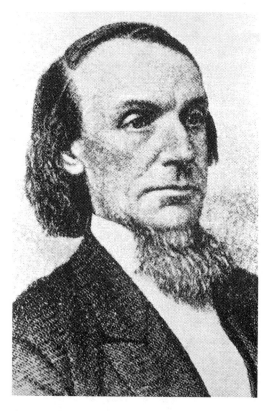

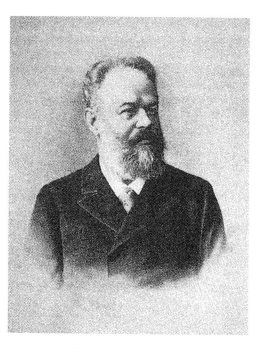

Figure 8.2 Carl Langenbuch.
Photograph provided by Dr Busso Maska, Lazarus
Hospital, Berlin.

Figure 8.1 John Stough Bobbs.
From Robinson J O: *The Biliary Tract*. Austin, Silvergirl,
1985.

surgeon but also six of the eight medical witnesses
of the operation. Bobbs was a Pennsylvanian of
Dutch extraction. He trained at Jefferson Medical
College in his home state and served as medical
officer in the Civil War. He went on to become
Foundation Professor of Surgery in Indianapolis.

It was not for another decade that further operations to remove stones from the gall bladder were
reported by Marion Sims (1813–1883), Theodor
Kocher (1841–1917) of Berne, William Williams
Keen (1837–1932) in Philadelphia and Lawson Tait
(1845–1899) in Birmingham. It was only after many
years that John Bobbs received the world-wide
accolade of a surgical first.

The operation of cholecystotomy, although
simple and safe and, indeed, occasionally carried

out today, had the disadvantages of recurrent
infection, residual stones and often a persistent discharging biliary fistula. The first surgeon to remove
the gall bladder was Carl Johann Langenbuch
(1846–1901) (Figure 8.2) in 1882. He had already
performed the first nephrectomy for a kidney
tumour in 1877. Langenbuch was born in Kiel
and graduated from its university. At the age of
only 27 he was appointed surgeon to the Lazarus
Hospital in Berlin and died in harness in 1901
from peritonitis due to a ruptured appendix.

Langenbuch tackled the problem of extirpation
of the gall bladder in a scientific manner in the
post-mortem room. He noted that elephants and
horses do not possess this organ (nor do rats or
pigeons!) and therefore concluded that man, too,
could do without it! The operation he devised in his
cadaver experiments was carried out through a T-
shaped incision; the transverse limb was placed

along the inferior margin of the liver and was joined to the longitudinal incision along the lateral margin of the rectus muscle. The cystic duct was ligated with silk 1–2 cm from the gall bladder and the gall bladder was then dissected free from the liver bed. Having satisfied himself with these preliminary studies, the time came for the living experiment. The patient was a man aged 43 suffering from severe gall stone symptoms with intense attacks of pain and jaundice over many years; indeed, he had reached the stage where he could no longer manage without morphine. The operation was performed exactly in the manner of the procedure devised in the autopsy room and the inflamed gall bladder with its contained two small cholesterol stones was removed. The patient made a satisfactory recovery and after a couple of months had gained nearly 14 kilograms. He had required no morphine since the operation. Langenbuch argued strongly in favour of removal of the gall bladder rather than draining it. He wrote:

I believe, therefore, that I may state that the extirpation of the gall bladder, performed by me for insidious cholelithiasis, after preceding ligation of the cystic duct, may be regarded as the less dangerous and more effective method, as well as for most other diseased processes of this organ.

Removal or drainage of the gall bladder, of course, could not deal with the problem of calculi in the bile ducts themselves. Lawson Tait recommended crushing the stones with forceps covered with rubber tubing while Kocher advised crushing them with the fingers, fragments being allowed to pass into the duodenum. However, there would be obvious disadvantages that small fragments of stones could be left behind and form a nidus for recurrent calculi. In 1889 two surgeons, on either side of the Atlantic and within three weeks of each other, opened the common bile duct and removed the stones. Robert Abbe (1851–1928), attending surgeon at St Luke's Hospital, New York, removed an impacted stone in a strictured common duct, which he drained through a separate incision in the hepatic duct. The patient, a lady aged 36 who was deeply jaundiced, made a perfectly smooth

recovery and four years later was delivered of a son. Three weeks after Abbe's operation, J Knowsley Thornton in London removed two impacted stones from the common duct, again with recovery of the patient. The operation of choledochotomy was thus established. By the beginning of the 20th century, gall bladder surgery was becoming a routine procedure. Arthur Mayo Robson (1853–1933), surgeon at the General Infirmary at Leeds, who later moved to London and whose most famous protegé was Berkeley Moynihan (see Figure 8.16), was able to report in the *British Medical Journal* of 1903 that he had never lost a patient after any operation for gall stones in the absence of malignant disease or the deep jaundice of cholangitis. His mortality when operating on deeply jaundiced patients with cholangitis was only 1.7%.

Gastric surgery

Today, cancer of the stomach is common, about seventh in the list of killing malignancies in the Western world, but in the 19th century it led the field. The first attempt to resect a tumour at the pylorus was carried out in 1879 by Jules Péan (1830–1898) (Figure 8.3) of Paris. His patient died on the fifth post-operative day. In 1880 Ludwig Rydigier (1850–1920) of Culm, Poland (Figure 8.4), performed the second gastrectomy in history but his patient died only 12 hours post-operatively. Meanwhile, in Vienna at the Surgical University Clinic of the Allgemeines Krankenhaus, Theodor Billroth (1829–1894) (Figure 8.5) had his assistants work out the technical details of the procedure of gastric resection in the animal laboratory. They were able to demonstrate that survival was undoubtedly possible and eliminated the question of whether or not the gastric juice would dissolve the sutures or the healing tissues at the anastomosis between the gastric stump and the duodenum. Billroth wrote: 'No insurmountable obstacles to partial excision of the stomach exist either on anatomical, physiological or operative grounds. It must succeed'.

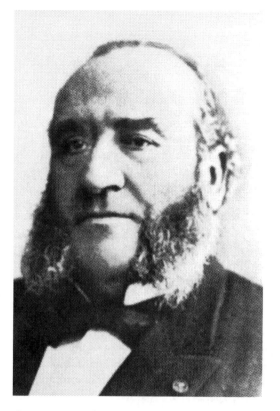

Figure 8.3 Jules Péan.
Photograph provided by Professor Louis Hollender, Strasbourg.

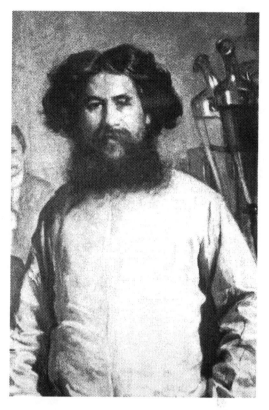

Figure 8.4 Ludwig Rydigier.
Photograph by the author of the portrait in the Surgical Clinic, Copernicus Academy of Medicine, Cracow.

In January 1881, Billroth's assistant Anton Wölfler (1850–1917) (Figure 8.6), a Czechoslovakian who was later to become Professor of Surgery in the University of Prague, asked his chief to see a 43-year-old patient, Thérèse Heller, who had all the features of a malignant obstruction of the gastric outlet. She was bedridden, wasted and continuously vomiting, with a thin rapid pulse and an obvious tumour to feel in the upper abdomen. The patient knew only too well that, untreated, her end could not long be delayed, and she readily agreed to what was, in fact, an experiment. Billroth knew of Péan's unsuccessful attempt at gastrectomy but, at this stage, had not heard of Rydigier's failure. The operation was planned in great detail. The stomach was carefully lavaged and nutrient peptone

enemas were given. The operation was carried out on January 29th under chloroform anaesthesia and strict antiseptic technique. Wölfler was the assistant. The abdomen was opened through a transverse incision and a large infiltrating carcinoma was revealed which involved more than one third of the distal portion of the stomach (Figure 8.7). The blood vessels along the greater and lesser borders of the stomach were ligated. A great anxiety was whether or not the stump of the stomach would pull over sufficiently to reach the duodenum, but once the healthy tissues were divided about one inch along the stomach side of the growth, the cut ends could indeed be brought together. The oblique wound in the stomach was sutured from below upwards until the opening was just big enough to fit the

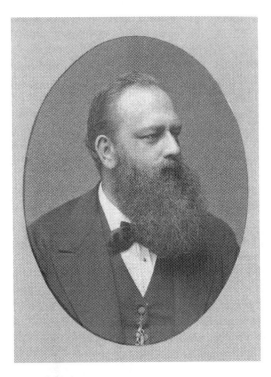

Figure 8.5 Theodor Billroth.
Royal College of Surgeons of England.

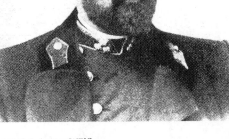

Figure 8.6 Anton Wölfler.
From Herwitz A, Degenshein G: *Milestones in Modern Surgery*. Philadelphia, Harper and Row, 1958.

duodenum and altogether some 50 sutures of silk were employed. The operation lasted 1½ hours and examination of the excised specimen revealed that the pylorus was so narrowed by the growth that it could just admit the shaft of a feather (Figure 8.8). Much to everyone's delight there was no weakness or vomiting and very little pain after the operation. The wound healed well and Billroth wrote in his report on February 4th:

The course so far is already sufficient proof that the operation is possible. Our next care, and the subject of our next studies, must be to determine the indications, and to develop the technique to suit all kinds of cases. I hope we have taken another good step forward towards securing unfortunate people hitherto regarded as incurable or, if there should be recurrences of cancer, at least alleviating their sufferings for a time.

The brave lady died of diffuse metastases in the liver and omentum only four months later, but the news that a successful partial gastrectomy had been performed served as an immense stimulus to the surgery of the alimentary tract, which blossomed rapidly from that date. By 1890, Billroth and his team had performed 41 gastric resections for cancer with 19 successes.

Theodor Billroth was one of the great surgical giants of all time. Qualifying at the University of Berlin, he trained under Bernard Von Langenbeck (1810–1887), who is regarded as one of the founders of modern German surgery. At the age of 31, Billroth became Professor of Surgery at Zurich and seven years later took up his appointment in Vienna. Here, he founded one of the greatest schools of surgery where he carried out pioneering work in experimental studies, surgical pathology and operative surgery. He pioneered excision of tumours of the bladder and the bowel, carried out the first laryngectomy for cancer in 1873 and performed a hindquarter amputation. He founded the modern concept of reporting the total clinical experience of the department to include operative mortality, complications and five-year follow-up. However, he sounded a warning note: 'Statistics are like women, mirrors of purest virtue and truth or like whores, to use as one pleases!'

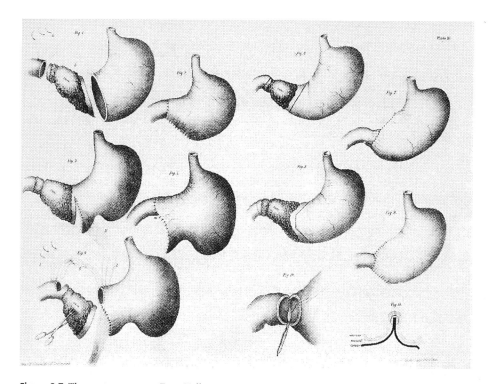

Figure 8.7 The gastrectomy on Frau Heller.
From Billroth T: *Clinical Surgery. Extracts from the Reports of Surgical Practice between the years 1860–1876.* London, The New Sydenham Society, 1891.

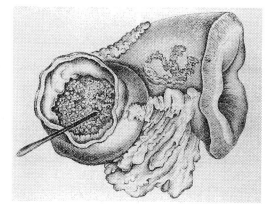

Figure 8.8 The resected specimen of stomach. Note that only a fine probe can be passed through the obstructing tumour.
From Billroth T: *Clinical Surgery. Extracts from the Reports of Surgical Practice between the years 1860–1876.* London, The New Sydenham Society, 1891.

Billroth's protégés included Vincenz Czerny, Carl Gussenbauer and Johannes von Mikulicz. Vincenz Czerny (1842–1916), who became Professor of Surgery at Heidelberg, performed the first total hysterectomy by the vaginal route in 1879 and developed a technique of intestinal anastomosis. Carl Gussenbauer (1842–1903) helped with the dog experiments on gastric resection and succeeded Billroth to his Chair in Vienna. Johannes von Mikulicz (1850–1905) became Professor of Surgery in Breslau. He developed techniques of pyloroplasty, colectomy as a two-stage procedure and thyroidectomy. He was first to use the electric oesophagoscope in 1881 and devised a technique for reconstruction of the oesophagus after resecting its cervical portion for cancer. We have already noted that Anton Wölfler, Billroth's first assistant at the time of the early gastrectomies, became Professor of Surgery in Prague and pioneered the operation of gastroenterostomy. Anton von Eiselberg (1860–1939), Billroth's last great pupil, became Professor of Surgery in Vienna in 1901. He himself was a great teacher and produced no less than nineteen chiefs of surgical departments.

Another facet to Billroth, which is perhaps less well known, was his life-long association with music. As a student, his only talent was for music, which he wished to pursue professionally. However, his mother, widow of a Lutheran pastor, insisted that he study medicine, although he continued to play the piano and to compose. In Zurich, Billroth first became friendly with Johannes Brahms and this continued when both moved to live in Vienna. Nearly all Brahms' compositions were first tried out at the home of Billroth. Who knows what he might have achieved if his mother had not made him study medicine! Billroth is buried in the Central Cemetery in Vienna, not far from the graves of Beethoven and Schubert and the monument to Mozart.

What of the two surgeons whose pioneer gastrectomies ended in failure? Jules Péan, surgeon at the St Louis Hospital in Paris, was a versatile surgeon who had already published the first successful elective removal of the spleen. This was carried out in 1867 at an exploratory operation in a girl of 20 whose suspected ovarian tumour proved to be an enormous splenic cyst. Péan devised forceps for the compression of arteries which incorporated in the handles a ratchet to lock them in position. These were later modified by Spencer Wells, but in France these instruments are still termed 'les pinces de Péan'. Péan died suddenly of pneumonia while still busily engaged in his enormous private practice. Ludwig Rydigier went on to become Professor of Surgery at Cracow and is regarded as the father figure of modern Polish surgery, founding its Association of Surgeons. In November 1881 he performed the first successful gastrectomy for a benign gastric ulcer and went on to detail the indications for gastric resection in cases of pyloric stenosis, haemorrhage and cancer.

The first successful total removal of the stomach for cancer was performed by Carl Schlatter (1864–1934) of Zurich in 1897 and was reported the fol-lowing year in *The Lancet*. The duodenum was closed and a loop of small intestine brought up and anastomosed to the oesophagus. The patient died of metastases in the lymph nodes and pleura a year later.

The now quite commonly diagnosed condition of hypertrophic pyloric stenosis of infants was poorly recognised until the Danish paediatrician, Harald Hirschsprung (1830–1916), described post-mortem examinations on two infants who had died of this disease. In spite of its almost certain fatality, physicians were reluctant, if not vehemently opposed, to advise operation for its relief. Over the years, reports appeared from time to time of attempts to relieve the obstruction by various techniques using various forms of pyloroplasty or gastrojejunostomy. In 1907, Pierre Fredet (1870–1946) of the Pitié Hospital, Paris suggested a new operation in which the serous and muscular coats of the pylorus alone were cut longitudinally, the mucosa being left intact, and the muscle then sutured together. This procedure was taken up by Wilhelm Weber (1872–1928) of Dresden. In 1911, Conrad Ramstedt (1867–1963), a German military surgeon, greatly simplified the operation. He wrote in his report of his first case:

When in September 1911 I was first confronted with an operation for pyloric stenosis, I decided to perform a partial pyloroplasty according to Weber. During the operation I noticed, after section of the firmly contracted, almost bloodless and hypertrophied muscular ring, that the wound edges gaped markedly. I had the impression that the stenosis was already overcome. Nevertheless I sutured the incision transversely in order to complete the Weber pyloroplasty. The tension of the wound edges was, however, very great and the sutures cut through so that the union of the wound edges in the opposite direction was incomplete. I therefore covered the suture area with a tag of omentum for protection. The child is cured. Today, about one year after the operation, he had developed as well as any child of his age.

In the second case, Ramstedt decided to leave the incision gaping; it was a complete success.

This simple procedure of merely dividing the thickened muscle ring at the pylorus (pyloromyotomy) remains the standard operation today

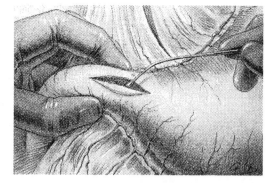

Figure 8.9 Ramstedt's pyloromyotomy operation. From Sir Frederick Treves, *The Student's Handbook of Surgical Operations*. London, Cassell, 1930.

(Figure 8.9). Since the introduction of the Ramstedt operation, the mortality of this condition has fallen to practically zero. However, in spite of much research, the aetiology of the condition remains something of a mystery.

Surgery of the large intestine

It is interesting that two common diseases of the large bowel in the Western world today – diverticula of the colon and its complications and ulcerative colitis – were rarities up to the early years of the 20th century.

Diverticula of the colon are easy enough to recognise (Figure 8.10). Indeed, as a first year medical student in 1943, with no knowledge at all of pathology, I noted a peculiar collection of saccules along the borders of the sigmoid colon in the cadaver that I was dissecting. I pointed these out to my Professor of Anatomy, Sir Wilfred Le Gros Clark (1895–1971), who said 'those are called diverticula; a diverticulum means a way-side house of ill repute and well do they deserve the name'. I was therefore amazed when some years later I looked up the old textbooks to find no description of this obvious condition until that of Jean Cruveilhier (1791–1874), Professor of Descriptive Anatomy in Paris, who wrote in 1849:

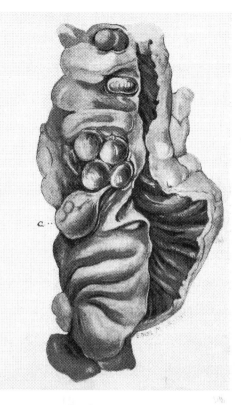

Figure 8.10 Maxwell Telling's illustration of diverticula of the sigmoid colon. *British Journal of Surgery*, 1917.

We not infrequently find between the bands of longitudinal muscle fibres in the sigmoid a series of small, dark, pear-shaped tubers, which are formed by herniae of the mucous membrane through the gaps in the muscle coat.

Cruveilhier noted that these sacs could be irritated by faecal matter and that this might lead to inflammation and perforation. The first account in the English language was given by Samuel Habershon (1825–1889), physician at Guy's Hospital, who wrote:

Pouches of the colon sometimes become of considerable size . . . these pouches are the result of constipation, the muscular fibres become hypertrophied, but their effort to propel onward their contents leads to these minute hernial protrusions.

He noted also that these pouches do not appear to produce any symptoms or lead to any dangerous results.

To the clinicians and pathologists of the 19th century, these diverticula were curiosities and, indeed, Sir Arthur Keith (1866–1955) just before the First World War could collect only seven specimens in the museum of the Royal College of Surgeons in London and the museums of the London Medical Schools. However, by 1917, Maxwell Telling (1874–1938), a physician at the General Infirmary, Leeds, was able to review no less than 324 examples of colonic diverticula and gave a good account of the complications of this condition. The first resection of the sigmoid colon for diverticulitis appears to have been performed by James Rutherford Morison (1853–1939), Professor of Surgery in the University of Durham in 1903. The patient was a male aged 60 who was thought to be suffering from obstruction of the colon due to carcinoma. The resected specimen showed what Morison termed 'sacculitis'. The anastomosis leaked and the patient died two days post-operatively.

Today, in the Western world, diverticula of the colon represent the commonest pathological condition of the large bowel and at present affect approximately 30–40% of the elderly population. We can only conclude that this condition is associated with the low roughage diet of the modern so-called civilised world. In much of Africa and Asia, in populations who still maintain a high bulk diet, the condition remains a rarity.

Non-contagious diarrhoea of a chronic type has been recognised for centuries although the name 'ulcerative colitis' dates only from the middle of the 19th century. Thomas Sydenham (1624–1689), who served as a cavalry officer under Cromwell in the Civil War before becoming a London physician, described the 'bloody flux' in 1666. Prince Charles, the Young Pretender, developed bloody diarrhoea following his defeat at the Battle of Culloden in 1746; surely a fact that would delight those psychiatrists who believe in a psychosomatic cause for colitis. However, the first good description of ulcerative colitis was given by Samuel Wilks (1824–1911) and Walter Moxon (1836–1886) of Guy's Hospital in their *Pathological Anatomy*. They clearly differentiated this condition from febrile epidemic dysentery and wrote:

We have seen a case attended by discharge of mucus and blood where, after death, the whole internal surface of the colon presented a highly vascular, soft, red surface, covered with tenacious mucus or adherent lymph, and here and there showing a few minute points of ulceration; the coats were also much swollen by exudation into the mucous and submucous tissues. In other examples there has been excessive ulceration, commencing in the follicles, spreading from them to destroy the tissues around, thus producing a ragged, ulcerated surface.

In the standard textbook of the late 19th century, William Osler's (1849–1919) *The Principles and Practice of Medicine* published first in 1892, there are only three paragraphs dealing with ulcerative colitis and the description is poor – thus he states 'There is never blood or pus in the stools'. (Diverticula of the colon, by the way, are not even mentioned.)

The early treatment of ulcerative colitis was entirely non-specific and comprised a wide variety of anti-diarrhoeal medications. It was not until the 1940s that the first specific drug treatment, sulphasalazine, was introduced, and followed by the use of corticosteroids in the 1950s. Early surgical attempts at treatment included appendicostomy, first performed by Robert Weir (1838–1927) at the Roosevelt Hospital, New York, as a means of irrigation of the colitic bowel and indeed this procedure was carried out right up to the Second World War using a wide variety of irrigation fluids. Attempts to put the colon to rest by means of an ileostomy were first used by John Young Brown (1865–1919) of St Louis in 1913. Ileostomy certainly provided total faecal diversion but was associated with a high mortality since it was so often carried out only when the patient was almost moribund. It was also found that, even after prolonged rest, closing the ileostomy was almost invariably followed by a flare-up of the colitis. Moreover, until Bryan Brooke (1915–1998) of Birmingham introduced his spout ileostomy and efficient appliances were devised, the life

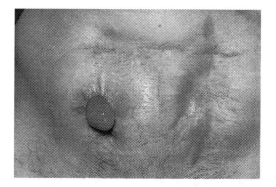

Figure 8.11 A Brooke spout ileostomy. The patient had undergone numerous previous operations for inflammatory bowel disease.

of the ileostomy patient was a miserable one indeed (Figure 8.11). As with efficient medical treatment it was only during the 1940s that the concept of resection of the diseased colon, first as a staged and then as a one-stage colectomy, together with excision of the rectum, began to be performed. In recent years a wide variety of procedures have been introduced to obviate the need for a permanent incontinent stoma. These include the ileorectal anastomosis, the Koch pouch and now the ileo-anal anastomosis with pouch.

The future must lie with determination of the aetiology (or aetiologies) of ulcerative colitis and its prevention or specific treatment. No doubt future generations will be just as amazed that the surgeons of today have to remove the whole of the large bowel because its mucosa is inflamed as present young surgeons view the surgical treatment of pulmonary tuberculosis in the pre-antibiotic era.

Cancer of the large bowel

In the pre-anaesthetic era, the most that could be offered to a patient with large bowel cancer was to relieve obstruction by means of a proximal stoma. The first attempt at this was performed by Pillore of Rouen in 1776; the patient was a wine merchant with large bowel obstruction due to a scirrhous tumour at the colo-rectal junction. The distended caecum was exposed through a transverse incision,

opened and fixed to the margins of the wound with a couple of sutures. The operation produced great relief of the obstruction but the patient died on the 28th post-operative day because of necrosis of a loop of jejunum produced by the large amounts of mercury, amounting to 2 lb in weight, which had been given in the original conservative attempts to overcome the obstruction. Pierre Fine (1760–1814) of Geneva carried out the first successful transverse colostomy in 1797. The patient, a woman aged 63 with a rectosigmoid obstructing growth, lived for three and a half months before dying of ascites.

A number of successes were reported of the formation of an 'artificial anus' in infants with imperforate anus, but the next successful case in an adult was reported from the United Kingdom by Daniel Pring (1789–1859), a surgeon of Bath. His patient was a woman aged 64 who had complete obstruction due to a growth in the upper rectum. He operated on July 7th 1820 and recorded the case in the *Medical and Physical Journal* the following year. Prior to recourse to the operation, he carried out every other measure he could think of, and an account of these makes interesting reading:

All the medical resources of art were afterwards exhausted in fruitless attempts to procure evacuations. Salts, senna, aloes, colocynth, jalap, scammony, gamboge, elaterium, calomel were given in their largest doses and variously combined; castor oil was also given in doses of three ounces and as vomiting was by no means frequent, these medicines were commonly retained. Injections of every sort and by different means were also administered; they were sometimes retained for about half an hour to the amount of four to six ounces and were then forcibly expelled. It was attempted to pass a flexible catheter beyond the obstruction, through which clysters might be thrown into the bowels above the seat of it . . . she was once bled without any relief to her symptoms and when all other means had failed, some large doses of laudanum were given, without any reasonable expectation on the supposed possibility of the existence of spasm.

With regard to the inconvenience of a colostomy, Pring wrote:

It may be worthwhile to observe that the inconveniences of an anus in this situation are not such as to have any cause to regret for having to submit to the operation; on the contrary, so far from her having any reason to lament this circumstance, I believe myself that it has afforded her of a moral as well as a physical advantage; for she is now at no loss for an interest, and is provided for something to think of for the rest of her life.

Cold comfort, indeed, even for a phlegmatic English woman!

Cancer of the colon

Jean Francis Reybard (1790–1863) of Lyon incredibly performed a successful resection of a sigmoid colonic growth with immediate anastomosis of the ends of the bowel in 1823 without an anaesthetic; the patient, a man of 29, survived for a year. However, it awaited the development of general anaesthesia and the introduction of antiseptic surgery before a flood of reports of resections of large bowel tumours was reported. In 1879, Vincenz Czerny (see page 97) successfully resected a colonic growth with end-to-end anastomosis, and in the same year Theodor Billroth (Figure 8.5) performed a colonic resection and brought the proximal end of the bowel out of the abdominal wound as a colostomy. By the end of 1899, the number of reported resections had risen to 57, with 19 operative deaths, a mortality of 37%. The majority of these fatalities were due to peritonitis, the infection taking place either during the conduct of the operation, or from leakage or necrosis of the suture line some five to ten days after surgery. It was soon appreciated that resection and anastomosis of the colon, especially its left half, was much more dangerous than the same procedure elsewhere along the alimentary canal and surgeons turned their attention to the solution of this danger.

An early approach was excision of the tumour with exteriorisation. Initially, this comprised exteriorisation of the loop of colon containing the tumour. At the second stage the protruding growth was removed, and at the third operation the resulting colostomy was closed. The first successful case was reported by Walter Heineke (1834–1901) of Erlangen, Germany. In 1895, Frank Thomas Paul

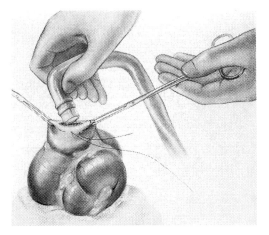

Figure 8.12 Insertion of a Paul's tube into the large intestine.

(1851–1941), of Liverpool, published his technique in which he exteriorised the affected loop, sutured a glass tube into the bowel above and below the site of the tumour and then immediately excised the growth (Figure 8.12), thus reducing the operation to a two-stage procedure. Johannes von Mikulicz-Radecki (1850–1905), Professor of Surgery in Breslau, popularised this procedure on the continent of Europe and was able to show a reduction in operative mortality in his own cases from 43%, when he attempted primary anastomosis, to 12.5% for the exteriorisation technique, which subsequently came to be termed the Paul–Mikulicz operation.

Frank Paul had a career which was typical of the surgeons of his era who commenced their work in pre-Listerian days and who went on to experience the almost miraculous differences produced by antiseptic and aseptic methods. When he was appointed Resident Medical Officer at the Liverpool Royal Infirmary in 1875 he described his hospital work thus: 'Erysipelas, septicaemia, pyaemia and hospital and gas gangrene were rampant. One out of three ovariotomies and excisions of the breast died of sepsis. Most of the surgeons of that time operated in a dirty frock coat'.

After serving 20 years on the staff of the Royal Infirmary he wrote, in contrast to his early experiences: 'It was a very wonderful 20 years in which the safety of operations increased astoundingly. In my last years I did over 1,000 consecutive breast cases without a death and in appendix cases, with the exclusion of five hopeless cases already suffering from general peritonitis, also 1,000 consecutive recoveries'.

Undoubtedly, the Paul–Mikulicz operation represented a considerable advance in making colonic surgery safe. Its disadvantages were difficulty of the procedure when applied to bulky tumours or growths in the non-mobile segments of the large bowel, and the fact that adequate resection of the areas of lymphatic drainage was impossible. Indeed, local recurrence in the wound was not uncommon. Safe modern surgery, of primary resection with immediate anastomosis of the large bowel, depended first on the development of efficient techniques of bowel suture, then on the importance of operating on decompressed bowel with, as an ancillary, knowledge of the risks of primary resection in the face of large bowel obstruction, and the importance of blood supply at the anastomosis.

Cancer of the rectum

With its vivid local symptoms and its ready detection by the insertion of the finger into the fundament, rectal cancer was well known to the ancients but, of course, until comparatively recent times its treatment was entirely palliative – warm baths, emollient enemas, and dilatations of the malignant tumour with bougies were employed. The first surgeon to amputate the rectum for cancer was Jacques Lisfranc (1790–1847), surgeon at La Pitié Hospital in Paris in 1826; three years later he had performed nine such operations. His procedure comprised an oval perianal incision, dissection of the distal rectum and its amputation above the growth. This resulted, of course, in the formation of an uncontrollable perineal colostomy. In 1874, now with the advantage of aseptic technique and anaesthesia, Theodor Kocher (1841–1917) (see Figure 13.2) of Berne performed preliminary closure of the anus with a purse-string suture in order to prevent faecal contamination of the wound. He was also able to increase the extent of the operation by opening the peritoneal cavity from below with more adequate mobilisation of the rectum.

In 1885, Paul Kraske (1851–1930) introduced his operation of sacral resection of the rectum, exposure being achieved by removing the coccyx and lower sacrum. The peritoneum was freely opened from below, the pelvic colon mobilised and brought down and, following removal of the tumour, an end-to-end anastomosis was carried out to the rectal stump. If the growth was too low to make this possible, a sacral colostomy was established. The Kraske operation became extremely popular on the continent of Europe. It had the disadvantage of a high rate of anastomotic breakdown but had the advantage of a relatively low mortality and reasonable survival results. One review of nearly 1000 such operations gave a mortality of 11.6% and 30% survival after five years.

It was J P Lockhart-Mummery (1875–1957) of St Mark's Hospital, London, who was responsible for the development of an effective technique of perineal resection of the rectum in 1907. A preliminary laparotomy was performed and a loop colostomy fashioned. The perineal stage could be performed at once but was more usually delayed for ten days and was carried out in the semi-prone position. The rectum was mobilised, the peritoneum opened from below and the superior rectal vessels were tied and divided as high as possible. The colon was then divided in the upper part of the wound and the blind stump closed. The peritoneum was sutured with catgut, leaving the stump of sigmoid colon on the wound side of the pelvic diaphragm. The author stated that the operation should not take more than 45 minutes, the patient should be out of bed in 14 days and usually able to return home in three weeks. The operation had the disadvantage of leaving a blind stump of colon distal to the colostomy which might leak but it was a relatively adequate cancer operation and had the advantage, in the days of fairly primitive anaesthesia and rarity of blood transfusion, of being relatively simple to perform and with a low

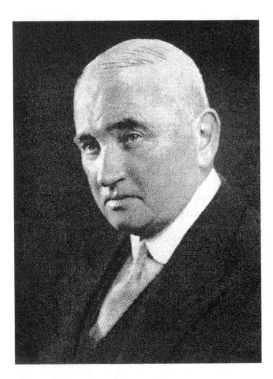

Figure 8.13 Ernest Miles.
Royal College of Surgeons of England.

mortality, in the region of 10%. Up to the 1930s, it was probably the most commonly employed technique in the USA and the United Kingdom.

Removal of the rectum by a combined abdominal and perineal operation was first performed by Czerny (see page 97) in 1884. This was not a planned procedure, but had to be carried out because an attempted sacral excision was found to be impossible to complete from below. It was Ernest Miles (1869–1947) of the Royal Cancer Hospital (later the Royal Marsden) and the Gordon Hospital who first performed this procedure electively in 1907. Miles (Figure 8.13) was disturbed by the high rate of early recurrence in his own experience of the perineal method of rectal excision. Careful post-mortem examinations of patients dying with this disease convinced him of the importance of wide and extensive excision of the rectum, anal canal, the levator ani muscles and the draining lymph nodes. The first patient was a house painter aged 55. After

the abdominal part of the operation had been performed, the patient was turned on the right side for the perineal procedure. The cavity of the pelvis was packed with gauze and a small tube drain placed in the lower part of the wound. The disadvantage of this procedure at first was the high mortality. In Miles' first 62 cases, there were no less than 22 deaths, although this was reduced in his third 100 cases to 13 fatalities. This mortality was greatly reduced with the introduction of modern anaesthesia, routine blood transfusion and antibiotics.

The penalty of these procedures, of course, is the permanent colostomy. Nowadays, tumours other than those at the distal end of the rectum or of the anal canal itself are treated by resection with anastomosis as low down as the anorectal ring. The introduction of the stapling gun has greatly increased the popularity of this operation.

The acute abdomen

Until surgery could be carried out without undue haste and in comparative safety, most of the causes of acute abdominal pain remained something of a mystery and were labelled 'ileus' or 'abdominal passion'. When patients died with advanced peritonitis, the extensive changes found at autopsy often disguised the exact locus of the original disease. Once the abdomen could be opened surgically, in what Berkeley Moynihan (1865–1936) (see Figure 8.16) called 'the pathology of the living', the pathology revealed in the operating theatre elucidated the causes and, in many cases, the cure of many of these emergencies. In this chapter some of the highlights of this period will be described.

Appendicitis

Lorenz Heister (1683–1758) (see Figure 6.7) must be given the credit of being the first to recognise the appendix as the site of acute inflammation. In 1755 he described these changes at a post-mortem:

I found the vermiform process of the caecum praeternaturally black, adhering closer to the peritoneum than usual. As I was now about to separate it by gently pulling it asunder the membranes of the process broke . . . and discharged two or three spoonfuls of matter . . . this instance may stand as a proof of the possibility of inflammation arising and abscesses forming in the appendicula as well as in other parts of the body.

For more than a century following this, there were occasional autopsy reports of gangrene and perforation of the appendix with local abscess or with general peritonitis, but most cases remained unrecognised or were given the vague diagnosis of 'typhlitis', 'perityphlitis' or 'iliac passion'.

The first person to report removal of at least part of the appendix was Claudius Amyand (1680–1740), surgeon first at Westminster and then at St George's Hospitals. This case was reported at the Royal Society in 1736; the patient, a boy of 11, had a right scrotal hernia associated with a discharging sinus. This was explored and found to contain the appendix perforated by a pin. A ligature was placed around the shaft of the appendix, the perforated portion and the imprisoned pin amputated and the patient made a satisfactory recovery.

The first successful operation for drainage for an appendix abscess was performed in 1848 by Henry Hancock (1809–1880) of Charing Cross Hospital, London. His patient was a lady of 30 in her eighth month of pregnancy. She developed abdominal pain, miscarried on the fourth day and developed a tender mass in the lower right abdomen. She was seen by Hancock on the twelfth day of the illness when she had a distended, tender abdomen, the symptoms and signs being particularly marked in the right lower quadrant. Hancock suspected inflammatory trouble around the caecum or appendix and prescribed opium and poultices. Two days later, her condition was much worse and there was a distinct mass to feel. By now her condition was desperate. An anaesthetic was given and an incision made 'inwards from the spine of the ilium just above Poupart's ligament'. When the abdomen was opened, very offensive pus and bubbles of gas escaped, followed a couple of weeks later by two faecoliths which Hancock postulated had escaped by ulceration from the diseased appendix. From

that time, her improvement was rapid and she made a good recovery. Hancock wrote:

I know of no instance on record where the abdomen has been opened under the circumstances detailed above, for it should be borne in mind that in this case there was neither redness nor fluctuation nor any external signs indicative of circumscribed abscess of the part . . . it may be premature to argue from the results of one case, but I trust that the time will come when this plan will be successfully employed in other cases of peritonitis terminating in effusion, and which usually end fatally.

However, so fixed was the idea that it was hopeless to interfere once peritonitis was established within the abdominal cavity that Hancock's advice was ignored for some 40 years.

Surprisingly, it was a physician and not a surgeon whose teachings led to the early treatment of acute appendicitis. Reginald Fitz (1843–1913) (Figure 8.14) published a review of 257 cases of perforating inflammation of the appendix in 1886 in which he showed quite clearly that abscesses in the right iliac fossa were in the main due to appendicitis and not to inflammation around the caecum. Not only did he give a clear description of the pathological and clinical features of appendicitis but he also pointed out the importance of surgical treatment. His summary is as true today as when first written:

In conclusion the following statements seem warranted; the vital importance of the early recognition of perforating appendicitis is unmistakable. Its diagnosis, in most cases, is comparatively easy. Its eventual treatment by laparotomy is generally indispensable. Urgent symptoms demand immediate exposure of the perforated appendix, after recovery from the shock, and its treatment according to surgical principles. If delay seems warranted, the resulting abscess, as a rule, intraperitoneal, should be incised as it becomes evident. This is usually on the third day after the appearance of the first characteristic symptom of the disease.

Fitz was a graduate of Harvard and carried out postgraduate studies in Vienna and Berlin. By the age of 35 he became Professor of Pathological Anatomy at Harvard, was later visiting physician at the Massachusetts General Hospital and at the age of 49 was appointed Professor of Medicine at

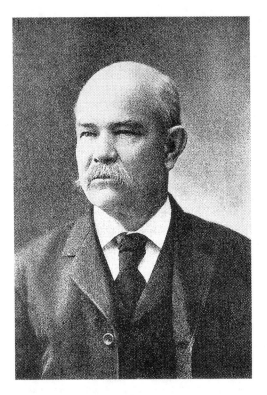

Figure 8.14 Reginald Fitz.
From Ellis H: The 100th birthday of appendicitis. *British Medical Journal* 1986; 293, 1617.

Harvard. Today he should be remembered not only for his work on appendicitis but for his equally valuable work on the clinical features and pathological changes of acute pancreatitis.

Fitz's advice was taken up rapidly in the United States. Although Robert Lawson Tait (1845–1899) of Birmingham as early as 1880 operated on a patient with a gangrenous appendicitis and removed the appendix with a successful result, he did not record the case until 1890. It remained for Thomas Morton (1835–1903) of Philadelphia to be the first correctly to diagnose appendicitis, drain the abscess and remove the appendix with recovery and to publish the case in 1887.

The sudden great advance in the early diagnosis and operative treatment of appendicitis in America was largely due to the example and teaching of a number of surgeons, particularly Charles McBurney and John Murphy. Charles McBurney (1845–1913), Surgeon in Chief at the Roosevelt Hospital, New York, described 'McBurney's point' the point of maximum tenderness in acute appendicitis, and devised the muscle-splitting incision which is still employed for appendicectomy more often than any other approach. John B Murphy (1857–1916) (see Figure 14.22) of Chicago, who was incidentally the first surgeon to perform successful suture of a divided femoral artery, made a special point of insisting that there is a regular sequence of symptoms in a typical case of appendicitis: pain around the umbilicus, vomiting, and pain shifting to the right iliac fossa (Murphy's sequence).

On the continent of Europe and in the United Kingdom the operation for removal of the inflamed appendix was slower in being adopted. Frederick Treves (1853–1923) (Figure 8.15) of the London Hospital did much to popularise the operation in England and by 1901 he had performed 1000 appendicectomies. On June 24th, 1902, two days before the coronation, Treves drained the appendix abscess of King Edward VII. The patient recovered and went though the full ceremony of his delayed crowning seven weeks later. Treves, the serjeant surgeon, was made a baronet. As can be well imagined, this royal operation did much to draw the general public's attention to the disease.

Perforated peptic ulcer

Perforation of a gastric or duodenal ulcer into the peritoneal cavity gives rise to sudden severe symptoms and usually leads to fatal peritonitis unless the perforation is closed. Unsuccessful attempts at repair were made by Mikulicz in 1884, Czerny in 1885 and subsequently by a number of other surgeons. The first success was achieved in 1892 by Ludwig Heusner (1846–1916), under considerable difficulties and by candlelight, in Barmen (now Wuppertal), Germany. The patient, a man aged 41, had perforated 16 hours previously; the hole was only found after careful search high up along the lesser curve of the stomach. The patient recovered

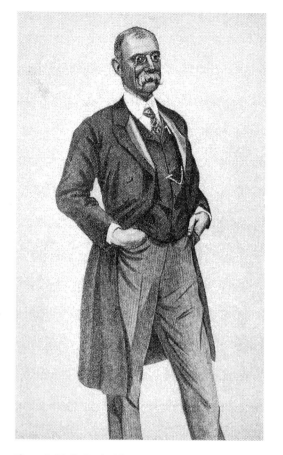

Figure 8.15 Sir Frederick Treves.
Cartoon by 'Spy'.

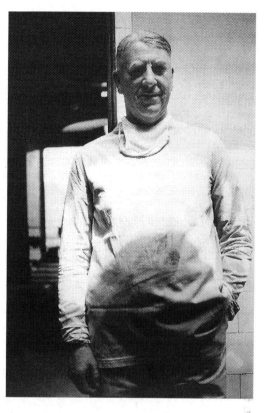

Figure 8.16 Sir Berkeley (later Lord) Moynihan
photographed in very bloodstained operating clothes at
the General Infirmary at Leeds.
Institute of Orthopaedics, London.

although subsequently a left-sided empyema required drainage. Five months later, Hastings Gilford
(1861–1941) of Reading operated on a patient with
a perforated ulcer who only survived one week. In
1893 Gilford operated on a second patient who survived after a stormy convalescence. The case was
not immediately published so the credit for the first
published successful operation for perforated gastric
ulcer in England must go to Thomas Herbert Morse
(1877–1921) of Norwich who reported the successful
repair of a perforated gastric ulcer near the cardia
in a girl of 20 in 1894.

The successes of Heusner and Morse quickly
became known and operation for suture of perfor-

ated ulcer was almost at once adopted at every
major centre. When operations for perforated gastric
ulcer first began to be performed, duodenal ulcer
was a comparatively rare condition. It was Berkeley
Moynihan (1865–1936) (Figure 8.16) who first made
the condition of duodenal ulcer well known in 1901
in his book on *Diseases of the Stomach*, written jointly
with Mayo Robson. In this he was able to collect only
51 cases of operation for perforated duodenal ulcer,
of which a bare nine had recovered. Of his two personal cases, one was successful. Moynihan was to
become one of the great teachers of surgery of his
time. His father had won the Victoria Cross in the
Crimean War as a sergeant and, most unusually in
those days, was commissioned from the ranks. He

was trained and spent the whole of his career at the General Infirmary at Leeds and was appointed to its staff in 1896. He pioneered many of the modern operations of the stomach, biliary system, intestines and pancreas, and his textbook *Abdominal Operations*, which first appeared in 1904, made his name known on both sides of the Atlantic. More than anyone else at the time, he preached the importance of gentle, unhurried but purposeful surgical craftsmanship. A visiting French surgeon, after watching Moynihan's meticulous haemostasis, is reported to have remarked 'Is then your English blood so precious?' Moynihan created the Association of Surgeons of Great Britain and Ireland, launched the *British Journal of Surgery* and was an effective President of the Royal College of Surgeons. He was created Baron Moynihan of Leeds in 1929 when, until then, the only other surgeon to have been elevated to the peerage was Joseph Lister (see Figure 7.15).

Intussusception

With its vivid manifestations of blood-stained mucus passed per rectum, a palpable abdominal mass and, in late cases, a prolapsing mass to be felt in the rectum or even to be seen extruding through the anal verge, it is not surprising that intussusception in children was one of the earliest forms of intestinal obstruction to be specifically recognised. Treatment was expectant, with efforts to reduce the intussusception by enemas or by the passage of rectal bougies. Surgeons were encouraged to continue these efforts by occasional reports of successes and by still rarer examples where spontaneous cure of the infant resulted from the passage per rectum of the gangrenous segment of strangulated bowel. The first successful operation for reduction of an intussusception in an infant was performed in 1871 by Jonathan Hutchinson (1828–1913) (Figure 8.17) who published a detailed report of a case in 1874. In this paper he meticulously tabulated 131 previous case reports, which makes sad reading indeed. His patient was a female child aged two years who presented with all the classical features of the condition. He wrote:

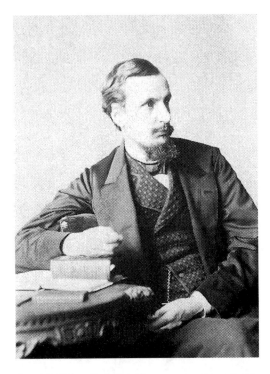

Figure 8.17 Jonathan Hutchinson as a young surgeon. Royal College of Surgeons of England.

My experience of several other somewhat similar cases, all of which have resulted in death, after patient and repeated attempts by the injection method, did not encourage me to expect success in this. It was very evident from the child's condition, that unless relief were afforded she would not live long and I therefore felt justified in telling the parents that although an operation would be, in itself very dangerous, yet I thought that it afforded the only chance. They begged me to give the child a chance if I thought it was one, and we accordingly determined to lose no time.

The child having been taken up into the operating theatre, chloroform was administered and I then opened the abdomen in the median line below the umbilicus and to an extent admitting of the easy introduction of two or three fingers. I now very readily drew out of the wound the intussuscepted mass, which was about six inches long. I found that the serous surfaces did not adhere, and that there was no difficulty whatever in drawing the intussuscepted part out of that into which it had passed. . . . Having completed the reduction I put the bowel back into the abdomen, and closed the wound with harelip pins and

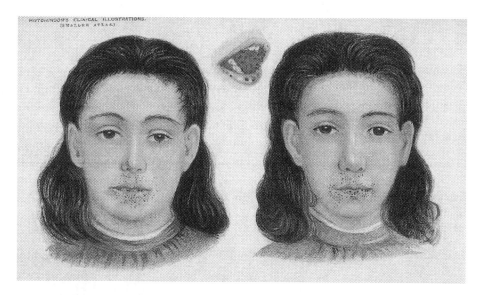

Figure 8.18 Identical twins with pigmented cutaneous spots. From *Hutchinson's Archives of Surgery* of 1891.

interrupted sutures. The operation had been an extremely simple one, and had not occupied more than two or three minutes. ... The child recovered without having ever showed the slightest symptom of peritonitis, and left the hospital in excellent health about three weeks after the operation.

The operative treatment today remains the same as that described by Jonathan Hutchinson, although nowadays many early cases can be reduced satisfactorily using a contrast enema under X-ray control.

Sir Jonathan Hutchinson, surgeon at the London Hospital, was a remarkable clinical observer. He described the stigmata of congenital syphilis, which included the peg-top incisor teeth (Hutchinson's teeth), and he described the increasing dilatation of the pupil in cases of extradural haemorrhage (Hutchinson's pupils), the mask-like facial appearance of tabes dorsalis (Hutchinson's facies) and half a dozen dermatological conditions. He published ten volumes of *Archives of Surgery* between 1889 and 1900, the entire contents of which were written by him. In the 1891 volume is a remarkable report and illustration of identical twin sisters aged nine, who, at the age of three, had developed identical

black pigment spots on their lips and inside the mouth (Figure 8.18).

In 1919, Frederick Parkes-Weber (1863–1962), a London physician, noted a follow-up on these girls, one of whom had died following an operation for intussusception 11 years after Hutchinson's original observation. Perhaps Hutchinson's name should be given eponymously to the syndrome of cutaneous pigment spots associated with intestinal polyps and intussusception described by the Dutchman John Peutz (1886–1957) in 1921 and by Harold Jeghers (1904–1990) in 1949.

The ruptured spleen

The spleen is the viscus most commonly damaged in closed abdominal injuries, particularly with a severe crushing blow to the left lower chest or the abdomen. Although spontaneous healing may occasionally occur, untreated the majority of patients with this injury will die of exsanguination. Rather surprisingly, therefore, there seemed in the pioneer days of abdominal surgery to be a diffidence by surgeons to open the abdomen in this condition and to remove the ruptured spleen. This was in spite of the fact that Jules Péan (see Figure 8.3) had performed a successful elective splenectomy in 1867 in a girl of 20 suffering from an enormous splenic cyst. The first two unsuccessful attempts to be recorded were reported in 1892 by Sir William Arbuthnot Lane (1856–1943) (see Figure 10.8) of Guy's Hospital. The first was a boy of 15 who fell off a brougham, landed on its pole and was operated on by Lane shortly afterwards. The pulped spleen was removed but the patient died five hours later. The second was a boy of four who received a blow on the abdomen from the pole of a carriage. Splenectomy was performed for the completely ruptured spleen, but the child survived only a few hours. The following year Friedrich Trendelenburg (1844–1924), Professor of Surgery in Leipzig, reported a further unsuccessful splenectomy for trauma and indeed published two further fatal cases. Reading these case reports suggests that, had blood transfusion been available, these patients might well have survived.

It fell to Oskar Riegner (1844–1910), Chief Surgeon at the All Saints Hospital in Breslau, to have the distinction of performing the first successful splenectomy for closed splenic trauma in 1893. His patient was a 14-year-old labourer who fell two floors from scaffolding, striking his abdomen on a board. By the next day he had become increasingly pale with a pulse of 120 and with a distended painful abdomen, which was dull in the left flank. At operation about one and a half litres of blood poured out of the abdomen and the spleen was found to have been completely severed, its lower half lying free within the abdomen. The splenic vessels were tied and the upper half of the spleen excised. In the days before blood transfusion, normal saline was infused subcutaneously into each of the arms and thighs. His recovery was complicated by gangrene of the left foot, which required amputation, but he left hospital, complete with an artificial limb, five months after surgery.

It was not until two years later that Sir Charles Alfred Ballance (1865–1936) carried out the second reported successful splenectomy for closed trauma

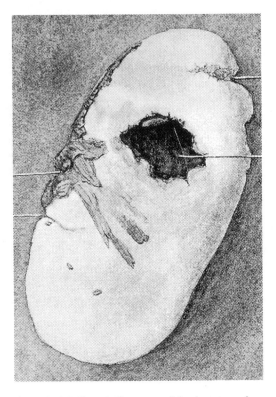

Figure 8.19 Ballance's first successful splenectomy for trauma; rupture of the spleen from a cricket ball. From *Trans Clin Soc* 1896; 29, 77–104.

(Figure 8.19). This took place at St Thomas' Hospital in London on a schoolboy aged ten who had been struck by a cricket ball on the left side of the abdomen five days before admission. Today, of course, delayed rupture of the spleen is well recognised. Ballance described the shifting dullness in the right flank and fixed dullness in the left, which he claimed occurred in haemorrhage from the spleen. This rather doubtful physical sign is often referred to as 'Ballance's sign'. I, personally, have never elicited it.

Ruptured ectopic pregnancy

Until 1883 a ruptured ectopic pregnancy was a death sentence. In his book on extrauterine pregnancy published in 1876, Dr John Parry wrote: 'Here is an

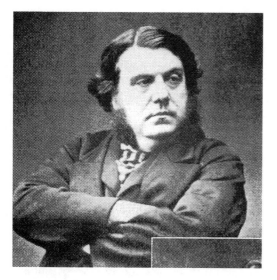

Figure 8.20 Robert Lawson Tait.
Royal College of Surgeons of England.

accident which may happen to any wife in the most useful period of her existence, which good authorities have said is never cured; and for which, even in this age when science and art boast of such high attainments, no remedy either medical or surgical has been tried with a single success'.

When we read that eminent authorities were advising the use of electric shocks, the injection of narcotic materials into the sac, and copious and frequent bleeding, one is hardly surprised at the rate of failure. Parry himself went on to suggest that the only remedy would be to open the abdomen and either to tie the bleeding vessels or to remove the sac entirely.

The first surgeon to perform a successful operation of the kind recommended by Parry was Robert Lawson Tait (1845–1899) (Figure 8.20) of Birmingham, and it is interesting that the suggestion that he should operate came from a general practitioner. The dramatic story involves three successive cases described vividly in Tait's own words:

In the summer of 1881 I was asked by Mr. Hallwright to see with him in consultation a patient who had arrived by train from London in a condition of serious illness

diagnosed by Mr. Hallwright as probably haemorrhage into the peritoneal cavity from a ruptured tubal pregnancy. The patient was blanched and collapsed, the uterus was fixed by a doughy mass in the pelvis and there was clearly a considerable amount of effusion in the peritoneum. I agreed with Mr. Hallwright as to the nature of the lesion. This gentleman made the bold suggestion that I should open the abdomen and remove the ruptured tube. The suggestion staggered me and I am ashamed to say that I did not receive it favourably . . . I declined to act on Mr. Hallwright's request and a further haemorrhage killed the patient. A post mortem examination revealed the perfect accuracy of the diagnosis. I carefully inspected the specimen which was removed and I found that if I had tied the broad ligament and removed the ruptured tube I should have completely arrested the haemorrhage and I now believe that had I done this the patient's life would be saved.

The second opportunity came eighteen months later, in the summer of 1883, when Tait was consulted by Mr Spackman of nearby Wolverhampton with a similar case. The patient was clearly dying, but Tait operated; it was the first occasion when an active surgical attempt was made to save a life under such circumstances. As Tait records:

We got her to bed alive and that is all that can be said . . . I thought very much about this case for it was a bitter disappointment. I thought I should achieve a triumph and I had only a failure.

He resolved then that in any future case he would ignore the bleeding, go for the source of the haemorrhage, the broad ligament, tie it at its base and then remove debris and clots at leisure. The next patient presented herself on March 1st, 1883. Tait was consulted by Dr Page of Solihull, a suburb of Birmingham, with a patient who had a fixed mass in the pelvis and whose menstruation had been arrested for about three months. She had a high pulse, an elevated temperature, and was in great pain. Tait writes:

I advised abdominal section and found the abdomen full of clot. The right fallopian tube was ruptured and from it a placenta was protruding. I tied the tube and removed it. I searched for, but could not find, the foetus and I suppose it got lost among the folds of intestine and there was absorbed . . . The patient made a very protracted convalescence but she is now perfectly well.

Within a year Tait had operated on three additional patients; four years later, in 1888, he was able to report 39 cases with only two deaths, including his first attempt.

Tait, a remarkable man, was one of the fathers of abdominal surgery. We have already noted earlier in this chapter that he was the second surgeon to carry out a cholecystotomy (1879) and the first to diagnose and successfully remove an acutely inflamed appendix (1880). He was a pupil of the great Sir James Young Simpson, Professor of Obstetrics in Edinburgh, who introduced chloroform into midwifery and surgery in 1847 (see Figure 7.9). Tait bore a striking resemblance to his professor, and indeed there were rumours that he was Simpson's natural son. Apart from the resemblance there seems to be little evidence to support this gossip, which secretly amused Tait.

He qualified in 1866, moved to Birmingham at 25 years of age, and spent the rest of his active life there until his death from uraemia due to renal stones at the early age of 54. Apart from his work on ectopic pregnancy, Tait pioneered the surgery of ovarian cysts and tumours, closely following on the early work of Sir Thomas Spencer Wells (1818–1897) of the Samaritan Hospital, London, in this field. His surgical skill is shown by the publication in 1886 of 137 consecutive cases of ovariotomy performed without a death.

Tait was a short, stout man with a magnificent head, a thick bull neck, corpulent body, pudgy legs, and small hands and feet; he was described as having the body of Bacchus and the head of Jove. His voice could be soft and musical; he would sing sweetly and yet, when in a rage, would roar like a lion. Many observers commented on his marvellous rapidity and dexterity as a surgeon. His technique was simplicity itself. He operated in small nursing homes with the patient laid on a plain wooden table. He would remove his jacket, roll up his sleeves, and scrupulously prepare his hands with soap and water. The patient's abdomen would be carefully cleansed, first with turpentine and then with soap and water, and the instruments were sterilised by boiling; Tait was thus one of the

pioneers of aseptic rather than antiseptic surgery and indeed he attacked Listerism as not only unnecessary but dangerous. The contributions of this surgeon are best summed up by William Mayo who said: 'The cavities of the body were a sealed book until the father of modern abdominal surgery, Lawson Tait, carried the sense of sight into the abdominal cavity'.

Obstruction due to post-operative adhesions

There was a downside to the new abdominal surgery – a novel abdominal emergency. Adhesions are almost invariable following a laparotomy and, once abdominal surgery commenced, it was not long before cases of small bowel obstruction due to post-operative bands and adhesions were reported. Thomas Bryant (1828–1914) of Guy's Hospital reported the first example in 1872 – a fatal case following removal of an ovarian cyst. William Battle (1855–1936) reported a second fatal case in 1883; this occurred four years after an ovariotomy. Today, post-operative adhesions account for some three-quarters of all cases of small bowel obstruction in the Western world.

'Visceroptosis'

Now that inspection of the abdominal viscera was possible at operation, surgeons found, to their surprise, that the position of the organs was often quite different to the findings in the cadaver, especially in the preserved bodies of the dissecting room. A still further surprise followed the discovery of X-rays by Wilhelm Roentgen (1845–1923), Professor of Physics at Wurzburg, in 1895 and then the X-ray visualisation of the abdominal organs by contrast material, first by using bismuth sulphate introduced by Walter B Cannon (1871–1945) at Harvard Medical School, in 1897. The spleen, kidneys and in particular the stomach and intestines were often situated in a lower plane than described in the anatomical textbooks. Some of these appearances, in fact, were brought about by the weight of the contrast material in the stomach and bowel with the

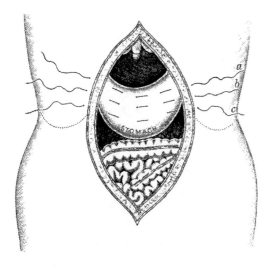

Figure 8.21 Rovsing's gastropexy for 'ptosis of the stomach'.
Thorkild Rovsing 1862–1927, Professor of Surgery, Copenhagen.

patient in the upright position but the rest, as we now know, simply represented normal biological variation. However, what can only be described as a 'non-disease' came into existence – 'visceroptosis'.

Even that shrewd clinician, Berkeley Moynihan (see Figure 8.16) wrote in his textbook *Abdominal Operations*:

The circumstances which are generally present are these; there is a weakening of all the natural supports of the viscera; the peritoneal ligaments are long, lax, and unequal to their burden, and the abdominal wall in its lower part is pushed forwards, bulging in characteristic fashion; a passive dilatation of any part, or of all parts of the alimentary canal may be present. The patient complains chiefly of a sense of a heavy weight, of dragging and of weariness in the abdomen. There is often nausea and sometimes vomiting; there are fullness, flatulence, eructations. The bowels act irregularly, and constipation is always a prominent feature. The patient is almost always a neurasthenic of a most pronounced type. An examination will disclose the circumstances mentioned above – a laxity of the supports and consequently an undue mobility of all the organs in the abdomen.

He did, however, point out later in the chapter: 'The existence of these various forms of ptosis does not always, does not indeed often, entail the association with them of any disturbance of health'.

Large numbers of patients were fitted with ptosis corsets to support the viscera. If this failed, however, thousands of patients, mostly neurotic women, were subjected to major abdominal operations in which the stomach, liver, kidneys and bowel were hitched up (gastropexy, hepatopexy, nephropexy, etc.) and various peritoneal bands, which we now know are perfectly normal, carefully divided. Meanwhile the gynaecologists were busy at work putting the pelvic organs back into their 'normal' position. These operations persisted well into the 1920s and can still be seen in illustrations of textbooks of those times (Figure 8.21).

Urological surgery

The new era saw major advances in the surgery of the urinary tract (see also Chapter 12). An important landmark was the first successful planned nephrectomy, carried out by Gustav Symon (1824–1876) in Heidelberg in 1869. However, this was not the first time the kidney had been removed; in the same decade at least four inadvertent nephrectomies had been performed, all with fatal results, on the mistaken diagnosis of the mass being ovarian in three cases and a liver cyst in the fourth.

Symon's patient was a woman of 46 who had undergone removal of an ovary 18 months previously by another surgeon, who inadvertently excised a length of left ureter. The patient developed an abdominal urinary fistula and also a ureterovaginal fistula, so her life with double incontinence together with urinary infection was becoming intolerable. Symon made four attempts to improve her condition by conservative surgery, all of which failed. He realised that only removal of the kidney would cure her. Before doing so, he performed the operation on 30 dogs to assure himself that the procedure was compatible with perfect health and he also practised the operation in the post-mortem room, in particular to study efficient ligation of the renal pedicle. Post-operatively, the patient developed ileus, wound infection and pneumonia and the wound took months to heal completely, but fortunately she was restored to full health.

Following this, the operation of nephrectomy became comparatively common for a wide variety of indications, including stone, tumour and tuberculosis, but it remained a formidable operation. Thus Samuel Gross (1837–1889) of Jefferson Medical College, Philadelphia, in a review of 233 collected cases in 1885, found an overall mortality of 45%. That of the lumbar approach was 37% while that of the abdominal route was 51%. By the way, after his untimely death, Gross' widow married Sir William Osler, later Regius Professor of Medicine in Oxford.

Prostatectomy

Cases of urinary retention had been treated by catheterisation by the ancient Chinese and Egyptians and by the Indian surgeons Susruta and Charaka. Prior to the advent of prostatectomy, the patient with retention from prostatic disease was condemned to a life of self-catheterisation, being taught to carry out the procedure himself three or four times daily. In 1827, after removal of a stone by suprapubic cystotomy, Jean Amussat (1796–1856) in Paris observed a firm rounded mass, which must have been the enlarged middle lobe of the prostate, projecting from the bladder neck. This he removed with scissors, with relief of the patient's obstructive symptoms; this operation probably represented the first partial prostatectomy. However, the era of suprapubic prostatectomy awaited the twin benefits of anaesthesia and antisepsis. Early pioneers were William Belfield (1856–1929) of Cook County Hospital, Chicago, who, in 1886, performed the first planned operation when he avulsed a pedunculated middle lobe by this approach. In 1887 Arthur Fergusson McGill (1850–1890) of the Leeds General Infirmary was able to report three cases of suprapubic prostatectomy described as 'removing with scissors and forceps that portion of an enlarged

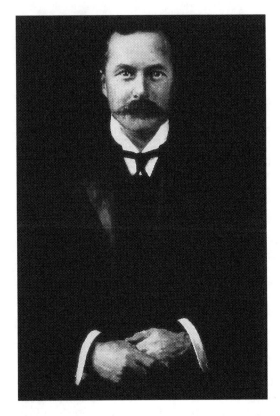

Figure 8.22 Sir Peter Freyer.
Portrait at the Institute of Urology and Nephrology, London.

prostate which prevents the flow of urine'. Of some interest was that his assistant at his first operation was a young student, Berkeley Moynihan (see Figure 8.16). By 1890 McGill was able to record 33 such operations performed by himself and his colleagues in Leeds. In 1895, Eugene Fuller (1858–1930) of New York reported six successful cases of prostatectomy in which there is no doubt that he attempted complete enucleation of all diseased tissue. A suprapubic tube was placed in the bladder and a second soft rubber tube was passed through the perineum into the bladder, for drainage.

Despite the work of Belfield, McGill and Fuller, the operation of suprapubic prostatectomy gained relatively little support and it remained for Sir Peter Freyer (1852–1921) (Figure 8.22) to popularise the

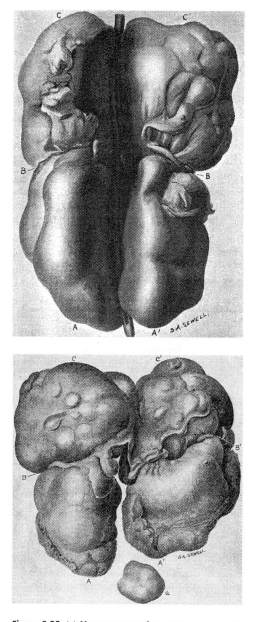

operation in a series of papers and monographs, so that today suprapubic enucleation of the prostate with bladder drainage through a large suprapubic tube (probably one of the reasons for Freyer's undoubtedly good results) is eponymously entitled 'the Freyer prostatectomy' (Figure 8.23). Freyer claimed, quite wrongly, that he and only he had introduced total removal of the gland and indeed claimed that the essential feature of his operation was that he removed the whole prostate and its capsule from its adventitial sheath. Both these claims were patently not true and the journals of the time were filled with the acrimonious claims and counter-claims of Freyer, Fuller of New York, the Leeds Group and others. However the publicity given to the operation by the controversy, as well as Freyer's numerous lectures, articles and books, made the operation widely known and did Freyer himself little harm. Indeed, during the controversy, he quoted Sidney Smith who wrote 'that man is not the discoverer of any art who first says the things; but he who says it so long and so loud and so clearly that he compels mankind to hear him'.

Freyer was a colourful character. He qualified from Queen's University, Belfast, in 1874 with Gold Medal, served in the Indian Medical Service as a Colonel and became particularly skilled in the use of the lithotrite (see Chapter 12) in the crushing of bladder stones. Successful operations with this instrument upon Bahadur Ali Khan, the Rajah of Rampur, were rewarded with a lakh of rupees and a magnificent present of jewellery. He returned to London in 1896 and was soon appointed to the staff of St Peter's Hospital, London, then, as today, the only specialised urological hospital in the United Kingdom, now the Institute of Urology. He was a skilful and speedy surgeon and his excellent results attracted a large private practice. In 1920 he reported a series of 1625 prostatectomies with a mortality of only 5%.

The Freyer prostatectomy remained popular until quite recently; indeed, as a house surgeon in Oxford in 1948 I assisted my chief at many of these operations. Although Hugh Young (1870–1945) of Baltimore perfected the perineal prostatectomy in 1903, the operation, although quite popular in the USA, did not compete with the suprapubic

Figure 8.23 (a) Upper aspect of an enormous prostate, weighing 10½ ounces, removed from a patient aged 75. The catheter indicates the position occupied by the urethra. Portion A, A1, B, B1, lay in the bladder; B, B1, C, C1 outside the bladder between the pubic arch and the rectum. (b) Showing under aspect of the same prostate; an adenoma detached from the prostate.
From Freyer P J: *Clinical Lectures on Stricture of the Urethra and Enlargement of the Prostate.* London, Baillière, Tindall and Cox, 1902.

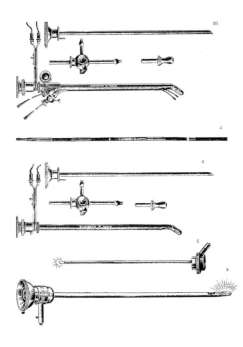

Figure 8.24 Max Nitze's cytoscope and accessories (patented in Vienna 1877 and published 1879).

approach elsewhere in the world. It remained for Terence Millin (1903–1980) to bring in his operation of retropubic prostatectomy, which he first performed in 1945, to replace the transvesical approach. It had the obvious advantages of leaving the bladder intact, efficient closure and good healing of the prostatic capsule and a much shorter and more comfortable post-operative course.

Give surgeons their due: they rapidly adapt advances in technology to their armamentarium. The discovery of X-rays, for example, was applied within weeks to the diagnosis of fractures and localisation of foreign bodies. The development of an effective small electric light bulb enabled one of the fathers of modern urology, Max Nitze (1848–1906), Professor of Urology in Berlin, to construct an electrically lighted cystoscope in 1877 that revolutionised urological diagnosis (Figure 8.24). By 1911, Hugh Young used a cystoscope with a punch attachment to perform a transurethral prosta-

tectomy. Control of bleeding was a problem until John Caulk (1881–1938) substituted the electric cautery for the knife so that bleeding could be controlled by coagulation of divided blood vessels. Nowadays, the use of fibreoptic instruments has seen the almost entire replacement of open prostatectomy by the transurethral cystoscopic operation (the transurethral prostatectomy or TUR), with its low morbidity and short patient stay.

Neurosurgery

We have already noted in the first chapter of this book that trephination of the skull was among the earliest operations and was carried out in widely different loci throughout the world. We have described the efforts of both civilian and military surgeons to deal with head wounds and skull fractures. However, as in so many other branches of surgery, elective operations upon the central nervous system had to await the modern era before they could be developed. It was Sir William Macewen (1848–1924) (see Figure 10.16) of Glasgow who first successfully removed a cerebral tumour, in 1879. The patient was a girl of 14 who presented with a left supraorbital mass and developed severe right-sided Jacksonian fits while being observed on the ward. At operation, a meningioma arising from the dura, adherent to the skull and extending into the orbital cavity was removed. Post-operatively the patient had further convulsions on the fifth day, but after that made a smooth recovery.

Macewen must be regarded as one of the founding fathers of neurosurgery. In 1876 he diagnosed a cerebral abscess in the left frontal lobe of a boy of 7 and advised surgery. This was refused, but at autopsy the diagnosis and localisation were brilliantly confirmed. Three years later, and in the same year that he performed his successful excision of the brain tumour, he accurately localised and successfully evacuated a subdural haematoma. By 1893, he had operated on 24 cases of cerebral abscess with no less than 23 recoveries, a marvellous record which can hardly be equalled today.

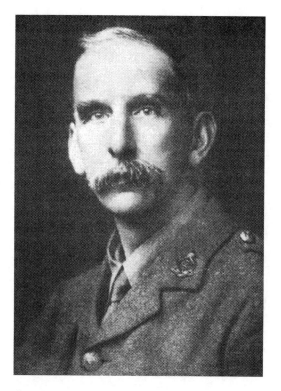

Figure 8.25 Sir Victor Horsley (as Colonel in the RAMC). Royal College of Surgeons of England.

Sir Victor Horsley (1857–1916) was the first surgeon to remove a spinal tumour. The year was 1887; the patient, a retired army officer, was admitted to the National Hospital for Nervous Diseases, Queen Square, under the care of the neurologist Sir William Gowers (1845–1915) with paraplegia, retention of urine and severe painful flexion spasms of the lower limbs. Gowers diagnosed a spinal tumour compressing the cord at the level of the fifth thoracic vertebra. Horsley, who had only been put on the staff at the hospital the year before, was called into consultation and operated within three hours of seeing the patient because of the obvious urgency of the condition. A laminectomy of the fourth to the sixth thoracic vertebrae was performed and revealed nothing, but higher exploration and opening the dura demonstrated an almond-sized tumour

which was indenting the spinal cord and was completely removed. The patient made a full recovery and died of other causes 20 years later. The pathology report on the specimen described it as a 'fibromyxoma'. Horsley (Figure 8.25) also pioneered the difficult cranial operation of excision of the trigeminal ganglion in the treatment of trigeminal neuralgia ('tic doloureux') – attacks of dreadful facial pain localised to one or other of areas of distribution of the divisions of the fifth cranial nerve. At Queen Square he carried out surgery for brain tumours, cerebral abscesses and focal epilepsy. Horsley was a remarkable man. A brilliant graduate of University College Hospital, London, he was soon appointed to its surgical staff in addition to his duties at Queen Square. He had wide interests in surgery, physiology and public health – he was a strong advocate of abstinence from alcohol. In the First World War he was appointed consultant surgeon in the Middle East and died suddenly while serving in Mesopotamia, perhaps from heat stroke or else paratyphoid fever, which was rampant at that time. He lies buried in the British war cemetry at Amara.

The founder of neurosurgery in the United States is recognised to have been Harvey Cushing (1869–1939) (Figure 8.27 and see also Figure 9.27), and his contributions to the surgery of head injuries in the First World War are detailed in Chapter 9. Trained by William Halsted at Baltimore, where he commenced his neurosurgical work, Cushing was appointed Surgeon-in-Chief at the newly built Peter Bent Brigham Hospital in Boston in 1912. Here he developed his meticulous technique, which passed into standard neurosurgical practice. Before the First World War he published important work on the surgery of trigeminal neuralgia and tumours of the brain and of the pituitary. Cushing was an accomplished artist; his books and articles were illustrated by his own superb drawings (Figure 8.26). On his return to civilian life after the war, he went on to produce massive studies on brain tumours.

From his earliest days in neurosurgery, Cushing realised the vital importance of haemostasis in dealing with the vascular tissues of the scalp, skull

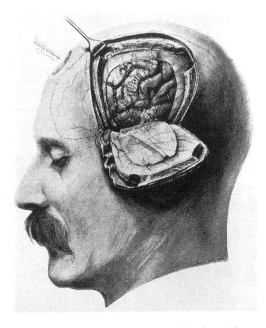

Figure 8.26 An example of Harvey Cushing's artistic skill. The exposed motor area of the brain in a man with focal epilepsy secondary to a bullet wound in the speech area.
From Cushing's chapter in Keen's *System of Surgery*, published in 1908.

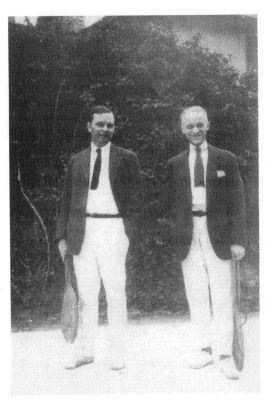

Figure 8.27 Walter Dandy (on the left) with his rival in surgery and tennis, Harvey Cushing.
From *Harvey Cushing, a Biography*, John Fulton Oxford, Blackwell Publications, 1946.

and the brain itself. He showed that scalp bleeding could be controlled by infiltration with adrenaline combined with traction with a series of artery forceps applied to the skin edges. In 1910, he introduced silver clips, to which his name is still applied, that could be used to occlude meningeal and cerebral vessels. Suction was introduced to deal with severe bleeding, especially deep within the brain substance. However, it was his introduction of the use of diathermy in 1926 that was the most important of these innovations.

The first occasion on which Cushing used diathermy (operating on a highly vascular meningioma) has a particular fascination for me because his assistant at the time fainted. This was none other than Hugh Cairns (1896–1952), who later was my Professor of Surgery at Oxford. At that time he was a young Australian veteran of the Gallipoli

landings in the First World War, where he had fought against the Turks as a private in the Australian army. He later served in France as a Junior Medical Officer. Obviously, the smell of coagulating brain tissue proved too much for him at that historical operation in 1926. Indeed, Cairns used to say that Gallipoli and the Battle of the Marne were nothing compared to working as Cushing's assistant.

One of Cushing's bright young men in his days at the Johns Hopkins was Walter Dandy (1886–1946) (Figure 8.27). Dandy served as Cushing's research assistant in 1910, then as his assistant resident from 1911 to 1912, but their very different personalities clashed then, as they did for the rest of the careers of both these outstanding neurosurgeons. When

Cushing moved to Boston in 1912, taking with him most of his staff, Dandy was left behind, but was soon on the staff at Johns Hopkins where he soon established himself as a brilliant innovator and a superb and, in contrast to Cushing, rapid operator. In 1922 he reported his technique of complete removal of an acoustic neuroma, (a fairly common tumour of the eighth, auditory, cranial nerve). Before that time Cushing had advocated an incomplete intracapsular removal of the growth. He was the first to perform the operation of clipping the feeding artery to obliterate a Circle of Willis aneurysm on the inferior aspects of the brain. He carried out fundamental research on the secretion and circulation of cerebro-spinal fluid and devised procedures to treat hydro-cephalus. Dandy developed the first radiological technique for visualising radiologically intra-cerebral pathology. This involved the injection of air as a contrast material into the ventricular system of the brain (ventriculography), which at the time was an enormous advance in the diagnosis of focal lesions within the skull. At first this brilliant innov-ation was opposed by Cushing, who believed that it would distract neurosurgeons from trying to make an accurate diagnosis by clinical examination only!

Caesarian section

The early history of Caesarian section (see Figure 5.9) is shrouded in myth and mystery. The origin of the very name itself has various interpretations. The story that Julius Caesar was delivered by this means is highly improbable, since his mother, Aurelia, was alive and well at the time of his invasion of Britain in 55 BC! In 715 BC Numa Pompillius, King of Rome, enacted a law in which burial of a dead pregnant woman was forbidden until the fetus had been removed, so that mother and child could be buried separately. The *lex Regia* (Royal Law) later became the *lex Caesarea* – a more likely explan-ation of the term.

There are numerous references to this procedure in ancient myths and made by classical writers. Ovid, the Roman poet, describes how Aesculapius,

god of Physic, was delivered by this means, the surgeon being none other than the great Apollo himself (Figure 8.28). The well-known Shake-spearian quotation from *Macbeth*:

Tel them Macduff was from his mother's womb
  Untimely ripped

is probably derived from Holinshead's *The Chron-icles of England, Scotland and Ireland* of 1577 – another myth!

The term itself appears first to have been used in print in a book by Francis Rousset, physician to the Duke of Savoy, published in 1581 and entitled *Enfantement Caesareinne* in which he advises the operation to be performed on the living mother and records seven case reports that he had collected which purported survival of the mother. Other surgeons were more cynical. Ambroise Paré (see Figure 9.4) in his *Textbook of Surgery*, published at about the same time, even though he had heard of a successful case, strongly criticised the operation.

Most of the early accounts were of operations carried out after the death of the mother in an att-empt to save the child, but there were also reports of women in obstructed labour operating on them-selves or being delivered thus by the desperate husband. More recently, showing that such indeed could have been true, there have been eye witness accounts of the operation being performed in primitive communities. Robert Felkin MD, in 1884, published a vivid description in the *Edinburgh Medical Journal* of a Caesarian section he had observed in Uganda, performed by a native practi-tioner. The patient, a primipara aged 20, was first intoxicated with banana wine. The wine was then used both to bathe the girl's abdomen and the surgeon's hands. A midline incision was made from the pubis to the umbilicus. The assistant cauterised the bleeding vessels with a red-hot iron. The uterus was incised, the baby and then the pla-centa delivered, and the abdominal wound brought together with seven metal spikes passed through the edges of the wound and tied together with string. Felkin left 11 days later, at which time both mother and child appeared well. Reading this report, one

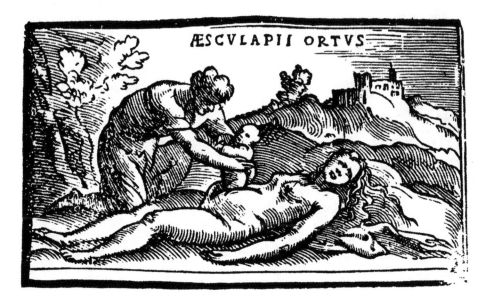

Figure 8.28 Aesculapius being delivered from his mother Coronis by Apollo. Woodcut from Alessandrio Beneditti's De Re Medicine 1549.

can easily imagine similar operations taking place, sometimes with equally happy results, over the centuries (Figure 8.29).

It seems that the first successful Caesarian to be performed in the British Isles was performed by a skilful but illiterate midwife, Mary Donally, in Claremont, Ireland, in 1738. The patient, Alice O'Neale, aged 33, was a farmer's wife who had already had several children. She had now been in labour for 12 days. The midwife opened the lower abdomen and the uterus with a razor and delivered a dead child. She then held the wound edges together while a neighbour ran a mile to fetch a tailor's needle and thread with which the midwife closed the cut in the abdominal wall. The mother recovered but, as was almost invariable in early successful attempts at abdominal surgery, she developed a large ventral hernia.

William Smellie (1697–1763) (Figure 8.30) of Lanark, Scotland, and then London, regarded as the father of British midwifery and a pioneer in the use of the obstetrical forceps, published his *Treatise on the Theory and Practice of Midwifery* in 1752. As might

be expected from this experienced and pragmatic obstetrician, he took a sound and commonsense approach to the subject of Caesarian section. The operation might be employed in obstructed labour when it was impossible to insert the hand vaginally into the pelivis, when the woman was strong and when no other means was available of saving either mother or child. Alternatively, it might be employed when the mother had expired and there was a chance of saving the infant. His personal experience appears to have been limited to three cases – all performed after death of the mother from haemorrhage caused by placenta praevia. In all cases the child was dead.

Smellie quotes, like other contemporary writers, the success of Mary Donally. Of course, the standard practice in those days in the management of an obstructed labour was to perform a destructive operation, craniotomy, on the fetus and then to deliver the parts piecemeal.

Apparently the first Caesarian operation with maternal survival to be performed by a medical practitioner in this country was not until 1793, although it was not recorded till 1798. This was

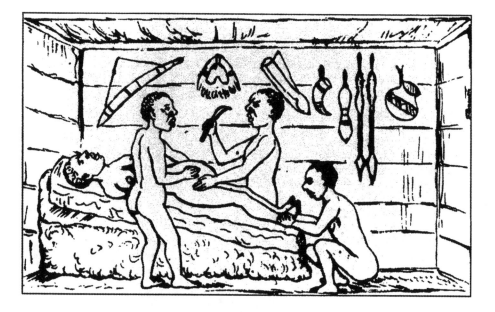

Figure 8.29 Drawing by Robert Felkin of a Caesarian section he witnessed in Uganda. Edinburgh Journal of Medicine, 1884.

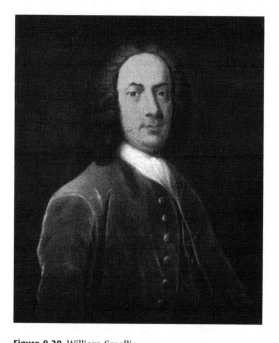

Figure 8.30 William Smellie.
Portrait in the Royal College of Surgeons of Edinburgh.
(Reproduced by kind permission.)

performed by a surgeon named Hawarden in Wigan, Lancashire. His patient, aged 40, had had several children previously but now had a grossly deformed pelvis as result of a severe fracture. After the patient had been in labour for three days, Hawarden was summoned. He opened the abdomen through a five-inch incision to the left of the midline and delivered a dead fetus. The mother survived.

That wise obstetrician James Blundell (1790–1877) of Guy's' Hospital (see Figure 9.29), whom we have already met as the father of clinical blood transfusion, speculated in his published lectures in 1832 whether the dangers of Caesarian section – haemorrhage and sepsis – might not be considerably reduced by removal of the uterus after delivery of the child. This speculation was based on his successful performance of a vaginal hysterectomy on a woman with a totally prolapsed uterus some months after she had delivered. As we shall see, this idea was taken up with enthusiasm four decades later and was first carried out the year before he died.

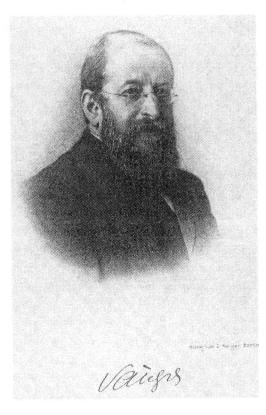

Verlag von S. Manger, Berlin

Figure 8.31 Max Sanger.

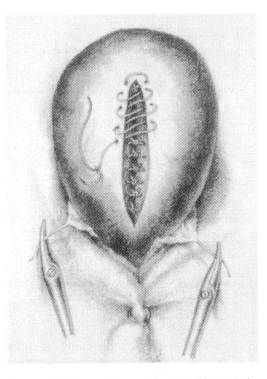

Figure 8.32 "Classical" Caesarian section. The vertical incision through the body of the uterus is sutured, as first advocated by Max Sanger.

The introduction first of anaesthesia and then of antiseptic surgery (see Chapter 7) rendered the operation at last painless and certainly safer. Initial indications were principally for the delivery of women with obstructed labour due to pelvic deformity or obstruction from an ovarian or other pelvic tumour. The great danger was still sepsis from the uterus – contaminated as result of the prolonged labour, often with repeated pre-operative vaginal examinations, which almost always resulted in an infected birth canal. Eduardo Porro (1842–1902), Professor of Obstetrics at Pavia, Italy, dissatisfied with the high mortality of the operation, devised a new procedure in 1876 – first proposed, as we have noted above, by Blundell. Immediately after delivering the child, a ligature of wire or elastic was placed around the neck of the uterus. The body

of the uterus, together with the tubes and ovaries, was excised and the cervical stump exteriorised – the operation of Caesarian section and hysterectomy, or Porro's operation. His first patient was a 25-year-old dwarf who also had rickets and who was in her first pregnancy. The operation was carried out under chloroform, using strict aseptic precautions. . Both mother and child survived – the first maternal survival from Caesarian section in Pavia. The operation resulted in a distinct improvement in maternal mortality and enjoyed a period of popularity.

Lawson Tait of Birmingham (see Figure 8.20) was first to suggest this operation for haemorrhage from placenta praevia and carried this out successfully in 1898 for a multipara with severe haemorrhage and a rigid closed cervix. He was able to report seven Porro

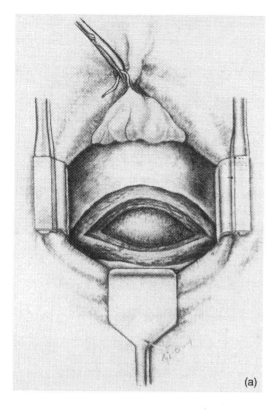

(a)

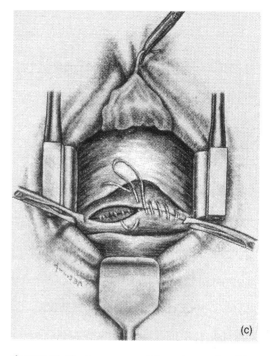

(c)

Figure 8.33 The lower-segment Caesarian section: (a) a transverse incision is made through the thin lower segment of the gravid uterus; (b) the baby's head is being delivered, here with the aid of obstetrical forceps; (c) the uterine incision is sutured.

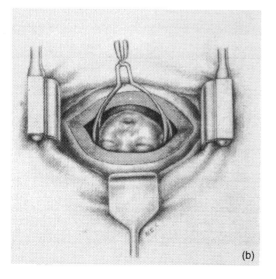

(b)

operations with a single maternal death. A major advance was made by the German gynaecologist Max Sanger (1851–1903) (Figure 8.31), who introduced suturing of the uterine incision instead of leaving it as a gaping wound, with post-operative bleeding from the incision being a common – and often lethal – complication (Figure 8.32). He also advocated early intervention in the difficult case, before the mother become exhausted and septic. Sanger's advice was soon adopted as standard, and again maternal mortality dropped.

The next important step was the introduction of the lower-segment Caesarian section (Figure 8.33). In this procedure, the uterine incision is made transversely through the much thinner lower segment of the uterine wall. This is much less vascular than the body of the uterus, easier to suture, and greatly reduces the risk of rupture of the uterus in any subsequent vaginal delivery. It was first performed successfully for both mother and child by T G Thomas (1831–1903) at the College of Physicians and Surgeons, New York, in 1878. His patient was a crippled dwarf with gross pelvic contraction.

It was popularised in the United Kingdom by John Munro Kerr (1868–1960) of Gasgow and Sir Eardley Holland (1879–1967) of the London Hospital, who both reported excellent results in 1921, and the modern operation of Caesarian section was firmly established.

9

The surgery of warfare

Mankind has always been subject to injury; the earliest surgeons were no doubt those men and women who were particularly skilled in binding up the contusions, lacerations, fractures, perforations and eviscerations of their fellows (Figure 9.1). Since man is undoubtedly the most vicious and aggressive of all animals, much of this trauma was inflicted in battle, and warfare has therefore played an important part in the development of wound management. Indeed, it has been said that the only thing to benefit from war is surgery.

Until the introduction of gunpowder into warfare in the 14th century, war wounds were inflicted mainly by knives, swords, spears, arrows and various blunt weapons such as the mace and cudgel. The sharp weapons would produce penetrating and lacerating injuries, the blunt instruments would produce severe contusions. The early surgeons well recognised that some injuries were going to prove almost invariably fatal. These comprised penetration of a vital structure, such as a perforating wound of the skull, chest or abdomen, or haemorrhage from a major blood vessel. However, if the victim survived the initial injury, he was very likely to live. This was because these lacerated and contused wounds produced little tissue destruction and thus allowed the natural powers of the body's healing to cure the victim. So the surgeon became skilled at dressing and bandaging wounds and splinting fractures. The various ointments employed, although probably usually ineffective, at least did little harm. Haemorrhage would be treated by pressure on the wound or the use of the cautery. The technique of tying the bleeding artery, a device introduced by the Alexandrian surgeons around 250 BC and described by the Roman writer Celsus in the 1st century AD, appeared to have been forgotten.

The medieval surgical textbooks often carried an illustration of a 'wound man' which showed the various injuries the surgeons of the Middle Ages might be called upon to treat; we can guess quite accurately which would prove successes and which would be almost certainly lethal (Figure 9.2).

The invention of gunpowder

Gunpowder appears to have been invented in China and was used in the manufacture of fireworks and probably also in cannons. It first appeared in Europe in the 14th century and it is well documented that cannon were employed in the Battle of Crécy in 1346 when Philip VI of France was defeated by Edward III and his longbowmen. The introduction of firearms completely changed the pathology of war wounds. The gross tissue destruction produced by the musket ball and cannon provided a wonderful medium for the growth of bacteria, especially anaerobic microbes, those that thrive in the absence of oxygen and which grow on dead tissues. These include the organisms that produce tetanus and gas gangrene. Thus dreadful wound infection and gangrene of a type not previously seen were encountered by surgeons treating these war wounds. Now this, of course, was centuries before our knowledge

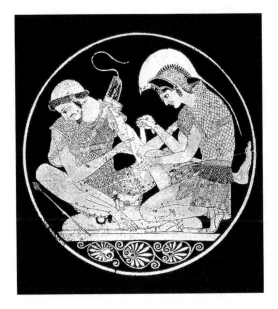

Figure 9.1 Achilles bandages the arm of Patroclus during the Trojan Wars 1200 BC.
From a painting on an ancient Greek vase.

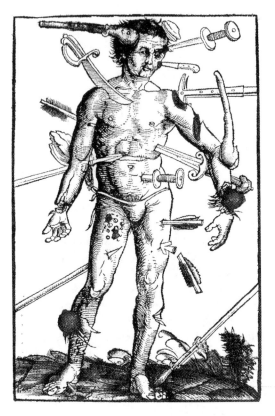

Figure 9.2 A 'wound man'.
From Hans Gersdorff: *Feldbusch der Wundarztney*. Strasburg, 1517. Courtesy of Mr J Kirkup FRCS.

of the bacterial causation of wound infection. It was not unreasonable, therefore, for military surgeons to conclude that these awful complications were due to the poisonous nature of the gunpowder itself. The solution was obviously to destroy the poison and this was done by means of a red-hot cautery or by the use of boiling oil poured into the wound. The great popularity of the latter method was undoubtedly due to the writings of the Italian surgeon Giovanni da Vigo (1460–1525), whose surgical treatise entitled *A Compendious Practice of the Art of Surgery* was first published in Rome in 1514 and went through more than 40 editions in many languages; it greatly influenced the surgical thinking of his time. Of course, we now know that this practice had the opposite effect to the one desired. The red-hot cautery (Figure 9.3) and the boiling oil in fact destroyed more tissue than the missile itself and aggravated an already serious situation, as well as inflicting untold torture upon the poor soldier victim.

We now come to one of those great landmarks that punctuate surgical history; a surgeon who, through his example and writings, greatly influenced progress in the management of wounds. Ambroise Paré (1510–1590) was born in the little town of Laval in the Province of Maine (Figure 9.4). His father was probably Valet de Chambre and barber to the local squire and he may thus have obtained some interest in the work of the barber-surgeons. Paré's sister married a barber-surgeon who practised in Paris and his elder brother was a master barber-surgeon in Vitré. Paré may have begun the study of surgery with his brother and it is certain that he did work with a barber-surgeon in the provinces before coming to Paris at the age

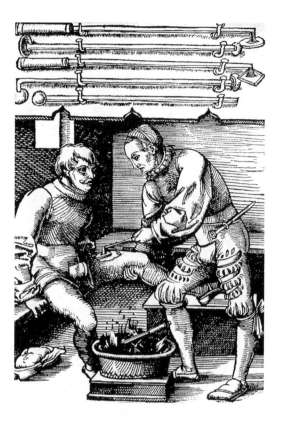

Figure 9.3 Cauterisation of a wound of the thigh.

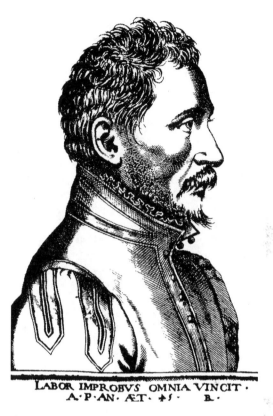

LABOR IMPROBVS OMNIA VINCIT ·
A · P · AN · ÆT · 45 ·   B ·

Figure 9.4 Ambroise Paré, aged 45.
From Geoffrey Keynes: *Apologie and Treatise of Ambroise Paré*. London, Falcon, 1951.

of 22 as an apprentice barber-surgeon. He was soon appointed compagnon-chirurgeon, roughly equivalent to house surgeon today, at the Hôtel Dieu, that immense medieval hospital and the only one in Paris at the time, where he worked for the next three or four years and must have gained a great experience in that repository of pathology.

Perhaps because he could not afford to pay the fees for admission to the ranks of the barber-surgeons, Paré started his career at the age of 26 as a military surgeon. In those days, there was no organised medical care for the humble private soldiers of armies in the field. Surgeons were attached to individual generals and to other important personages, and might, if they wished, give what aid they could to the common soldiers in their spare time. Otherwise the troops had to rely on the rough

and ready help of their companions or of a motley crowd of horse-doctors, farriers, quacks, mountebanks and camp followers.

Paré was appointed surgeon to the Mareschal de Montejan, who was Colonel-General of the French infantry. This, his first of many campaigns, took him to Turin, and it was here in 1537 that he made his fundamental observations on the treatment of gunshot wounds. He soon realised that the accepted method of treating these injuries with boiling oil did more harm than good and substituted a more humane and less destructive dressing. Here is his description of what today might well be called one of the earliest controlled surgical experiments. How many of us have carried out some new untried treatment and have shared Paré's experience of being unable to sleep and have come into the ward to see how a patient is before anyone else is around, with pulse racing, to see whether the treatment we have carried out has been a brilliant success or a disastrous failure?

I was at that time a fresh-water surgeon, since I had not yet seen and treated wounds made by firearms. It is true I had read in Jean de Vigo in his first book of *Wounds in General* Chapter 8, that wounds made by firearms are poisoned because of the powder. For their cure he advised their cauterisation with oil of elders mixed with a little theriac. To not fail, this oil must be applied boiling even though this would cause the wounded extreme pain. I wished to know first how to apply it, how the other surgeons did their first dressings, which was to apply the oil as boiling as possible. So I took heart to do as they did. Finally, my oil was exhausted and I was forced instead to apply a digestive made of egg yolk, rose oil and turpentine. That night I could not sleep easily, thinking that by failure of cauterising, I would find the wounded in whom I had failed to put the oil dead of poisoning. This made me get up early in the morning to visit them. There, beyond my hopes, I found those on whom I had used the digestive medication feeling little pain in their wounds, without inflammation and swelling, having rested well through the night. The others on whom I had used the oil I found feverish, with great pain, swelling and inflammation around their wounds. Then I resolved never again to so cruelly burn the poor wounded by gunshot.

Paré also went on to show that bleeding after amputation of a limb should be arrested not by the terrible method of the red-hot cautery, but by simply tying the divided blood vessels. Ligation of blood vessels was known to the ancients, and Paré's only claim, as he makes quite clear in his own writings, was that he was the first to apply this technique in performing amputations. He first employed the ligature in amputation of the leg in 1552 at the siege of Danvillier but did not publish his technique until 1564 when he wrote: 'wherefore I must earnestly entreat all surgeons that leaving this old and too cruel way of healing they will embrace this new, which I think was taught me by the special favour of the sacred Deity, for I learned it not of my masters nor of any other, neither have I at any time found it used by any'.

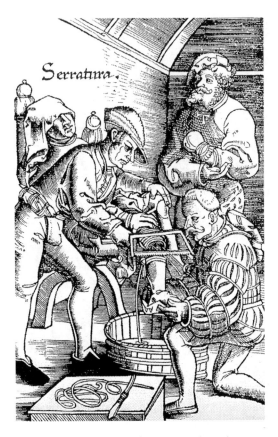

Figure 9.5 A below-knee amputation in the 16th century. Note the patient in the background who has had his left hand amputated.
From Hans von Gersdorff: *Feldbuch der Wundartzney.* Strasburg, 1517.

A description by Paré of one such case is worth repeating here:

In the year 1583, the tenth day of December, Toussaint Posson, having his leg all ulcered and all the bones carried and rotten, prayed me for the honour of God to cut off his leg by reason of the great pain which he could not longer endure. After his body was prepared I caused his leg to be cut off four fingers below the patella by Daniel Poullet, one of my servants, to teach him and to embolden him in such works, and there he readily tied the vessels to stay the bleeding without application of hot irons [Figure 9.5]. He was well cured, God be praised, and is returned home to his house with a wooden leg.

So here was Paré at the age of 73 passing down his skill and experience to his apprentices, a tradition we still see today as surgeons teach their residents in the operating theatre.

Paré went from fame to fame and dominated the history of surgery in the 16th century. He was a veteran of no less than 17 military campaigns and surgeon to four successive kings of France. However, his practice continued to embrace the humblest soldier as well. He died at the age of 80 in Paris as he had always lived, a simple, humble man. In his very first campaign he ended his description of the treatment of a gunshot wound of the ankle with perhaps his most famous phrase, 'I dressed the wound and God healed him'.

The most notable English surgeon of the 16th century was Thomas Gale (1507–1587), whose long life corresponded closely to that of Ambroise Paré and indeed he is known as 'the English Paré'. He combined his military career with his civilian practice in London and eventually succeeded Thomas Vicary (see Figure 5.2) as Master of the Company of Barber Surgeons. He served in the army of Henry VIII and was present at the siege of Montreuil in 1544. Later he was Serjeant Surgeon to Elizabeth I. Gale was a prolific author who published in English; his most famous publication was his *Certaine Workes of Chirurgerie* (1563) which contained a section on 'wounds made with gunshot' in which he denied the traditional misconception that gunpowder was itself poisonous. He decried the poor quality of men pretending to be surgeons in the military; these included tinkers, cobblers and sowgelders, who treated wounds with grease used to lubricate horse's hooves, shoemaker's wax and the rust of old kettles.

Over the next two and a half centuries, until the revolution effected by anaesthesia and antisepsis (see Chapter 7), there was essentially little change in the surgery of warfare. Many surgeons gained much practical experience on the battlefield, some later achieving great fame. For example, John Hunter (1728–1793) served at Belle Isle and Portugal during the Seven Years War, and Sir Charles Bell (1774–1842) attended the wounded after Waterloo.

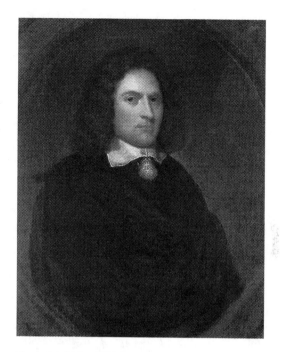

Figure 9.6 Richard Wiseman. Royal College of Surgeons of England.

A number of surgeons made their careers in military or naval service and rendered important contributions by their experience and writings.

Among the most colourful of the military surgeons was Richard Wiseman (?1621–1676), whose life reads more like a novel than the biography of a distinguished surgeon (Figure 9.6). We do not even know the exact date or place of his birth and know nothing of his parentage, which indicates that he was probably illegitimate. In 1637 he was apprenticed to Richard Smith, a surgeon, and following this he may have served in the Dutch Navy. At the beginning of the Civil War in 1645 between the Cavaliers of Charles I and the Roundheads of Oliver Cromwell, Wiseman was appointed surgeon to a Royalist battalion and was present at the battles of Taunton and Truro. With the defeat of his troops, Wiseman escaped and worked in exile in France and the Low Countries as a surgeon.

1649 saw the trial and execution by decapitation of Charles I. The following year, his son, now

Charles II, left Holland and landed with his followers in Scotland. He was accompanied by Richard Wiseman, who acted as surgeon at several bloody battles, including the battle of Dunbar, but the Royalists were finally defeated in 1651 at the battle of Worcester. Charles, after many adventures, managed to escape to the continent but many of his followers, including Wiseman, were captured and spent many months in prison at Chester. On his release Wiseman practised as a surgeon in London but was imprisoned again for some months. In 1654, his practice now in ruins, he left for Spain and served in the Spanish navy. On the restoration of Charles II in 1660, Wiseman was appointed his Surgeon. Five years later he was elected Master of the Company of Barber-Surgeons and in 1672 he was appointed Serjeant Surgeon to the King. He was now a sick man, probably from pulmonary tuberculosis, but in 1676, the year of his death, he published his major work by which he is remembered to this day. The *Several Chirurgical Treatises* recalls Wiseman's wide surgical experience afloat and ashore in both military and civilian practice. He quotes no less than 600 cases from his personal experience. The work is logically arranged and is particularly detailed in the sections devoted to injuries. He stressed that the decision to amputate a limb should be made promptly, when the patient would be less sensitive to pain. He wrote: 'In the heat of fight, whether it be at sea or land, the chirurgeon ought to consider at the first dressing, what possibility there is of preserving the wounded member; accordingly if there would be no hope of saving it, to make his amputation at that instant, while the patient is free of fever'.

Typical of Wiseman's vivid writings is this case report in his section on wounds on the brain:

At the siege of Melcombe-Regis, a foot-soldier of Lieutenant-Colonel Ballard's by the grazing of a cannon-shot, had a great part of his forehead carried off, and the skull fractured into many pieces and some of it driven with the hairy scalp into the brain. The man fell down as dead, but after a while moved and an hour or two after, his fellow soldiers seeing him endeavour to rise, fetched me to him. I pulled out the pieces of bone and lacerated flesh from amongst the brain in which they were entangled, and dressed him up with soft folded linen dipped in a Cephalick Balsam, and with emplaster and bandage, bound him up supposing I should never dress him any more. Yet he lived 17 days and the 15th day walked from that great corner fort over against Portland by the bridge which separates Weymouth from Melcombe-Regis only led by the hand of someone of his fellow soldiers. The second day after he fell into a spasmus, and died, howling like a dog as most of those do who have been so wounded.

Presumably he died of tetanus.

The Napoleonic Wars

The Napoleonic Wars produced two outstanding French surgeons, Percy and Larrey. Pierre François Percy (1754–1825) served as Surgeon in Chief with the French army in Spain. He was the first to introduce into any army a trained corps of field stretcher bearers for the skilled transportation of wounded to surgical aid. His system was universally adopted by the French army in 1813.

Although vast numbers of surgeons, from every European country, were engaged in dealing with the carnage of the Napoleonic Wars (1792–1815), one stood out as the greatest military surgeon since Ambroise Paré; he was another Frenchman, Dominique Jean Larrey (1766–1842) (Figure 9.7). At the tender age of 13 he became apprenticed to his brother, a surgeon in Toulouse. On qualification, he joined the French navy in 1787 and served as a ship's surgeon along the coast of Newfoundland. He returned to France a few months before the revolution of 1789. In 1792, Larrey was posted to the Army of the Rhine, and from then on was engaged in almost continuous active military duties until Waterloo in 1815, where he was seriously wounded. He served all over Europe, in Egypt, Syria and Russia, in a total of 25 campaigns and 60 battles. He was Chief Surgeon to the Imperial Guard, Surgeon in Chief to the Imperial Army and Professor of Surgery at the army medical school at Val-de-Grâce in Paris. After the Napoleonic War, Larrey became Surgeon Inspector to the army and Chief Surgeon at

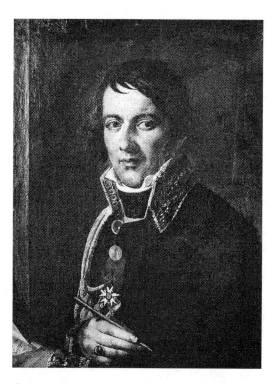

Figure 9.7 Dominique Jean Larrey, portrait attributed to Mme. Benoit.
From Dible J H: *Napoleon's Surgeon*. London, Heinemann, 1970.

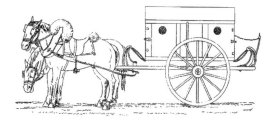

Figure 9.8 Larrey's light ambulance.
From Dible J H: *Napoleon's Surgeon*. London, Heinemann, 1970.

the Invalides, continuing to serve military medicine in his care of the army veterans until his retirement at the age of 72.

Larrey's contributions to military surgery were primarily his organisational skills. He insisted on getting his special surgical teams near the front line to ensure early surgery for the wounded and stressed the rapid evacuation of wounded men by means of his specially designed light horse-drawn vehicles which he named his 'flying ambulances' (Figure 9.8). He laid emphasis on the desirability of immediate amputation for seriously damaged limbs. His work constituted the foundation of the present concepts of military surgery.

It should be noted that the word 'ambulance' in French has a different connotation and means a field hospital attached to the army and moving with it, not the conveyance used for transportation of the wounded.

In the midst of all Larrey's wartime duties, he published his massive *Memoirs of Military Surgery*, which were promptly translated into English! In it, he writes:

When a limb is so much injured by a gun-shot wound that it cannot be saved, it should be amputated *immediately*. The first 24 hours is the only period during which the system remains tranquil, and we should hasten during this time, as in all dangerous diseases, to adopt the necessary remedy. In the army many circumstances force the necessity of primitive amputation: first the inconvenience which attends the transportation of the wounded from the field of battle to the military hospitals on badly constructed carriages; the jarring of these wagons produces such disorder in the wounds, and in all the nerves, that the greater part of the wounded perish on the way, especially if it be long, and the heat or cold of the weather be extreme. Secondly, the danger of remaining long in the hospital. This risk is much diminished by amputation. It converts a gun-shot wound into one which is capable of being speedily healed, and obviates the causes that produce the hospital fever and gangrene. Thirdly, in case the wounded are of necessity abandoned on the field of battle, it is then important that amputation be performed, because when it is completed, they may remain several days without being dressed and the subsequent dressings are more easily accomplished. Moreover, it often happens, that these unfortunate persons do not find surgeons sufficiently skilful to operate, as we have seen among some nations whose military hospitals were not organised like ours.

Not only had Larrey great organisational and teaching skills, he was also a brave soldier and a capers, which saved us, since the cavalry could not follow over broken ground and I was fortunate enough to gain our rearguard ahead of the English dragoons. I ultimately reached Alexandria with my patient on my shoulders and effected his cure there. The General has been living in France in retirement for many years.

Larrey was wounded and left for dead at the battle of Waterloo, captured by the Prussians and sentenced to be shot. Just before the time of his execution he was fortunately recognised by a German surgeon who had attended his lectures and who interceded for him. He was brought before the Prussian Commander, Marshall Blücher, whose son had been wounded, captured by the French and treated successfully by Larrey. Not surprisingly, Blücher cancelled the death sentence.

At the battle of Borodino in the Russian campaign of 1812, Larrey performed no less than 200 amputations in a 24-hour period. He described his own technique for the rapid disarticulation of the arm at the shoulder joint (Figure 9.9). Here is a typical Larrey case report from his memoirs:

At the latter engagement [the battle of Wagram 1809] the first who was brought to my ambulance was General Daboville, then Colonel of light artillery. A large ball had carried away part of his right shoulder and fractured the scapulo-humeral articulation. A large portion of the pectoralis major, the deltoid and latissimus dorsi muscles were torn away and the acromion and extremity of the clavicle were fractured. The head of the humerus was broken into three pieces and driven into the axilla. One of them was wedged into the brachial plexus, and several of its nerves broken. The axillary artery was much distended and ready to break. His pulse was scarcely perceptible and he appeared to be in articulo mortis. Indeed, death seemed to approach so rapidly that I hesitated under the supposition that he could not live under the operation. But I resolved to go through with it, more with an expectation of relieving his pain than of seeing him survive. The operation was performed in a few minutes and to my great surprise succeeded completely. Had it been delayed in this case a few minutes longer, he never would have gathered the laurels which he deserved. He was placed on a miserable bed of straw, where he lay very quietly until he was sent to Vienna. During this period, he several times fell into syncope, and I was apprehensive he

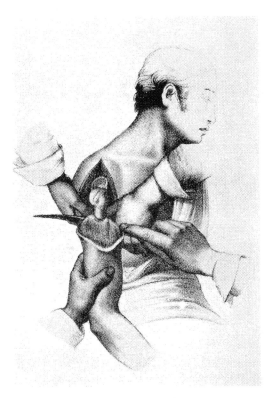

Figure 9.9 Larrey's method of amputation at the shoulder. From Dible J H: *Napoleon's Surgeon.* London, Heinemann, 1970.

skilful and rapid surgeon. At the battle of Alexandria in 1801 he operated on General Sylly in the field, then hoisted him on to his back and ran with him to escape the advancing enemy. In recalling this incident 40 years later Larrey wrote:

General Sylly had his left leg almost completely shot away at the knee joint, the limb being attached only by a few strands of ligaments and tendons. He was carried behind the line of battle to the ambulance of the centre but did not realise the seriousness of his wound on account of his state of extreme collapse from loss of blood . . . I performed the amputation in three minutes amidst the fighting, had just finished when we were charged by a body of English cavalry. I had barely time to hoist the patient onto my shoulders and carry him as quickly as I could towards our army, which had begun to retreat. I crossed a series of holes or ditches used for cultivation of

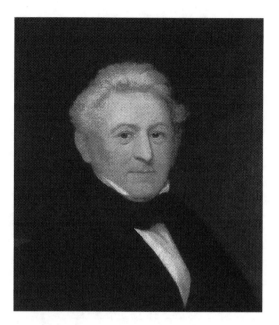

Figure 9.10 George James Guthrie.
Royal College of Surgeons of England.

could not support the fatigue of this short journey and he was therefore removed among the last. . . . His wound was very large but he continued calm and spoke with a more audible voice. The dressings were simple, and were performed under my own inspection. The Colonel's strength gradually returned and in a short time he could use light food and was cured perfectly in three months.

On the British side, one surgeon distinguished himself sufficiently to earn the title of 'the British Larrey'. This was George James Guthrie (1785–1856) (Figure 9.10). At the age of 16 he entered the army as a hospital mate but soon after this it became compulsory for such men to become medically qualified so Guthrie sat and passed the MRCS. This was followed by five years of military surgery in Canada and then six years as surgeon in the Peninsular campaign. Guthrie returned from civilian life to help deal with the wounded at Waterloo. He was present at numerous battles, for example, he cared for 3000 wounded after the battle of Talavera in Spain and even captured a French cannon single-handed. At the end of the

war, Guthrie published his *Gunshot Wounds*, in which, like Larrey, he advised early amputation where this was indicated, certainly within the first 24 hours of wounding. He served on the staff of Westminster Hospital, founded the Royal Westminster Ophthalmic Hospital and wrote *The Operative Surgery of the Eye* (1823), where he advised extraction of the lens in cataract surgery rather than 'couching' (i.e. displacing) it.

This quotation from Guthrie's *Treatise on Gunshot Wounds* gives an example of his pithy writing, based on his considerable experience:

A wound from a cannon-shot injuring the bones of the elbow joint demands immediate amputation, as the neighbouring parts are also generally injured. The operation being necessary, the patient should be placed upon a chair . . . if the surgeon has the slightest confidence in himself, and the assistants are good, no tourniquet should be applied, but the artery be compressed against the bone by two fore-fingers. For my own part, I never apply a tourniquet; and I believe if by any accident this assistant should fail, the operator can without difficulty compress the artery himself, so as to prevent any evil consequence, and not interrupt the operation; and in the first case in which I tried the operation on the arm, I had to compress the artery against the head of the humerus with the left hand, whilst I sawed the bone with the right.

The Crimean War

The Crimean War (1854–1855) was the first major campaign in which anaesthesia was employed. Apart from this, the war was a story of an ill-planned catastrophe on the part of the British Medical Services. The French, due no doubt to the lessons of Larrey, had the advantages of light ambulances to transport their wounded. The miserable sufferings of the British sick and wounded caused an outcry at home. Florence Nightingale (1820–1910) (Figure 9.11), a lady of good birth and education, who had trained in Germany and had set up a nursing home in London, organised a staff of women nurses for service at the military hospital at Scutari. The first things she requisitioned on

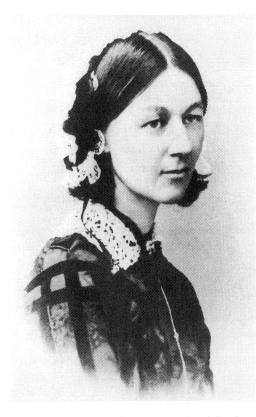

Figure 9.11 Florence Nightingale. Signed and dated photograph, 18th July, 1861.
Reproduced by courtesy of the Florence Nightingale Museum Trust, London.

her arrival were 300 scrubbing brushes. Returning to England after the war, she established the Nightingale School at St Thomas' Hospital and remained Superintendent of the School for the following 27 years. She is rightly regarded today as one of the founders of the nursing profession (Figures 9.12 and 9.13).

The greatest Russian military surgeon of the time was Nikolai Pirogoff (1810–1881), who trained in Moscow and became Professor of Surgery in St Petersburg. He served in many campaigns and in particular was Surgeon in Chief in the Crimea. Here he did equivalent work to Florence Nightingale, introducing skilled female nurses into his hospitals and emphasising the need for proper medical equipment for the wounded. He was early to adopt anaesthesia and devised a conservative amputation of the foot which still bears his name. He insisted that surgeons required a high standard of anatomical knowledge and published a remarkable atlas of anatomy in five volumes between 1852 and 1859. This contained a series of 200 plates depicting transverse sections through the body, obtained from cadavers which he froze in the snow!

A few years after the Crimean War, a young Swiss banker, J H Dunant, witnessed the bloody battle of Solferino between the French and Austrians in 1859. His description of the battle and the horrors of the neglected wounded, published in 1862, inspired the formation of the Red Cross.

The American Civil War

The American Civil War (1861–1865) saw the widespread use of anaesthesia; this was usually chloroform (because of the convenience of the small amount that needed to be employed), less often ether or a mixture of the two. William Morton himself, the dentist who introduced the use of ether (see Chapter 7), served as a civilian anaesthetist in the Union Army. He wrote in a letter to a friend in 1864:

When there is any heavy firing heard the ambulance corps, with its attendants, stationed close to the scene of the action, starts for the wounded. The ambulances are halted nearby, and the attendants go with stretchers and bring out the wounded. The rebels do not generally fire upon those wearing ambulance badges. Upon the arrival of a train of ambulances at a field hospital, the wounds are hastily examined and those who can bear the journey are sent at once to Fredericksburg. The nature of the operations to be performed on the others is then decided upon and noted upon a bit of paper pinned to the pillow or roll of blanket under each patient's head. When this has been done I prepare the patient for the knife, producing perfect anaesthesia in the average time of three minutes, and the operators follow, performing their operations with dexterous skill, while the dressers in their turn bound up the stumps.

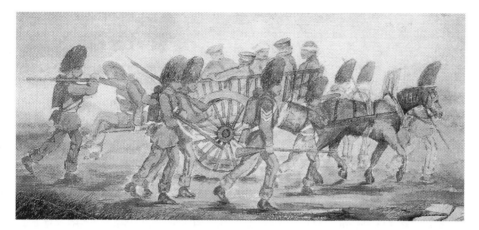

Figure 9.12 Watercolour by Captain Hedley Vicars of a scene from the Crimean War; wounded being transported after the battle of Inkerman. Vicars served in the 97th regiment of infantry; he was killed during an assault on the Russian trenches near Sebastopol on 22nd March, 1855.
Reproduced by courtesy of the Florence Nightingale Museum Trust, London.

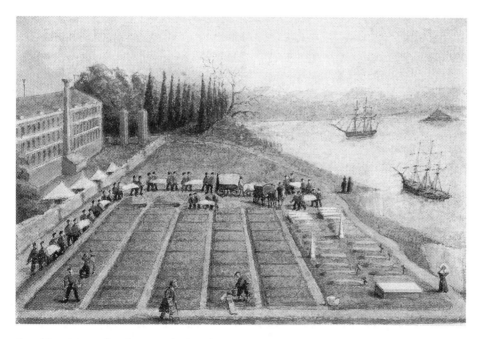

Figure 9.13 Watercolour by General Edward Wray of the burial ground at the General Hospital, Scutari, in April 1855. There were two British Army Hospitals at Scutari during the Crimean War, the Barrack Hospital and the smaller General Hospital. Scutari (the anglicised version of Uskudar), was a suburb on the Asian side of Constantinople. Major (later Lieutenant General) Edward Wray (1823–1892), a British artillery officer, was attached to the Turkish Army during the Crimean War.
Reproduced by courtesy of the Florence Nightingale Museum Trust, London.

Although the agonies of the surgeon's knife were relieved, mortality remained high, principally because of post-operative wound infection, with pyaemia, burrowing abscesses and secondary haemorrhage as infected ligatures around blood vessels loosened. The mortality for amputation of the lower limbs was 33.2%; at the thigh it rose to 54.2% and at the hip reached a fearful 83.3%.

It should be remembered that the deaths from battle were matched, indeed exceeded, in this war, as in all others up to well into the 20th century, by deaths from the medical diseases of crowding and of poor sanitation. Thus the Union forces in the American Civil War lost 96 000 in battle but 183 000 from diseases, of which dysentery featured highest on the list.

The Franco-Prussian War

The Franco-Prussian War (1870–1871) was the first major conflict after the publication of Lister's papers on the antiseptic treatment of wounds in 1867 (see Chapter 7). Although this was recognised by the German surgeons to be an important advance – more so than by their French and, indeed, their British counterparts at this time – Lister's technique for the most part was put into effect rather casually, wounds tending to be packed with whatever dressing was available. Lister himself published a short paper in the *British Medical Journal* in 1870, which gave excellent advice on the management of war wounds. This comprised meticulous cleansing of the wound by irrigation with carbolic acid, extraction of foreign material, spicules of bone, etc., ligation of blood vessels with sterilised catgut and then leaving the wound open, meticulously protected with a large antiseptic dressing. Towards the end of the war the British supplied both sides with the necessary material for Lister's method to be used. Although the experience of a number of hospitals that did use the antiseptic method helped to convince surgeons of the value of this technique, mostly it was ignored and the death rate for penetrating wounds remained high, even worse in fact in

many series than those published from the American Civil War. For example, at the battle of Metz, the German mortality for upper extremity wounds was 41% and for lower extremity wounds 50%, while penetrating injuries of the knee joint carried a 77% mortality. In most cases it was the old story of sepsis.

The Boer War

The Boer War (1899–1902), once again, placed a far greater burden on the physicians than on the surgeons. Enteric fever alone accounted for twice as many deaths among the British (over 8000) than occurred from Boer shot and shell. Sir Almroth Wright (1861–1947) produced a vaccine against the enteric fever organisms – typhoid, paratyphoid A and paratyphoid B (TAB) – which was shown to be highly effective. For example, during the siege of Ladysmith, the incidence of typhoid fever among 1705 inoculated soldiers was 2%, whereas among 10 529 uninoculated men the incidence was 14%. (In the First World War 90% of the troops were inoculated; the incidence of typhoid fever per 1000 strength was 2.35 cases compared with 105 cases in the Boer War.)

To the surgeon, the results of treatment of the wounded seemed highly satisfactory. Most wounds were caused by Mauser rifle bullets fired at considerable range, which produced relatively 'clean' wounds. Furthermore, the campaign took place over a terrain of sun-baked rock and sand, on which the risk of infection from dangerous soil and faecal organisms was minimal. Such injuries responded extremely well to basic Listerian antiseptic treatment. William McCormack (1836–1901), a surgeon at St Thomas', who had practical battle experience in the Franco-Prussian and the Russo-Turkish wars, was appointed Consultant Surgeon to the South African Field Force. As a result of his observations, he advised strictly conservative treatment for gunshot wounds of the abdomen, advice that, as we shall see, had disastrous consequences in the early days of the Great War a few years later.

His advice was no doubt based on the result of seeing patients at the base hospitals who had *survived* the immediate injury to the abdomen and subsequent several days of evacuation to the rear. Such patients, if still alive, had obviously sealed off their injury by this time and certainly would not have benefited from meddlesome surgical interference at this stage.

The Russo-Japanese War

During the Russo-Japanese war of 1904 excellent results were obtained by a pioneer woman surgeon, results that were to be largely ignored by the outside world. Princess Vera Gedroitz was a Russian surgeon who had studied medicine in Germany. She brought a well-equipped ambulance train close to the front line and was able to operate on battle casualties within a short time of wounding. Her policy of early surgery for penetrating wounds of the abdomen produced statistics far better than had previously been obtained. Although a princess, Gedroitz survived the Revolution and became Professor of Surgery in Kiev in the 1920s.

The First World War

In the early days of 'The Great War' (1914–1918), as it was called until the next world catastrophe, surgeons in the Royal Army Medical Corps (RAMC) in Flanders were amazed and horrified at the wounds they were called upon to treat. These surgeons were experienced men: the regular soldiers were often veterans of South Africa, the Territorials had extensive experience of major industrial accidents at home, and they were therefore familiar with the good results to be expected from routine antiseptic treatment of such wounds. Now they were seeing a different pathology, the effects of high explosive, high velocity missiles – machine-gun bullets, shell fragments, shrapnel – at close range on human tissues. Moreover, these wounds were heavily contaminated with the fertile and

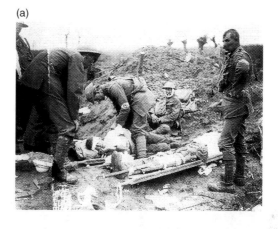

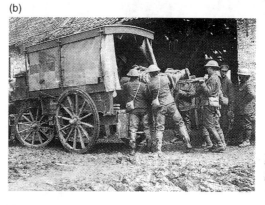

Figure 9.14 The primitive conditions at the Western Front. (a) A regimental Aid Post; first aid is given by the RMO, the regimental medical officer. (b) A horse-drawn ambulance of the Royal Army Medical Corps. Permission of Trustees, Imperial War Museum, London.

fertilised soil of Belgium and Northern France (Figure 9.14) and teemed with the anaerobic clostridial organisms of gas gangrene and tetanus, which found an ideal culture medium in devascularised soft tissues. Gas gangrene was more common than in any war previously documented (Figure 9.15) and tetanus complicated 8.8 per 1000 wounds. Pyaemia and erysipelas were common and secondary haemorrhage was a feared complication as ligatures sloughed off blood vessels in septic wounds. A compound fracture of the femur carried with it an 80% mortality.

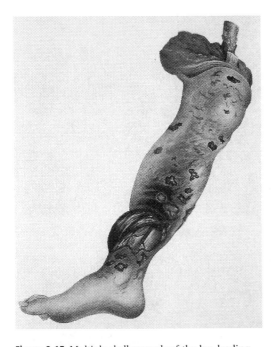

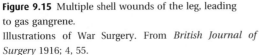

Figure 9.15 Multiple shell wounds of the leg, leading to gas gangrene.
Illustrations of War Surgery. From *British Journal of Surgery* 1916; 4, 55.

Strenuous attempts were made to improve the situation; antiseptic infusions were found not to be the answer but over the next year or so it became obvious that best results were obtained by early surgery at which excision of all dead and devitalised tissues from the wound could be carried out, together with removal of any foreign matter such as pieces of uniform. The wound was not closed but the skin approximated by a few loose stitches over a sterile dressing. Four or five days later, with the patient by now at a base hospital, the wound was inspected and, if healthy, the skin could be sutured. This technique, called delayed primary suture, was perhaps the greatest advance made in military surgery during the war and was a lesson that had to be re-learned in subsequent conflicts (Figure 9.16).

The need for early surgery was met by establishing advanced surgical units, manned by surgeons and anaesthetists and nursing sisters (the

(a)

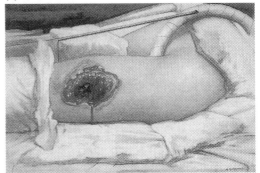

(b)

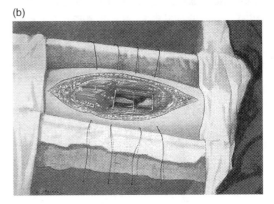

(c)

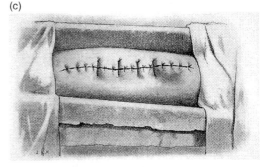

Figure 9.16 Stages of delayed primary suture. (a) Explosive exit wound in arm caused by rifle bullet 13 hours after infliction. Comminuted fracture of the humerus.
(b) Wound after excision of damaged muscle and cleansing of the fracture. Deep sutures of silk in position. (c) Closure of the wound. The wound healed by first intention.
Pictures and text from Fraser F: *Primary and delayed primary suture of gunshot wounds. A report of research work at a CCS, December 27, 1917–March 1st 1918.*

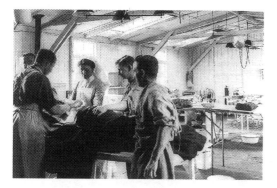

Figure 9.17 Operating theatre in a Casualty Clearing Station (C.C.S.), behind the line at the Battle of the Somme 1916. Note the 'QA', the Queen Alexandra's Nursing Service, sister; this is the closest to the front line that women reached in the Great War.
Permission of Trustees, Imperial War Museum, London.

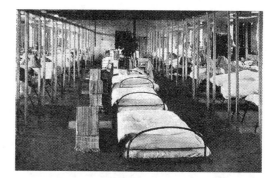

Figure 9.19 A ward dedicated to fractures of the femur. From Hurley V, Weedon SH: Treatment of cases of fractured femur at a base hospital in France. *British Journal of Surgery* 1919; 6, 351.

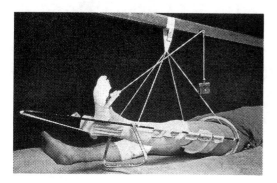

Figure 9.18 The Thomas splint used to treat a compound fracture of the femur.
From Max Page C, Le Mesurier AB: The early treatment of gunshot fractures of the thigh. *British Journal of Surgery* 1918; 5, 66.

nearest women were to get to the front line during the war), termed Casualty Clearing Stations (CCS) (Figure 9.17). These were situated six to nine miles from the front line and were designed to admit between 150 and 300 casualties at a time. The problem of the high death rate from compound fractures of the femur was addressed by Sir Robert Jones (1857–1933), an orthopaedic surgeon from Liverpool who had had considerable experience organising the casualty services in the construction of the Manchester Ship Canal. As Director General of military orthopaedics, he introduced the use of the Thomas Splint, invented by his uncle, Hugh Owen Thomas (1834–1891) to the Western Front (see Figures 9.18 and 10.2). Stretcher bearers were taught how to apply the splint blindfolded, so that they could immobilise the leg of a wounded soldier on the battlefield in the dark. (I have attempted to do this myself and I can confirm that it is very difficult!) Special wards were established to deal with this injury (Figure 9.19) and there was a satisfactory drop in mortality by the end of 1915.

Wound excision combined with tetanus prophylaxis given at the field ambulance reduced the incidence of tetanus to the region of 0.2 per 1000. Gas gangrene, however, was still encountered when there was delay in the wounded soldier receiving definitive surgery.

In the early days of the war, surgeons were directed to treat penetrating abdominal injuries conservatively, in line with the South African experiences. It soon became evident to the front-line surgeons that the results of such management were disastrous. At the base hospitals, the mortality for abdominal injuries was in the region of 80% and, of course, many more deaths had already occurred in the lines of evacuation. This is hardly surprising because of

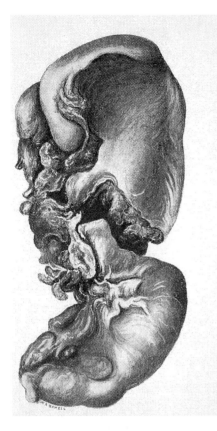

Figure 9.20 Lacerated bullet wound of spleen.
From Cuthbert Wallace A study of 1200 cases of gunshot wounds of the abdomen. *British Journal of Surgery* 1917; 4, 679.

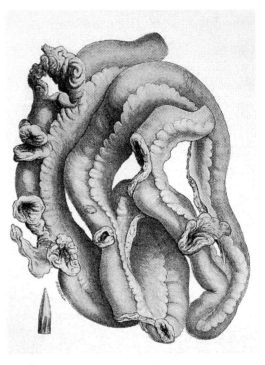

Figure 9.21 Multiple wounds of the small intestine as the result of a rifle bullet. The bowel was resected but the patient died a few hours later at the Casualty Clearing Station.
From Illustrations of War Surgery. *British Journal of Surgery* 1916; 4, 63.

the devastating effects of high explosive missiles on the abdomen (Figures 9.20 and 9.21). Impressed by these awful results, a group of young British surgeons, operating at the CCSs close behind the front line, were able to show that early intervention gave the patients with wounds of the belly their only reasonable chance of survival. The first notable success was that of Owen Richards, a professor of surgery who had been made a temporary Captain in the British Expeditionary Force. Early in 1915 he performed two successful resections for gunshot wounds of the small intestine (Figure 9.22). It was soon evident that early surgery was the only hope for such cases and even then, of course, in the

absence of antibiotics and effective fluid replacement and paucity of blood transfusions the mortality remained high: for the small intestine in the region of 65% and for the colon in the region of 59%. Perforations of the small bowel were sutured with drainage or resected if extensive. Perforations of the colon were sutured if small but otherwise usually exteriorised. Wounds of the stomach were sutured, as were wounds of the bladder, which were closed with catheter or suprapubic drainage.

One of the young British surgeons working at the CCSs was Major Gordon Gordon Taylor (1878–1960) (Figure 9.23) of the Middlesex Hospital, London. His speed and skill, particularly with the surgery of abdominal injuries, became a legend. He ended the

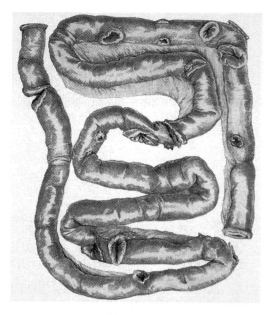

Figure 9.22 Portion of the small intestine showing 20 wounds produced by a fragment of shell. The piece of bowel, which is six feet in length, was successfully excised by Owen Richards March 18, 1915. This was the first successful case of bowel injury treated on the British front. The patient walked back with his intestines outside his abdomen because 'he wanted to die in his own lines'. Text and illustration from Gordon Taylor G: *Abdominal Injuries in Warfare.* Bristol, John Wright, 1939.

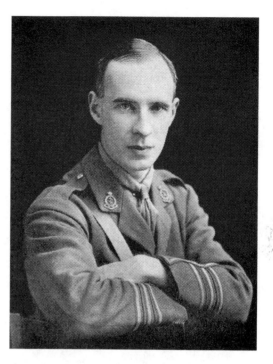

Figure 9.23 Sir Gordon Gordon Taylor as a Major in the RAMC in the First World War.
Royal College of Surgeons of England.

war as Consultant Surgeon to the Fourth Army and in World War II joined the Naval Medical Service as a Rear Admiral. At the outbreak of the Second World War he published a small book on abdominal wounds based on his war experience; this extract gives a striking example of the wartime surgery of penetrating wounds of the abdomen:

Private T. was admitted into a Casualty Clearing Station on September 18th 1918, with a severe wound of the abdomen. He came to operation eight and a half hours after being hit, and was found to have a hernia of shattered, strangled small intestine through a wound in the right hypochondrium; about 18 inches of bowel was thus prolapsed. The missile had then passed down between the internal oblique and transversalis muscles of the abdominal wall on the right side, and had struck against and

shattered the anterior part of the crest of the ilium. Thence its course was deflected again into the peritoneal cavity, and it had become impacted in the posterior surface of the right pubic bone, transfixing the bladder and impaling a coil of ileum against that bone. With such force had the projective been driven into the os pubis, that a considerable pull was required to dislodge it. The patient, when placed on the operating table, had a surprisingly good pulse of 96; but immediately the wound of entry was enlarged and the constriction of the neck of the prolapsed bowel thereby released, the pulse-rate rose to 130. The wound was filthy, and parietes and bowel alike were covered with grease and dirt. Four feet of badly damaged and perforated jejunum were resected, and other coils of jejunum and upper ileum were assiduously cleansed of grease and clothing. The coil of lower ileum impaled against the pubic bone was gangrenous and stinking, and a second resection of 2½ft was performed. The posterior wall of the bladder was sutured and a glove drain was passed down into the cave of Retzius towards the wound on the anterior vesical surface. Very wide excision of the

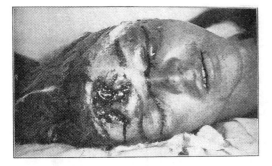

Figure 9.24 Severe orbito-frontal perforating wound from a rifle bullet. Patient died from gas encephalitis.
From Harvey Cushing: A study of a series of wounds involving the brain and its enveloping structures. *British Journal of Surgery* 1918; 5, 558.

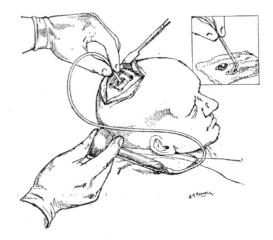

Figure 9.26 Cushing's technique of suction debridement of a cerebral wound track.

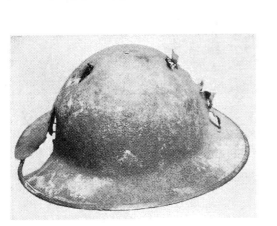

Figure 9.25 A British 'Tommy's' helmet. The subtitle reads: 'Showing seriously damaged helmet of patient with but lightly scored cranium'.
From Harvey Cushing: A study of a series of wounds involving the brain and its enveloping structures. *British Journal of Surgery* 1918; 5, 558.

damaged abdominal muscles was performed, after the peritoneum had been closed; a defect in the latter was filled in by a graft of fascia obtained from the anterior layer of the sheath of the rectus. The anterior end of the crest of the ilium was widely exsected, the wound was packed with gauze soaked in flavine, and frequent instillations with flavine through Carrel's tubes were enjoined. A transfusion of 900 cc of blood was given and the patient was treated by the usual resuscitatory measures. The gauze and Carrel's tubes were removed on the fifth day and skin was resutured. The patient was evacuated to the Base on the fourteenth day, and subsequently to England, February 7th 1919. Nearly 21 years later he is in good health.

Compound skull injuries were common, as men peered over the parapet of the trenches (Figure 9.24). Many lives were undoubtedly saved by the introduction of steel helmets to the armies confronting each other on the Western Front (Figure 9.25). Important work was carried out by Harvey Cushing (1869–1939) on the management of penetrating injuries of the brain. Cushing was one of the founding fathers of American neurosurgery, first in Baltimore and then in Boston. He taught the importance of meticulous excision of the wound and showed how a glass sucker could be used to debride pulped brain (Figure 9.26). Removal of the missile from the wound track was important and this was helped by the availability of X-rays at the CCSs. Cushing also pioneered the use of the electromagnet to remove metallic foreign bodies from the brain. Because of its excellent blood supply, the scalp wound could be closed by primary suture, but if there was extensive skin loss, Cushing introduced his rotation flap for closure of the scalp defect.

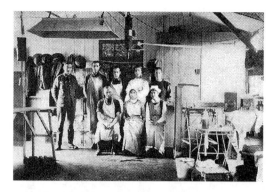

Figure 9.27 Harvey Cushing and his team at a Casualty Clearing Station in 1917. Cushing sits in the front row on the left.
From Cushing H: *From a Surgeon's Journal 1915–1918.* London, Constable, 1936.

Most of Cushing's experience came from his periods of intensive military surgery, first in the spring of 1915 with an American unit dealing mainly with French casualties. On his return to the USA, perhaps realising that American intervention in the war was inevitable, he set about organising a Base Hospital in Boston. He was sent to France again in May 1917 attached to the British Expeditionary Force (Figure 9.27). Throughout this period of military service, Cushing kept a meticulous, almost daily diary which he edited into a single volume (now long out of print). Today, his case reports read with great poignancy and illustrate, perhaps as well as any written account by any other surgical author, the horrors and futility of war:

Wednesday 15 August 1917

We nearly 'busted' on six cases in the twenty four hours since yesterday's note. We began at 8 p.m. on 'L/Cpl. Wiseman 392332; 1/9 Londons S.W. Frac. Skull', which interpreted means that a lance corporal of the 9th Londons had a shell wound. It went through his helmet in the parietal region, with indriven fragments to the ventricle. These cases take a long time if done carefully enough to forestall infection, and it was eleven o'clock before we got to 'Sgt. Chave, C.25912, M.G.C. 167-S.W. head and back-penet' according to his field-ambulance card. This sergeant of the Machine Gunners had almost the whole of his right

frontal lobe blown out, with a lodged piece of shell almost an inch square, and extensive radiating fractures, which mean taking off most of his frontal bone, including the frontal sinuses – an enormous operation done under local anaesthesia. We crawled home for some eggs in the mess and to bed at 2.30 a.m. – six hours for these two cases.

Friday 17 August 1917

We beat our record today with eight cases – all serious ones. A prompt start at 9 a.m. with two cases always in waiting – notes made, X-rays taken, and heads shaved. It's amusing to think that at home I used to regard a single major cranial operation as a day's work. These eight averaged two hours apiece – one or two very interesting ones. One in particular – a sergeant, unconscious, with a small wound of entrance in the vertex and a foreign body just beside the sella turcica. We have learned a new way of doing these things – viz., to encircle the penetrating wound in the skull with Montenovesi forceps, and to take the fractured area with the depressed bone fragments out in one piece – then to catheterize the tract and to wash it out with a Carrel syringe through the tube. In doing so the suction of the bulb is enough occasionally to bring out a small bone fragment clinging to the eye of the catheter. Indeed, one can usually detect fragments by the feel of the catheter; they are often driven in two or three inches.

In this particular man, however, after the tract was washed clear of blood and disorganized brain, the nail was inserted its full six inches and I tried twice unsuccessfully to draw out the fragment with the magnet. On the third attempt I found to my disgust that the current was switched off. There was nothing to do but make the best of it, and a small stomach tube was procured, cut off, boiled, inserted in the six inch tract, suction put on, and a deformed shrapnel ball (not the expected piece of steel shell) was removed on the first trial – of course a non-magnetizable object.

Tonight while operating on a Boche prisoner with a 'G.S.W. head' about 11 p.m. – our seventh case – some Fritz planes came over on a bombing raid, as they do almost every night nowadays – nowanights (which is it?). Of course all our lights were switched off, and we had to finish with candles. If we didn't do a very good job, it was Fritz's fault, not entirely ours.

The Boche prisoner, I may add, was a big fellow with a square head, badly punctured though it was. The case in waiting was a little eighteen year old Tommy from East London – scared, peaked, underfed, underdeveloped. He had been in training six months and was in the trenches for the first time during the present show – just ten minutes when he was hit.

Alexis Carrel: Visionary Surgeon

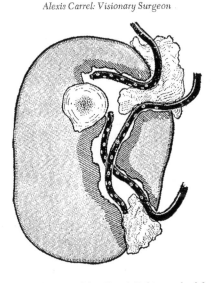

Figure 9.28 Diagram of the Carrel–Dakin method for irrigation of a massive penetrating wound of the thigh.

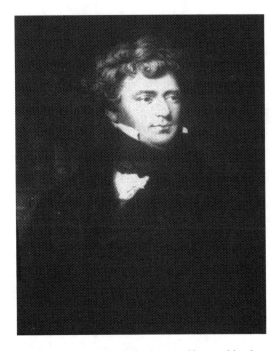

Figure 9.29 James Blundell, pioneer of human blood transfusion. Gordon Museum, Guy's Hospital.

Cushing's slow and meticulous neurosurgical technique came in for considerable criticism both from his British and American colleagues. It is true that during major battles many cases of head wounds died before they could be operated on. However, Cushing insisted that unless adequate surgery was carried out, the patient was probably better left untouched.

In spite of the pioneer work of Carrel (see Figure 15.4), who had shown how to suture blood vessels in the experimental laboratory, arterial reconstruction surgery was virtually unknown. Major arteries, if torn, were ligated and this led, especially in the presence of an associated fracture, to amputation in most cases – a finding made again in the Second World War. It was not, indeed, until the Korean War that arterial reconstruction became a possibility in military surgery.

A particularly serious problem was wound infection. After much experimentation, irrigation of the wound with hypochloride solution through multiple tubes (the Carrel–Dakin technique) was in common use. Its value probably lay more in the fact that careful drainage of the wound was performed rather than any effect of the irrigating solution itself (Figure 9.28).

Many fatalities of war were due to, or compounded by, severe blood loss. Sir Christopher Wren (1632–1723), the celebrated English architect, experimented with intravenous injections of various fluids in animals. Richard Lower (1631–1691) first transfused blood from one animal into the vein of another and later transfused blood from a sheep into a man, having been preceded in this experiment by a few months in 1667 by Jean Baptiste Denys (1625–1704). The first successful human blood transfusions for specific therapeutic purposes were carried out by James Blundell (1790–1877) (Figure 9.29). He trained at the United Hospitals of Guy's' and St Thomas's and continued his medical education in Edinburgh, where he graduated with an MD in 1813. He returned to Guy's to teach midwifery and became Professor of Physiology and Obstetrics in 1823. He practised and

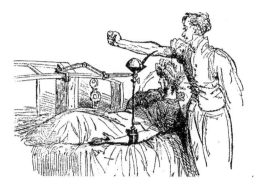

Figure 9.30 John Blundell's method of blood transfusion, 1829.

taught the importance of artificial respiration in the apparently stillborn baby and described a tracheal pipe, which he inserted by sliding the tube along his forefinger passed down to the entry of the larynx.

Blundell first carried out numerous experiments in blood transfusion in dogs. His first human experiment was 1818. This was in a man 'dying from inanition induced by malignant disease of the pylorus'. He improved after the transfusion, but 'died of exhausation' 56 hours later. Of the remaining nine cases documented, five were successful. The first of these was a woman dying of post-partum haemorrhage, who recovered after receiving a transfusion from her husband. His other successes were three further cases of post-partum bleeding and a boy in shock after amputation of the leg. The amounts transfused ranged from 4 to 14 ounces and the donors were either the patient's husband or the attending doctor. Blundell's equipment varied as the studies continued. One example, the 'gravitator', is shown in Figure 9.30.

The problem of clotting of the donor blood was solved in 1914 when it was found that sodium citrate was an effective anti-coagulant. A major complication of transfusion was encountered frequently when the transfused blood was rapidly destroyed in the recipient's circulation, often accompanied by shock and even death. This was shown by Karl Landsteiner (1868–1943) in 1900 to

be due to the presence of two complex agglutinating substances, A and B. This enabled him to divide subjects into four main groups (A, B, AB and O) and enabled transfusion of matched blood to be made. Landsteiner was awarded the Nobel Prize in 1930.

By 1914, transfusion of blood was well recognised but it was a tedious procedure and difficult to carry out under the wartime conditions of the CCSs, although transfusion with saline and with a solution of gum acacia in normal saline was often used.

Sir Geoffrey Keynes (1887–1982), surgeon at St Bartholomew's Hospital who was a CCS surgeon in Flanders, was an enthusiast in the use of blood transfusion. Donors were chosen by preliminary blood grouping of both patient and prospective donor, and donors were chosen from among the lightly wounded men. The inducement was an extra fortnight's leave. Keynes writes in his autobiography *The Gates of Memory*:

Transfusion naturally provided an incomparable extension of the possibilities of life-saving surgery. Trained anaesthetists were scarce, and often I dispensed with their services. A preliminary transfusion followed by a spinal analgesic enabled me to do a major amputation single-handed. A second transfusion then established the patient so firmly on the road to recovery that he could be dismissed to the ward without further anxiety. At other times I was greatly distressed by the state of affairs in one large tent known as 'the moribund ward'. This contained all the patients regarded by a responsible officer as being probably past surgical aid, since it was our duty to operate where there was reasonable hope of recovery, rather than to waste effort where there seemed to be none. The possibility of blood transfusion now raised hopes where formerly there had not been any, and I made it my business during any lull in the work to steal into the moribund ward, choose a patient who was still breathing and had a perceptible pulse, transfuse him and carry out the necessary operation. Most of them were suffering primarily from shock and loss of blood, and in this way I had the satisfaction of pulling many men back from the jaws of death.

The specialty of plastic surgery was created during the First World War. At first, little could be done for the dreadful deformities of face and jaw that

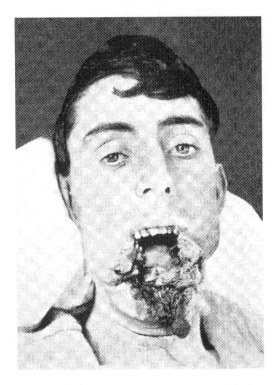

Figure 9.31 High velocity compound fracture of the jaw. From Kazanjian VH, Burrows H: The treatment of haemorrhage caused by gunshot wounds of the face and jaws. *British Journal of Surgery* 1918; 5, 126.

resulted from high velocity missiles (Figure 9.31). A young New Zealander in the RAMC, Harold Delf Gillies (1882–1960), an ENT surgeon, set up a special unit at the Cambridge Hospital, Aldershot, and later established a major hospital for this work at Queen Mary's Hospital, Sidcup. Here he developed a team of surgeons and dental surgeons from all over the Dominions and, starting from scratch, invented techniques such as the tubed pedicle flap, usually taken from the chest or the neck, to replace missing facial tissue. Bone grafts, usually from the iliac crest, were used to reconstruct shattered jaws.

The anaesthetists encountered two problems; how to anaesthetise a patient with a smashed face and how to keep the equipment away from the surgeon. Two young doctors, Stanley Rowbotham

(1890–1979) and Ivan Magill (1888–1986), who were to become leaders in the field, developed the technique of using a tube passed along the nose into the trachea (naso-tracheal intubation) through which the anaesthetic could be administered, a method which is now standard practice.

It is therefore easy, though amazing, to appreciate that, in four terrible years, enormous advances were made in orthopaedic, traumatic, abdominal, neurological and plastic surgery, and in resuscitation and anaesthesia.

The Spanish Civil War

The Spanish Civil War (1936–1939) was the first time in the Western world that massive civilian casualties were to be sustained from aerial bombardment, a foretaste of the horrors of the Second World War. Joseph Trueta (1897–1977), Professor of Surgery in Barcelona (Figure 9.2), preached the importance of thorough wound excision, then dressing the wound with gauze and immobilising the limb in plaster of Paris. This obviated the need for frequent dressings, a great advantage in the crowded hospitals with lack of skilled surgeons. Although the plaster casts smelled to high heaven, the patients remained well and comfortable and there were very few cases of gas gangrene or tetanus, since the wounds had an excellent blood supply and devitalised tissue had been removed. The disadvantage of this method was the slow healing of the wound, although this could be speeded by skin grafting (Figure 9.33). The wound was left untouched for between four and six weeks, and the plasters were changed every couple of months until the wound healed. In his own hands, Trueta's method gave excellent results. By the end of the war, he and his team had treated nearly 20 000 casualties with only four amputations and fewer than 100 deaths, although other, less experienced, surgeons had much less satisfactory results.

Towards the end of the war, when it was obvious that Franco's Nationalists were winning and that the future of people on the Government side, even

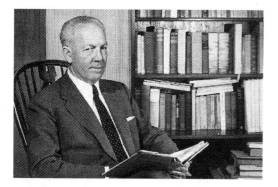

Figure 9.32 Joseph Trueta.
Photograph provided by Mr John Goodfellow FRCS.

(a)

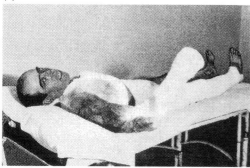

(b)

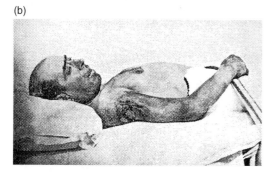

Figure 9.33 The Trueta technique, Spain 1936.
(a) Photograph at six days. Wounds of shoulder and femur produced in an air raid. Note that the plaster is blood-stained. The patient is comfortable. (b) Photograph taken after removal of the plaster on the 70th day.

eminent surgeons, would be in jeopardy, Trueta left Spain. He was put on the staff of the Wingfield–Morris Orthopaedic Hospital in Oxford, made great contributions to the training of allied surgeons in the Second World War and became Professor of Orthopaedic Surgery in Oxford. In 1955 he was the examiner for my Master of Surgery thesis – and passed me!

The Second World War (1939–1945)

Whereas surgery in the First World War produced important innovations, that of the Second World War consisted of consolidation and confirmation of the lessons of 1914–1918: the value of rapid evacuation, surgical units as near to the battle front as possible, early excision of wounds, delayed primary suture, effective immobilisation of injured limbs, early surgery of abdominal and chest wounds, meticulous care of head injuries and specialised units for plastic surgery. A surgeon from a Casualty Clearing Station on the Somme in 1916 would have felt very much at home in a Field Surgical Unit in Normandy in 1944.

It was in the ancillary aspects of the care of the wounded that enormous advances were made, in particular in blood transfusion and in the introduction of sulphonamides and, especially, of penicillin in combating wound infection.

By the end of the First World War, citrated blood was stored before major battles. By 1939, the Red Cross had organised a register of blood donors and it was well recognised that refrigerated citrated blood could be stored safely for up to a couple of weeks. Thanks to the organising genius of Brigadier Sir Lionel Whitby (1895–1956), the Royal Army Medical Corps entered the war with a fully operational plan. This enabled large quantities of stored blood and dried plasma to be available to both military and civilian casualties (Figures 9.34 and 9.35). Whitby himself had served as an officer, had been seriously wounded in 1918, and had received a blood transfusion before having a leg amputated through the thigh by Gordon Taylor (see Figure 9.23), who then

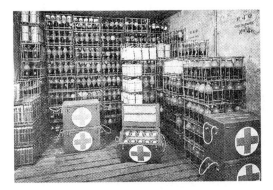

Figure 9.34 The Army blood bank at Bristol shortly after the D-Day landings in France, June 1944.
From Cope Z, ed.: *History of the Second World War Medical Series – Surgery*, 1953. Crown copyright; reproduced with permission of the Controller of Her Majesty's Stationery Office.

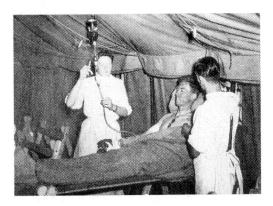

Figure 9.35 A blood transfusion taking place in a tented Casualty Clearing Station, Normandy 1944.
From Cope Z, ed.: *History of the Second World War Medical Series – Surgery*, 1953. Crown copyright; reproduced with permission of the Controller of Her Majesty's Stationery Office.

aided his patient's admission to his medical school, the Middlesex, as a student.

Since the work of Louis Pasteur on the bacterial basis of wound infection and of Joseph Lister on the antiseptic treatment of wounds, in which chemical agents were used to kill the contamin-ating bacteria, medical scientists dreamed of the possibility of an agent that would destroy invading microbes without damage to the patient's healthy tissues. Paul Ehrlich (1854–1915) of Frankfurt-on-Maine, Germany, synthesised the arsenical compound Salvarsan which was used clinically in 1911 as the first really effective drug against syphilis. It was Ehrlich who coined the term 'magic bullet' to mean a chemical bullet that would kill the organism but not the patient. Salvarsan was hardly the perfect bullet since it is a toxic drug with unpleasant side-effects.

The next major landmark in chemotherapy again came from Germany. Gerhardt Domagk (1895–1964) showed that the aniline dye Prontosil Rubra was highly effective against the much-dreaded spreading infections produced by streptococci, in spite of the disadvantage that the drug stained the patient, fortunately temporarily, a bright red colour. These important findings were published in 1935. Within weeks of this paper appearing, workers at the Pasteur Institute in Paris showed that it was the sulphanilamide moiety of the Prontosil molecule which was the active agent. The next few years saw a flurry of activity, both by the synthetic chemists and clinicians, in the development of new sulphonamide drugs. The effectiveness of these agents against many infections, such as pneumonia and puerperal fever (sepsis following childbirth), seemed almost miraculous. Sulphonamides were used during the Spanish Civil War and also in the Second World War in the treatment of major wounds and certainly reduced the risk of wound infections. However, they had the serious disadvantage of being ineffective in the presence of pus, i.e. once wound infection was established, and were also valueless in the treatment of gas gangrene and tetanus.

But what of the antimicrobial agents derived from fungi and bacteria, the antibiotics? Most people believe that the story begins with the description of penicillin by Alexander Fleming in 1928. In fact, the story goes back much further than this. In 1870, John Burdon Sanderson (1828–1905), while working as Medical Officer of Health in Paddington (he subsequently became Professor of

Medicine in Oxford), in numerous experiments showed that bacteria did not grow in culture fluid that contained visible mould. The publication of Sanderson's report stimulated Joseph Lister himself to begin a series of experiments in which he showed that urine which had a heavy growth of mould showed abnormal degenerate bacteria or the complete absence of micro-organisms and that the urine under these circumstances usually remained sweet-smelling. Aided by his brother Arthur, an expert mycologist, Lister identified the fungus as *Penicillium glaucum*. In 1884, Lister treated a nurse named Ellen Jones at King's College Hospital, London, who had a deep buttock abscess which was healing very slowly with an extract of a culture of this fungus. Unfortunately, Lister did not publish his methods or the results of using what was presumably crude penicillin. Numerous other reports appeared over the years, including one from Louis Pasteur himself in 1877, in which he reported that anthrax bacilli were inhibited in culture by unspecified bacteria and postulated that this might prove to be of clinical value.

Now to Alexander Fleming (1881–1955) and his place in the history of antibiosis. While working as a bacteriologist at St Mary's Hospital, London, in 1928, he made the observation that a culture plate of *Staphylococcus aureus*, a common cause of boils, abscesses and many other serious infections, contaminated by spores of a *Penicillium* mould showed lysis around the contaminating fungi. He made a detailed study of this phenomenon, named the agent produced by the mould 'penicillin', showed that a crude extract from the mould was remarkably active against a whole range of bacteria and published a report on this phenomenon in 1929. However, efforts by Fleming and his colleagues failed to concentrate and purify penicillin.

Ten years passed before Howard Florey (1898–1968), Professor of Pathology at the University of Oxford, and a young German Jewish refugee biochemist, Ernst Chain (1906–1979), determined to carry out a systematic study of the known naturally occurring antibacterial substances. A review of previous publications in this field naturally included

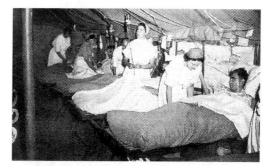

Figure 9.36 A tented CCS and Field Surgical Unit at the Sicily landings (1943). Penicillin was now available for local but not systemic treatment of wounds in the Services.
From Cope Z, ed.: *History of the Second World War Medical Series – Surgery*, 1953. Crown copyright; reproduced with permission of the Controller of Her Majesty's Stationery Office.

Fleming's paper of 1929 and, with the assistance of a team of dedicated young scientists, the difficult task of extracting penicillin from the mould of *Penicillium notatum* was carried out. In May 1940, enough penicillin was available for a crucial animal experiment which showed that the dry, stable brown powder prepared by a process of freeze-drying was highly effective in protecting mice given a lethal injection of *Staphylococcus aureus*. By the beginning of 1941, Florey had enough material to begin his first trial on human beings and, again, the results in patients with overwhelming bacterial infections were most encouraging.

It was obvious that penicillin was a potentially powerful weapon in both the treatment and prevention of infection in war wounds. Super-human efforts were made to increase the yield of penicillin in the 'factory' set up in the Pathology Department at Oxford. In 1941, with the USA in the war, production of penicillin was undertaken by a number of major American pharmaceutical companies. By the Sicily landings in 1943 (Figure 9.36), enough penicillin was available for extensive clinical trials, both as local treatment in the wound and by intramuscular injection; the results were excellent.

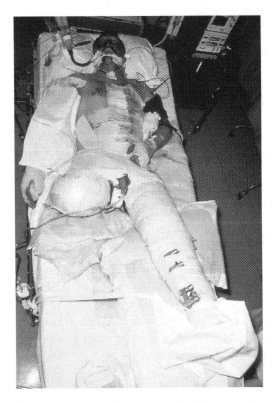

Figure 9.37 A victim of the Harrods bombing by the IRA 1984; multiple injuries including traumatic amputation of the right leg at mid thigh. Treated by wound excision and delayed primary closure.
Photographic Department, Westminster Hospital, London.

It was soon shown that the clostridia group of bacteria (those responsible for gas gangrene and tetanus) was highly sensitive to the drug. By the D-Day landings in Normandy in 1944 there was enough penicillin to allow its use for all casualties. The antibiotic era had well and truly commenced.

Subsequent wars have reinforced the lessons of the two Great Wars, lessons learned from the sufferings of countless millions of injured men and women. Significant advances continued to be made; for example, the development of sophisticated vascular surgery in the 1950s, using vein and synthetic grafts, enabled many extremities to be saved in the Korean and subsequent wars that would previously have required amputation.

These principles of treatment, of course, have been applied to the surgery of civilian trauma. The dreadful vascular injuries produced by 'knee-capping' carried out by terrorists in Northern Ireland, were treated along war-time principles, the damaged vessels repaired by grafts and limbs rarely lost. I was involved in treating casualties from four major terrorist 'incidents' at Westminster Hospital, London. Wound excision, immobilisation, antibiotics and delayed primary suture were carried out in every case and without a single example of wound infection (Figure 9.37). The only thing to benefit from war is surgery.

10

Orthopaedic surgery

The word 'orthopaedic' originated in 1741 when Nicholas André (1658–1742), Professor of Medicine in the University of Paris, published his book on the prevention and correction of musculoskeletal deformities in children entitled *L'Orthopédie*. This word was created from the Greek *orthos*, straight, and *paideia*, the rearing of children. The book's emblem, a straight pole supporting a bent tree trunk, is still used as a logo by a number of orthopaedic surgical societies (Figure 10.1).

Of course, a large part of the practice of orthopaedics today does concern children: fractures and dislocations, including birth injuries, congenital deformities such as spinal curvature (scoliosis), congenital dislocation of the hip and club foot, infectious diseases such as poliomyelitis and tuberculosis, as well as rare bone tumours of childhood.

The specialty of orthopaedic surgery is conveniently divided into the management of trauma to bones and joints, and the elective treatment of diseases of these structures.

Fractures and dislocations

The treatment of injuries of bones and joints goes back to the earliest days of surgery, since the most primitive of practitioners would have been called upon to bind up injuries and to splint fractures. The Australian Aborigines, until quite recently, took the adage 'splint the patient where he lies' quite literally: the relatives would take it in turn to hold the damaged limb still at the site of the accident until union occurred, a crude shelter being erected over both patient and human splint. Sir Grafton Elliot-Smith's Egyptian excavations have revealed fractures of 5000 years ago bound up in splints of bark, wrapped in linen and held by bandages (see Figure 1.4). The Hippocratic writings differentiate simple from compound fractures and describe the treatment of dislocations of the hip and of the shoulder (see Figure 3.2), while Celsus, the Roman encyclopaedist of the 1st century AD, gives instructions for setting fractures, their immobilisation by splints and the subsequent need for exercises following bony union. The earliest Anglo-Saxon medical writings refer to the treatment of fractures thus: 'If the shanks be broken, take bonewort, pound it, pour the white of an egg out, mingle these together . . . lay this salve on the broken limb and overlay with elm-rind apply a splint; again, always renew these until the limb be healed'.

All sorts of materials were used to immobilise the fracture. Splints of wood, cardboard and tinplate were employed. Hippocrates used a mixture of flour and gum; bandages were hardened with wax, starch, resin and egg white. For the most part these devices were clumsy, painful, inefficient and dangerous; gangrene, pressure sores and malunion appear to have occurred commonly even after relatively minor fractures. An article in *The Lancet* in 1835 condemned the large number of poor pieces of apparatus on the market:

Venerable fathers of surgery who have departed just look over your shoulders and see what a motley crew you have travelling behind you; carpenters with their boards

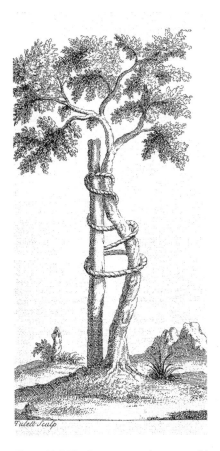

Figure 10.1 The bent tree trunk supported by a pole, from Nicholas André's L'Orthopedie, 1741. This emblem is often used to this day as a logo for orthopaedic associations.

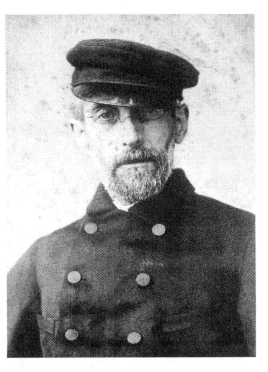

Figure 10.2 Hugh Owen Thomas. Royal College of Surgeons of England.

and glue; tea-trade makers with Japanned splints; iron-mongers with tin splints; blacksmiths with iron splints; Hindoos with cane splints (better to be applied to some backs than broken legs); sailors from the Arctic seas with whale-bone splints, milliners with pasteboard and bre-aches makers in the rear with straps and buckles to bind the broken ends of bones together.

Dominique Jean Larrey (1766–1842) (see Figure 9.7), that great military surgeon of the Napoleonic wars, invented the 'bandage inamovible' which consisted of compresses soaked in a mixture of egg white, lead subacetate and spirits of camphor held around the injured limb with a many-tailed bandage. For fur-ther reinforcement, he applied straw gutters, then covered the whole once more with his solution. This very solid dressing enabled easier transport and evacuation of the injured soldier. Plaster of Paris was used by the Arab surgeon Rhazes and by the Hindus, but it was the Dutch army surgeon Antonius Mathijsen (1805–1878) who introduced bandages impregnated with plaster of Paris in 1852. A practical war surgeon, he mentioned that if water was not available on the battlefield, urine was equally effective for moistening the plaster ban-dages. By the time of the Crimean and Franco-Prussian wars, plaster splints more or less in their modern form were in relatively common use.

One splint in particular deserves our attention, the Thomas splint. The story of Hugh Owen Thomas (1834–1891) (Figure 10.2) is one of the most inter-esting in the history of medicine. The son of a

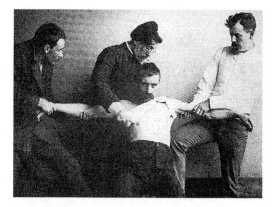

Figure 10.3 Hugh Owen Thomas reducing a dislocated shoulder; no anaesthetic is being used. The assistant on his right is Thomas' nephew, Robert Jones, later to become a distinguished Liverpool orthopaedic surgeon and to be knighted.

bone-setter, the whole of his professional life was spent in general practice in the slums of Liverpool, and he did more than anyone before him to advance the treatment of injuries and diseases of bones and joints. Thomas came from a family of unqualified bone-setters of Anglesey, whose secrets had been handed down from father to son for many generations. His father, Evan Thomas, was determined that his son should receive the benefits of a regular medical education and Hugh studied at Edinburgh and at University College, London, qualifying MRCS in 1857. He returned to Liverpool and soon gained a great reputation, with a vast practice among the poor of Liverpool and among the numerous seafarers returning to that city, many with severe injuries sustained weeks or even months before while at sea, where their only care had been from their shipmates and captain (Figure 10.3).

We shall consider later in this chapter Thomas' contributions to the management of chronic diseases of joints, but his splint was devised to solve the problem of efficient immobilisation of the lower limb, both in the treatment of fractures and of chronic bone disease. The splint used the ischial tuberosity of the pelvic girdle as a fixed point, and traction was applied by means of adhesive strapping

along the leg, which was then tied to the lower end of the splint. The work of Thomas might never have attained recognition had it not been for his nephew and pupil Sir Robert Jones (1858–1933) who introduced the use of the Thomas splint for the management of femoral shaft fractures in the First World War. The splint was at least partly responsible for the drop in the mortality of compound fractures of the femur from 80% in 1916 to 7.3% in 1918 (see Figure 9.18).

Thomas was a thin, dark, fragile little man. He had an accident while a student which resulted in a deformed eyelid and rather spoilt the expression of his face. He had indomitable energy, and worked from six in the morning until midnight, never taking a holiday. He was always dressed in a black coat, buttoned up at the neck, with a peaked naval cap tilted over his defective eyelid. He was seldom seen without a cigarette in his mouth. Although not recognised in his lifetime, Thomas is today acknowledged as a great pioneer in orthopaedic surgery.

An important contribution to fracture treatment was made by Percivall Pott (1714–1788) (see Figure 6.12), who showed that displacement of the bone fragments in a fracture is mainly due to tension of the surrounding muscles. These forces could be eliminated by placing the injured limb in a position that relaxes these muscles, thus enabling easier reduction and more certain immobilisation of the fracture. He gave an excellent description of fractures of the ankle, often still referred to as 'Pott's fracture' (see Figure 6.14).

Surgeons over the centuries were, of course, well familiar with the fact that a compound fracture was very likely to become inflamed and to suppurate, often with the demise of the patient. Amputation was commonly advised in all but the most minor of compound injuries. Joseph Lister's work (see Chapter 7) provided the basic understanding of the bacterial nature of such wound infection and provided the practical methods to overcome this. Surgeons before Lister avoided the idea of operative reduction of fractures because it was realised that operating on a closed fracture could, in fact, convert

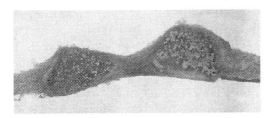

Figure 10.4 An old specimen of a transverse fracture of the patella. The widely separated bone fragments are joined by fibrous tissue.
Gordon Museum, Guy's Hospital.

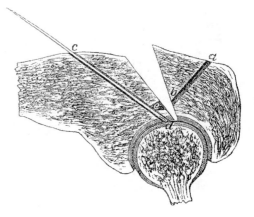

Figure 10.5 Joseph Lister's operation of wiring of a fractured olecranon.
From Lister J: An address on treatment of fractures of the patella. *British Medical Journal* 1883; 2, 855.

it into a 'compound' injury. Indeed, most would have regarded such a suggestion as being tantamount to malpractice. It was Lister himself who showed that, using antiseptic surgical techniques, it was safe to carry out operative reduction and fixation of a fracture. He himself reported successful wiring together of fractures of the patella and of the olecranon process of the elbow, where previously closed reduction and splinting of such fractures could only produce malaligned joint surfaces with the inevitable development of late arthritic change (Figure 10.4). Lister gave a detailed account of his technique and results in a lecture to the Medical Society of London, which was reported in the *British Medical Journal* of 1883 (Figure 10.5). He wrote:

In March 1873, my friend Dr Hector Cameron of Glasgow, recommended to my care at the Edinburgh Infirmary a case of ununited fracture of the olecranon. He reminds me that I had often expressed to him the opinion that the use of a metallic suture, antiseptically applied, . . . ought, in suitable cases, to be extended to the olecranon and patella. The patient was a man 34 years of age, who, five months previously, had received a blow from a policeman's baton on the left elbow. This occasioned great swelling which seems to have concealed the true nature of the case from a medical man who he first consulted. On admission, there was a considerable interval between the olecranon and the shaft of the bone; and although the limb was muscular, it was comparatively helpless, as he could not extend the forearm at all without the aid of the other hand. On the 28th of the month, I made a longitudinal incision, exposing the site of the fracture, and, at the same time, bringing into view the articular surface of the humerus,

and, having pared away the fibrous material between the fractured surfaces, I proceeded to drill the fragments, with a view to the application of the suture. The fracture was oblique from before backwards, as indicated by this diagram. I found no difficulty with the proximal fragment, in making the drill appear upon the fractured surface at a little distance from the cartilage (see b), but with the other fragment the obliquity of the position in which the drill had to be placed was so great that, instead of the end of the drill emerging at the fractured surface, as I had intended, I found it had entered into the substance of the humerus (d). I therefore withdrew the drill and substituted for it a needle (cd), passing the eyed end in first. Then, with a gouge, I excavated an opening (e) upon the fractured surface, opposite to the drill hole (b) on the other surface, until the needle was exposed. Withdrawing the needle, I introduced a silver wire in its place and I had no difficulty, by means of forceps passed into the excavation made by the gouge in drawing out the wire. I was then able to pass it through the other drilled opening and thus the two fragments were brought into apposition. The ends of the wire were twisted together and left projecting at the wound. Healing took place without suppuration or fever, and the wire was removed on the 19th of May, seven weeks after the operation. The wound made for its extraction soon healed, and the patient returned to Glasgow; and I afterwards had the satisfaction of learning that he was wielding the hammer in an iron ship building yard with his former energy.

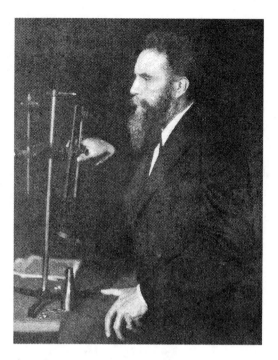

Figure 10.6 Wilhelm Konrad Roentgen.
Royal College of Surgeons of England.

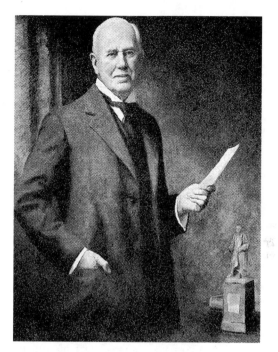

Figure 10.7 Sir William Arbuthnot Lane.
This painting hangs in the Medical School at Guy's.

In the same paper, Lister describes a second case of ununited fracture of the olecranon in which the patient had consulted no less than 18 other surgeons, all of whom advised against operation. Lister carried out an operation similar to the one described above with perfect success and goes on to say:

I have referred to a case of ununited fracture of the olecranon where 18 surgeons have been previously consulted. I trust no one here will suppose that I mention this circumstance for the purpose of glorifying myself. I mentioned it in order to emphasise what I believe, that by antiseptic means we can do, and are bound to do, operations of the greatest importance for our patients' advantage, which, without strict antiseptic means, the best surgeon would not be justified in recommending. How wise those 18 gentlemen were in counselling against operative interference, provided they were not prepared to operate strictly antiseptically, I think we must be all agreed. As regards the operative procedure in that case, it was of the most simple character; any first year student could have done the operation exactly as well as myself;

and, therefore, I trust I shall not be misunderstood by its being supposed that I came here to extol my own skill. That which justified me in operating in that case was simply the knowledge that strict antiseptic treatment would convert serious risk into complete safety.

The discovery of X-rays in 1895 by Wilhelm Roentgen (1845–1923) (Figure 10.6), Professor of Physics at the University of Würzburg in Germany, was almost immediately applied to the accurate diagnosis of fractures and provided a further impetus to the pioneers of open reduction, since it demonstrated that often anatomical reduction was not obtained by closed manipulation. Early innovators were Albin Lambotte (1866–1955) of Brussels, who devised a variety of screws, plates and metal bands, which he initially made himself, and also a technique for external fixation, and William Arbuthnot Lane (1856–1943) (Figure 10.7) of Guy's Hospital, London. Lane pioneered the use of screw fixation of fractures, which he commenced in 1893, and by 1905 he

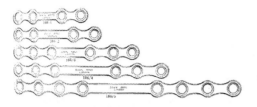

Figure 10.8 Lane's stainless steel plates for fracture fixation.

had introduced his special perforated stainless steel strips for plating fractures of the long bones (Figure 10.8). Of course, any infection in such instances would prove disastrous and, in other hands, there were many failures. Lane, however, insisted on the strictest asepsis in his theatres, the 'no touch technique'. For this he devised long artery and dissecting forceps so that, even in the deepest wound, the fingers that held them would not touch the wound edges. The sutures were never touched but were threaded using two pairs of dissecting forceps. This asepsis was combined with meticulous haemostasis and gentlest handling of the tissue. Much of his success was due to the fact that he was a brilliant technical surgeon.

Lane was such an interesting character that I must deviate from the subject of fractures to say more about him. He was the son of an army surgeon and entered Guy's Hospital at the early age of 16. He loved anatomy and was appointed a demonstrator while still a student. After qualifying he spent a further five years in the department of anatomy and liked nothing better than to demonstrate his prowess as a dissector. Indeed, the students would say 'don't let Lane touch your part or you will have nothing of it left'. He spent the whole of his professional life at Guy's and at Great Ormond Street, the hospital for sick children. He made important technical advances in many branches of surgery. He introduced exploration of the mastoid antrum in the treatment of chronic purulent otitis media (middle ear infection), devised an ingenious flap operation for the repair of cleft palate, was the first to treat septic thrombosis of the lateral sinus complicating mastoid infection by

ligature of the internal jugular vein and removal of the septic thrombus, was an early advocate of the use of saline for transfusion in haemorrhage, pioneered rib resection for chronic empyema in children and was the first to perform a successful cardiac massage, which was reported in 1902. The patient was a man of 65 undergoing appendicectomy:

During the trimming of the stump both pulse and respirations stopped together. Artificial respiration and traction on the tongue were performed without result. Then the surgeon introduced his hand through the abdominal incision and felt the motionless heart through the diaphragm. He gave it a squeeze or two and felt it restart beating.

The operation was completed and the patient recovered fully. Lane also devised the simple method of resuscitation in small infants by squeezing directly on the elastic chest wall.

Early in the 20th century, Lane started to become obsessed with the idea that chronic constipation produced toxaemia and was the cause of many of the ills of civilisation, ranging from migraine to rheumatism. He carried out total colectomies in patients suffering from such conditions. Fortunately, at a later date, Lane preached that one might keep the colon as long as it was maintained empty, and introduced the use of liquid paraffin, given in large doses by mouth. At least this was safer to the patient than having the whole of his colon removed! Naturally his views met with considerable opposition. Eventually, Lane took his name off the Medical Register in order to be able to address the public by lectures and through the Press on his ideas for health. He was indeed a pioneer in what we now call social medicine. He founded the New Health Society, whose principal aims were to teach the public the simple laws of health, to attempt to make fruit and vegetables abundant and cheap for the general public, and to encourage people to go back to the land, as well as, of course, keeping their bowels empty!

The risks of osteosynthesis, the open fixation of fractures, which include infection, delayed union and tissue reaction to the metal employed, created a long-standing debate between the conservative school, who would try where possible to use closed

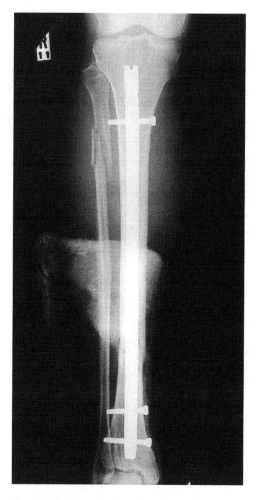

Figure 10.9 X-ray of a Küntscher intramedullary nail fixation of a fracture of the tibia. Westminster Hospital.

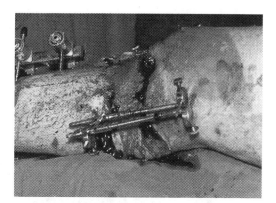

Figure 10.10 External fixators applied to a severe compound fracture of the tibia. An IRA bomb victim treated at Westminster Hospital, 1983.

methods, and those surgeons advocating open surgery. A leader of conservatism was Lorenz Böhler (1885–1973) of Vienna, who preached careful reduction of the fracture and strict immobilisation of the limb, combined with simultaneous exercises of all non-involved joints. His organisation methods at the Vienna Accident Hospital set an example for the development of specialist accident units world-wide.

Further advances included the development of non-reactive alloys such as vitallium to construct screws and plates, and the development of compression screws which allowed close apposition of the fracture surfaces. During the Second World War, Gerhard Küntscher (1900–1972) in Kiel, Germany, developed the intramedullary nail for fracture fixation (Figure 10.9). The difficulties of wartime communication meant that allied surgeons were unaware of this advance until they encountered returning prisoners of war who had had their fractures treated in this way. In recent years, external fixators have come into increasing use, particularly in the treatment of severely comminuted compound and multiple fractures – a technique first suggested by Lambotte nearly a century ago (Figure 10.10).

Fractures of the neck of the femur have always been a particular treatment problem because of the virtual impossiblity of holding the bone ends in continuity in all but impacted pertrochanteric fractures. Astley Cooper (1768–1841), in his *Treatise on Dislocations and Fractures*, was convinced that non-union was inevitable in this injury and advised disregarding the fracture and returning the patient to his normal life as far as the painful hip would allow. It remained for Marius Smith-Petersen (1886–1953) of Boston to devise a flanged nail to fix the fracture in 1925. This at first was performed by an

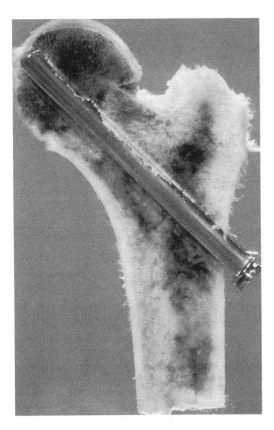

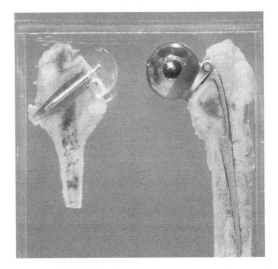

Figure 10.12 Prosthetic replacements of fractured femoral heads. Left: A Judet prosthesis; the patient was a male aged 80 who sustained a fracture of the femoral neck, in 1951. He died at home of a chest infection four months later. Right: A stainless steel Austin Moore prosthesis used to replace the femoral head in a pathological fracture secondary to a carcinoma of the thyroid in a male aged 83. He walked well post-operatively but died eight months later.
Specimens in the Gordon Museum, Guy's Hospital.

Figure 10.11 Autopsy specimen of a pinned hip fracture. The label reads: 'Female aged 53 had sustained a fracture of the neck of the right femur in a fall three weeks prior to her death. A Smith Petersen pin was inserted to stabilise the fracture but the patient died 13 days later from a pulmonary embolism'.
Gordon Museum, Guy's Hospital.

open operation until Sven Johansson (1880–1959) of Gothenburg, Sweden, introduced his drilling method for pinning the hip which avoided exposing the hip joint and which became a standard technique (Figure 10.11). Sub-capital fractures of the femoral neck, where it is almost certain that avascular necrosis of the detached head will take place, can now be treated by immediate replacement of the femoral head by means of a prosthesis (Figure 10.12).

Elective orthopaedics

Until the 19th century, little could be done for the halt, the lame and the crippled; the poor would drag themselves around the streets as beggars, the more fortunate would be confined to their bed or chair. Manipulations, irons and splints might be tried to correct the deformity but with only occasional success. Unqualified bone-setters, who were often quite skilled at dealing with fractures and dislocations, would also have a flourishing trade in massaging and manipulating patients with diseased bones and joints. They learned, from bitter experience, not to manipulate a 'hot' (and therefore inflamed) joint, where such interference would certainly be harmful.

The operative treatment of orthopaedic diseases was, of course, limited by the pre-Listerian risk of infection. Advanced tuberculous disease of bones and joints frequently required amputation of the limb; indeed, the very first major operation under ether anaesthesia was, in fact, amputation of the leg for tuberculosis of the knee (see Chapter 7). James Syme (1799–1870) (see Figure 6.31) advocated excision of the joint rather than amputation wherever possible and published, in 1831, a pamphlet on the subject entitled *Treatise on the Excision of Diseased Joints*. In it he wrote:

Though amputation is a measure very disagreeable both to the patient and to the surgeon, it has hitherto, with hardly any exception, been regarded as the only safe and efficient means of removing diseased joints which do not admit recovery. The idea of cutting out merely the morbid parts and leaving the sound portion of the limb, seems to have hardly ever occurred, or to have met with so many objections that it was almost instantly abandoned.

Of course, Syme was correct, although his cases were dogged by post-operative wound infection. Indeed, it is interesting that Syme's son-in-law, Joseph Lister (see Chapter 7), carried out a successful series of excisions of the wrist joint for tuberculosis using the antiseptic technique.

One of the early pioneers to attempt the correction of deformities by surgery was Jacques-Mathieu Delpech (1777–1832) in Montpellier, who carried out division of the tendo Achillis for club foot between 1816 and 1823. This involved an open operation and, presumably because of the almost inevitable infection, Delpech concluded that the operation was unjustified. Club foot continued to be treated by splints and manipulations. It is interesting that the poet Lord Byron suffered from this condition.

Delpech went on to publish an extensive study of bone and joint disease, *De L'Orthomorphie*, one of the earliest texts devoted to this subject. He was murdered by a mentally ill patient.

An important advance was made by George Friedrich Stromeyer (1804–1876) of Hanover, who set up a small hospital in that city for the treatment of bone and joint disease. In 1830 he treated a boy of 14 with club foot by manipulations for over a year without success. He then carried out the operation of division of the Achilles tendon, but not by open surgery: he introduced a narrow scalpel through a small stab wound behind the heel and passed it deep to the tendon, which was then divided – the operation of subcutaneous tenotomy. Division of the tendon allowed Stromeyer to manipulate the flexed ankle into its correct position and the tiny skin incision greatly decreased the chances of wound infection. The success of this case enabled Stromeyer to predict that other deformities could be amenable to this type of surgery, as indeed they were.

In 1836, a young English doctor, William John Little (1810–1894), who had qualified at the London Hospital four years previously, visited Stromeyer's clinic. Little had a club foot as a result of poliomyelitis at the age of two; he had been treated in the usual way with manipulations and splintage without success. He was naturally closely interested in this deformity and indeed was making it the subject for his MD thesis. He had come to the conclusion that clubbing of the feet was not caused by deformed bone growth, as had previously been thought, but resulted from a disordered action of the muscles. After watching Stromeyer at work, Little underwent his operation of subcutaneous tenotomy with considerable success. He stayed on at Stromeyer's clinic, learned his technique, wrote his MD thesis and returned to London, where he persuaded his friends to subscribe to a hospital for him. This became the Royal Orthopaedic Hospital, later the Royal National Orthopaedic Hospital, London, which is today a Mecca for orthopaedic surgeons. Whereas Stromeyer had only divided the Achilles tendon, Little advocated tenotomy for any tendon that was producing deformity; Stromeyer called him 'the apostle of tenotomy'. Little also published papers on other deformities, including knock-knee and scoliosis and described the spastic condition arising from birth injury of the brain, spastic diplegia, which is still known as Little's disease.

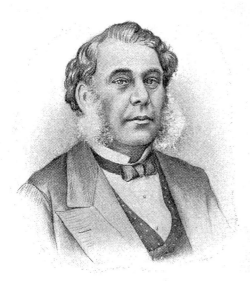

Figure 10.13 John Hilton.
Royal College of Surgeons of England.

Interestingly, Little failed in his ambition to get on the staff at the London Hospital as a surgeon; instead he switched to become a physician and was eventually elected to the staff of the London, but on the medical side.

In the pre-antibiotic era, tuberculosis of bones and joints accounted for large numbers of crippled children. Percivall Pott gave a good description of its most serious manifestation, involvement of the vertebrae (Pott's disease of the spine, see Figure 6.13) which was often complicated by adjacent tuberculous abscesses and which could result in paraplegia from spinal cord compression. John Hilton (1805–1878) (Figure 10.13), a surgeon at Guy's Hospital, delivered a course of lectures on rest and pain at the Royal College of Surgeons, England, in 1860 to 1862. These lectures were afterwards published in book form with the same title and can still be read with interest today. Hilton pointed out the importance of rest in the management of many

(a)

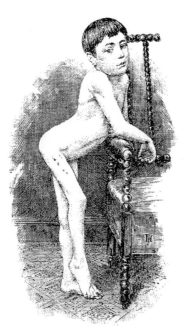

(b)

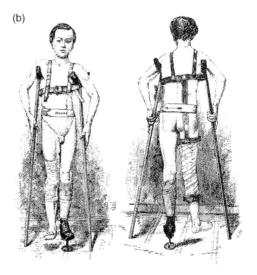

Figure 10.14 (a) Tuberculosis of the hip with gross flexion deformity. (b) The solution – the ambulatory Thomas hip splint with a patten on the sound side. Reprinted with permission from Thomas HO: *The Principles of Treatment of Diseased Joints*. Philadelphia, WB Saunders, 1883.

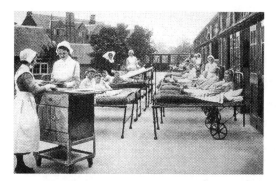

Figure 10.15 A long-stay children's orthopaedic ward in the 1940s. These hospitals were filled to capacity with victims of tuberculosis of bones and joints and of poliomyelitis.
Photograph provided by Mr MH Harrison FRCS, Birmingham.

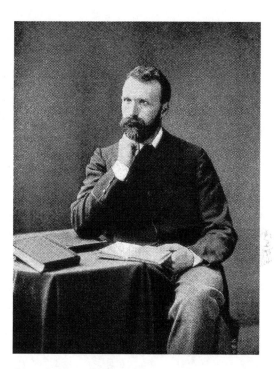

Figure 10.16 William Macewen.
From Comrie JD: *History of Scottish Medicine.* London, Baillière, Tindall and Cox, 1932.

chronic conditions. However, it was Hugh Owen Thomas, who we have already mentioned earlier in this chapter (Figure 10.2) who enunciated the importance of what he termed 'enforced, uninterrupted and prolonged rest' in the treatment of bone and joint tuberculosis. Immobilisation was continued until healing by fibrous ankylosis was achieved, the limb being now fixed in a position that allowed reasonable function. Immobilisation was accompanied by active use of unaffected limbs but the whole of the affected limb must be placed at rest. Thus, a tuberculous knee would be splinted the full length of the leg and a tuberculous hip joint would be treated by a splint which reached from the axilla to the foot, a patten being used so that the normal leg, thus 'elongated', would ensure non-weightbearing of the diseased joint (Figure 10.14).

Of course, all this was to be changed by the introduction of antibiotics; streptomycin was isolated by Selman Waksman (1888–1973) at Rutger's University, New Jersey, in 1943 and introduced into medical practice in 1948. As a medical student and newly qualified doctor, I was well familiar with orthopaedic wards filled with children being treated by techniques laid down by Thomas (Figure 10.15). Within a few years, such scenes would disappear from the hospitals of the Western world.

The introduction of antiseptic, and then aseptic, surgical techniques enabled not only rapid progress to be made in the operative surgery of fractures, but also allowed the development of what, until then, had been a risky experiment – the operative surgical correction of orthopaedic deformities. Sir William Macewen (1848–1924) (Figure 10.16), a student of Lister at Glasgow and later himself to become Regius Professor of Surgery at that University, was an early pioneer of aseptic surgery. Not only did he perform the first successful resection of an intracranial tumour (a meningioma in a girl of 14 in 1879) and the first successful pneumonectomy for tuberculosis in 1895, but he also pioneered the treatment of the gross deformities of genu valgum (knock-knee) and genu varus (bow-knee) (Figure 10.17) by dividing the tibia and straightening the leg – the operation of Macewen's osteotomy (1875). At first,

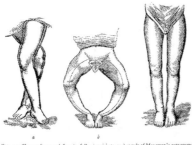

FIG. 104. Types of severe deformity following rickets, and result of Macewen's osteotomy
(a) and (b), two common types of deformity; (c) same case as (b), after operation
(W. Macewen, *Osteotomy*, London, 1880)

Figure 10.17 (a, b) Types of severe deformity of the knee following rickets: (a) genu valgum; (b) genu varus; (c) Result of Macewen's osteotomy in case (b). From Macewen W: *Osteotomy*, 1880.

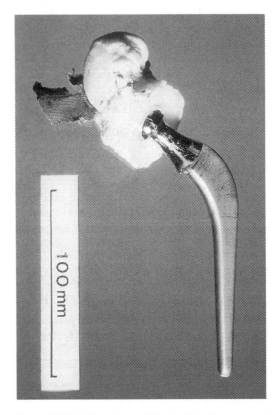

Figure 10.19 A Charnley total hip prosthesis removed at post-mortem many years later. The wire mesh in the acetabular cement was used to reinforce the weak inner wall of the pelvis.
Specimen in the Gordon Museum, Guy's Hospital.

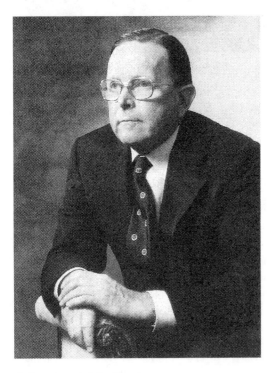

Figure 10.18 Sir John Charnley.
Royal College of Surgeons of England.

his instruments were an ordinary carpenter's chisel and mallet but he noted that the straight edge of the chisel did not produce an accurate cut in the bone and moreover the wooden mallet handle cracked with repeated sterilisation and use. He therefore developed a special bevelled osteotome and had his instruments made of polished steel. He performed his operation with such dexterity that visitors to his theatre, inspecting the X-rays on the screen, might well look round to see the patient being wheeled out, the operation having been accomplished. Osteotomy became a popular and useful operation

(a)

(b)

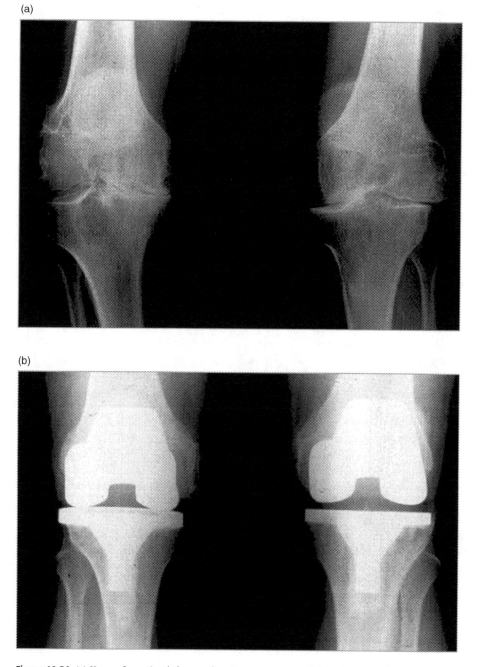

Figure 10.20 (a) X-ray of a patient's knees, showing gross osteoarthritis. (b) X-ray of the same patient after bilateral total knee replacements. (Case of Mr John Older FRCS.)

for treating other joint deformities, especially those resulting from ankylosis (fusion) of joints.

Macewen also pioneered the use of bone grafts, using fragments of bone removed at an osteotomy for a child with bow-legs to replace a segment of humerus which had been lost as a result of osteo-myelitis in a 4-year-old child. Thirty years later the patient was still at work with an excellent functioning arm. By 1911, Russell Hibbs (1869–1932) of New York had revolutionised the treat-ment of gross spinal deformities resulting from congenital scoliosis or tuberculosis by his spinal fusion operation. In 1915, Frederick Albee (1876–1945) of New York devised his well-known Albee graft. This is an autogenous graft taken from the shaft of the patient's tibia and implanted into a groove cut through several vertebrae above and below the diseased spinal segment.

Replacement of a diseased joint by a prosthesis, allowing movement to be restored, had long been a surgical dream. Themistokles Gluck (1853–1942) at the Kaiser und Kaiserin Krankenhaus, Berlin, in 1891 attempted to replace a diseased hip joint using an ivory ball and socket cemented and screwed into position but the apparatus was soon extruded.

Attempts by Philip Wiles (1899–1967) of the Middlesex Hospital in 1938 using a stainless steel ball and socket were also unsuccessful. Marius Smith Petersen (1886–1953) of Boston interposed a vital-lium cup between the bone ends of the hip in 1939, again with only temporary success. The brothers Judet (Jean, 1905–1995, and Robert, 1909–1980) in Paris replaced the diseased femoral head of arthritic hips with an acrylic head attached to a metallic stem which was passed along the neck of the femur (see Figure 10.12 left). This was a simple operation with brilliant early results, but unfortunately the metal stem fractured after a relatively short period of use. Moore and Thompson in the USA both used the Judet principle but replaced the femoral head with an entirely metallic head and shaft (see

Figure 10.12, right). This was satisfactory in the treatment of fractures of the neck of the femur but failed in arthritic disease when both sides of the joint were involved. It remained for George McKee (1906–1991) of Norwich and Sir John Charnley (1911–1982) (Figure 10.18) of Manchester to produce successful hip prostheses in the 1950s. Charnley's technique is still the most popular method in use today. This comprises a steel femoral head and neck, the neck being cemented into the upper shaft of the femur using acrylic cement, and a high density polyethylene cup which is cemented into the drilled out acetabulum (Figure 10.19). Much of the development of his prosthesis was carried out in Charnley's workshop at his home. Charnley was a perfectionist. He noted that occasional disastrous deep infection might occur following hip replace-ment operations, often resulting from common skin organisms, when the operation was carried out under normal 'aseptic' conditions. He obtained the co-operation of Howorth Air Engineering to pro-duce the first filtered air operating enclosure with elaborate 'space-age' suits for the surgeon and his assistants, which reduced the risk of operative infection to very low levels indeed. Charnley was the first practising orthopaedic surgeon to be elected a Fellow of the Royal Society.

In more recent years, highly successful prosthe-ses have been developed for other joint replace-ments, particularly of the knee (Figure 10.20) and the fingers.

Orthopaedic surgeons, like the urologists and gynaecologists, were quick to take up the develop-ment of fibre-optics for illumination. Arthroscopes, first for examination of joints and then for operative interventions, have made minimal interventional surgery possible for many joint conditions, notably removal of damaged cartilages and loose bodies from the knee and operations on a variety of shoulder lesions, particularly the supraspinatus syndrome.

11

Breast tumours

Much of today's surgery is concerned with the treatment of benign and malignant tumours. Indeed much of surgical history, especially in the past 100 years or so, is concerned with the development of techniques for the removal of organs affected by these diseases: resections of stomach, large bowel, lung and so on. It would take a book much larger than this to document the history of the surgery of all of the major tumours and I have selected the story of the treatment of tumours of the breast as a good example. The choice was a very simple one. After all, diseases of the breast have been studied and documented since the earliest days of surgery. Long before any surgeon could even dream of tackling other cancers, indeed before he was aware that many even existed, he could hardly fail to observe the growth, ulceration and spread of a breast cancer with the ultimate inevitable destruction of the patient. In Hippocrates we read: 'A woman in Abdera had a carcinoma of the breast and bloody fluid ran from the nipple. When the discharge stopped she died'.

Our knowledge of the Greco-Roman concept of cancer and its treatment is derived from the Roman encyclopaedist of the 1st century AD, Aulus Cornelius Celsus, whose *De Medicina* is a compendium of what was known of medicine at the time. He records the various methods of dealing with breast and other superficial tumours and with the poor prognosis of the disease:

There is not so great danger of a cancer, unless it be irritated by the imprudence of the physician. This disease generally happens in the superior parts, about the face, the nose, ears, lips and the breasts of women . . . some have made use of caustic medicines, others of the actual cautery, others cut them out with a knife. Nor was any person ever relieved by medicine, but after cauterizing, the tumours have been quickened in their progress and increased till they proved mortal; when they have been cut out, and cicatrized, they have not withstanding returned and occasioned death. Whereas, at the same time, most people, by using no violent methods to attempt the extirpation of the disease, but only applying mild medicines to soothe it, protract their lives notwithstanding the disorder, to an extreme of age.

Over the centuries, removal of the breast tumour by the knife, the cautery, a combination of the two or by means of caustics was carried out. Henri de Mondeville (1260–1320), for example, advocated the use of a paste made up of arsenic and zinc chloride. In those pre-anaesthetic days, amputation of the breast had to be performed as swiftly as possible. Wilhelm Fabry von Hilden (1560–1624), the leading German surgeon at the time, invented an instrument that constricted the base of the breast while an attached blade amputated the organ. He stressed the importance of ensuring that the tumour was mobile before he would operate. Scultetus (1595–1645) passed heavy ligatures through the base of the breast to serve as traction, amputated the breast with the sweep of a knife and then used the cautery to stop the bleeding. The full horror of this operation is vividly shown in his illustration of this procedure in his *Armamentarium Chirurgicum* (Figure 11.1).

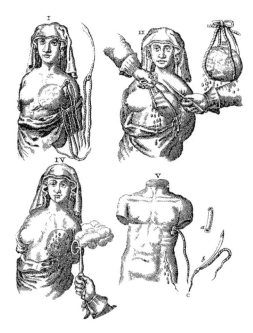

Figure 11.1 Seventeenth century amputation of the breast using the knife followed by the cautery. From Scultetus: *Armamentarium Chirurgicum*. Amsterdam, Jansson Waesberg, 1741.

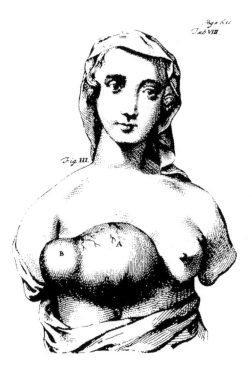

Figure 11.2 Massive tumour of the breast, probably an example of cystosarcoma phyllodes, submitted to mastectomy by Lorenz Heister, 1720.

The description by Lorenz Heister (1683–1758) of a mastectomy that he performed in 1720 gives us a vivid idea of what this operation comprised in those days. He discusses the careful pre-operative preparation, the mastectomy itself, performed at maximum speed, and the tedious post-operative dressings of the invariably suppurating wound (if the patient was lucky enough to survive the operation). His case report is interesting also because it shows that times have not changed all that much in the patient's attitude to cancer. So often there is an attempt to rationalise for a cause; his patient ascribed her tumour to cold air on the breast when she was in a sweat 16 years before the lump appeared and while she was pregnant. All too often patients put their faith in alternative medicine; his patient visited many quacks, who applied plasters, ointments and fomentations. Although Heister was convinced his patient had cancer, the description

of the tumour – its mobility, the colour of the overlying skin, the bosselations, the absence of secondary deposits in the axilla, and the long survival of the patient – suggests that the lesion was, in fact, an example of cystosarcoma phyllodes, a slowly growing benign tumour of the breast which may reach enormous proportions, although it may eventually turn malignant.

We have already met this extraordinary surgeon (see Figure 6.7). The illustration of his patient is shown in Figure 11.2 and his description of his case is as follows:

A farmer's wife came to me, the 21st or 22nd of January, 1720, from a neighbouring village, about a mile from Altdorff, with a very cancerous right breast; she was about forty-eight years of age, of a thin habit of body, and of a melancholic temperament, had been delivered of eight children; her breast was of a prodigious size, nearly as big again as her head, very hard, unequal, and deformed, and attended with severe pains. It was of a dark brown, red colour, like a mortified part, and here and there several large bloated veins appeared; the breast was not quite round, the left-side A, was as big as a large person's head, and next to it on the right-side B, such another substance adhered, of the bigness of a child's head, which extended itself to her right-arm as described in the figure.

Upon the inferior part of this large tumour, there were about twenty large excrescencies of a blackish colour, and of the size and form of the nipple, which I was not able to distinguish from them: these, added to the shocking aspect of the breast itself in general, rendered the appearance more horrid and frightful.

The woman was extremely weak and faint of herself, but the great weight of her breast, which weighed twelve pounds, was so troublesome when she walked, sat down, or lay in bed, pressing upon the thorax, that the respiration was so much affected, that it was with great difficulty she breathed at all; this rendered her yet more weak and faint. She complained too of a violent shooting pain in her breast, shoulders and back, which, by contracting the thorax, contributed to produce the great anxiety and oppression she complained of in breathing: I considered and examined every circumstance, reflected upon the uncommon magnitude of the breast, and finding the tumour moveable, without any adhesion to the ribs or sternum, for I could move it with ease from side to side, upwards and downwards, nor were the axillary glands enlarged or swelled, and as she complained of no other particular disorder, I could do no otherwise than inform her friends, that it was impossible for medicine to be of any use, and that there was no other method of cure but by amputation; and that this operation would of course be attended with danger, but that if she would submit to it, there were some hopes of a cure, and of preserving her life, for without taking off her breast, she would, in all probability, soon expire with the pain, continual restlessness, oppression, and weakness.

When she heard there were hopes of saving her life, she begged of me most earnestly to do whatever I thought necessary, and I accordingly promised to take off the breast very soon; but being desirous to know in what manner she became affected with this disorder, and how, from time to time, it had increased to the present enormous size, I enquired of her, and she related to me, that

about sixteen years before, during the time of her lying-in, being alone at home one day, and in a sweat, a person knocked at the door, rising, in this sweat, to see what he wanted, she perceived the cold air to strike upon the breast, and soon after observed an hard moveable lump, of the size of a hazel-nut, in the same breast, but without pain while in this state, so that she paid no regard to it, she had three children afterwards, who she suckled without perceiving the tumour to increase; but afterwards it increased gradually, and at the end of twelve years it was become as large as a hen's egg.

She now began to be apprehensive of the consequence, and had applied to many quacks, who had used, plaisters, ointments, fomentations, &c. to resolve or discuss the tumour or to bring it to a suppuration, but without success: it became bigger and bigger, till at length, her breast was as large as her head, and it began to be very painful, and the more it became enlarged, the more pain it gave her: still she applied to other people of this sort for relief, used what they advised for a time, but without any benefit, but, on the contrary, the breast grew worse.

About the end of November last, another quack came to her, and promised certainly to cure her, swearing that he could soften the tumour, and bring it to suppuration, and to that intent he applied emollient cataplasms for a month, which, instead of being serviceable, had increased the pain, and the smaller tumour B, on the right side of A appeared. She was now, by this treatment, rendered so weak that she was scarcely able to walk across the room; her breast before was quite round and equal, consisting of the single tumour only. In this miserable condition she was when she applied to me.

She also informed me, that since her first lying in, she had always been troubled with various tumours in her legs, which went off gradually with her menses, and both entirely left her about a year ago, when her breast became so large.

With regard to the cure of this terrible disorder, I conceived that there was indeed no great hopes, as the tumour was of such an enormous size, which in amputation, would require so large a wound, and as the woman herself was so greatly debilitated by the constant pains and length of time she had been afflicted, that she was not able to walk.

Celsus, that excellent Roman physician, has intimated to his successors, that, in dangerous cases, it is better to try a doubtful remedy, where the least hopes of success remains, than none . . .

I thought it advisable to proceed to the operation; not caring to defer it any longer, as the woman would become weaker and weaker, through the violence of the pain; much less could I think of putting off so considerable an operation till spring, as is customary in France, as the patient might die before the spring came, or so weak as not to be able to undergo the operation: for which reason, notwithstanding the days were short, and the weather the coldest in the year, I thought it would be dangerous to defer the operation till the spring; and accordingly, as necessity has no law, I fixed upon January 29th, for the day. I prepared everything in the morning for the operation, the necessary instruments, namely a knife, of my surgery; which, though pretty large, I chose for the purpose, as the breast was extremely large, and as with a large knife I could take it off more expeditiously.

I afterwards ordered such remedies to be got ready as were necessary to stop the bleeding . . .

A linen compress to be dipped in the spiritus terebinthinae, and applied to the divided arteries; pledgets of lint strewed with the astringent powder; bovist; of diachylum plaister, spread upon linen, twelve slips a foot and an inch broad, and another piece a foot square; quadrangular soft linen-cloths folded, two rollers six yards long, and four fingers broad. I had also, in readiness, the cauterizing irons to apply to the arteries if they should bleed too violently. I ordered also the assistant-surgeon to have ready heated a quart of beer, adding three ounces of butter to it, to dip the largest bolsters in, to apply over all the other dressings, as Helvetius, in a treatise on haemorrhages, recommends this application in amputations of the breast, as of great use in preventing inflammations . . .

The whole apparatus being in readiness, I now proceeded to the operation; placing the patient in an arm-chair in the middle of the room, and standing on the right-side, somewhat backwards, that I might make the incision at the inferior part with greater convenience, which is different from the common method: I then desired an assistant to extend her right-arm and raise it up, at the same time pulling it backwards; another assistant kept her head fixed: a third stood before, who I directed to hold the diseased breast with both hands, to raise, and, at the same time, to pull it towards him, that I might with greater ease, divide it from the subjacent muscles: a fourth assistant stood on my side with the instruments and dressings, and the fifth held the cordial medicines.

I now encouraged her to behave with resolution, and taking hold of her breast with my left-hand, applied the knife to the inferior part with my right-hand, cut through the integuments, and directed the assistant who held the breast, to pull the breast towards him; I carried on the incision by the direction of the finger of my left-hand, till the breast was extirpated, which was performed in a minute. [Figure 11.3]

The arteries, after the amputation, bleeding briskly, I applied to them compresses dipped in oil of turpentine, directing the assistants to make a compression upon them with their fingers: then I applied to the rest of the wound, the pledgets of lint strewed with the astringent powder, and over this a large piece of bovista, till the whole wound was covered thickly with it; over these, bolsters of tow, strewed with the astringent powder, which I redirected to be gently compressed by the hands of the assistants, till the bleeding stopped: while these dressings were applying, I gave the patient some of the cordial julep, and held the spirit for smelling to, under her nose; by which means she was kept from fainting.

The dressings I fixed with the twelve long slips of plaster, and over these I laid the large square compress, and over this two more large compresses, wetted with the hot beer and butter, and fixed the whole with a two headed roller.

After the dressing she repeated the cordial, and was put to bed. I ordered an assistant to sit by her bed-side, to compress the dressings with his hand extended, to prevent fresh bleeding, and desired the assistants to relieve each other every two hours.

I weighed the breast afterwards, and found it to weigh twelve pounds. A few hours afterwards the blood forcing its way through the dressings, I ordered another compress to be applied, and fixed with a roller in the manner of the first, which stopped the bleeding quite . . .

Heister then goes on to describe the prolonged period of dressing the wound, which inevitably suppurated, and finally concludes:

The regimen I directed this woman to observe, was, for the first fortnight thin soup and jellies; afterwards, when she had a better appetite, I permitted veal, boiled prunes, apples and pears, and eggs boiled soft; for ordinary drink, besides the vulnerary infusion prescribed above, I suffered her to drink small beer, when thirsty; at meals, as above mentioned, I allowed her a glass of wine, and in another fortnight, permitted her to drink some Altdorff strong beer. I advised her to keep herself quiet. She was regular as to stools and urine during the whole time; and, by the end of March, had recovered her strength so well as to be able

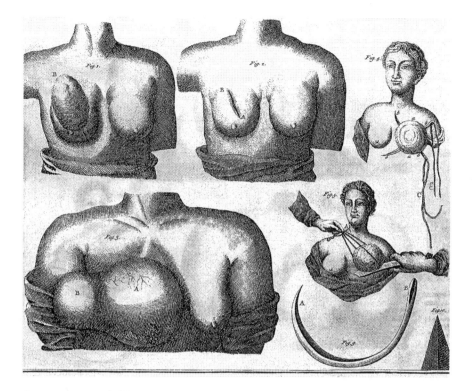

Figure 11.3 Heister's mastectomy.
From his Medical, *Chirurgical and Anatomical Cases*, English edition, 1755.

to get up and walk about, was brisk and cheerful, had a good appetite, and complained of no pain all the month of April. When I went to Helmstadt, I left directions with the surgeon to dress it with the dry lint and empl. saturninum only, till it should be healed; and a little time afterwards I was informed that she was perfectly cured, and enjoyed a good state of health. She lived several years afterwards. This cancerous breast was the largest ever extirpated or described by authors.

Reading descriptions such as this of mastectomy in the pre-anaesthetic era, it is not surprising that surgeons, as well as quacks, tried every conceivable non-surgical procedure in an attempt to treat cancers of the breast. Thus Alfred Velpeau (1795–1867), who held the Chair of Clinical Surgery in the Faculty of Medicine in Paris, gives an extensive list of remedies or medicines for breast cancer in his *A Treatise on the Diseases of the Breast and Mammary Region*, published in 1854 which include: repeated application of leeches, cure by hunger, hemlock, iron, ammoniacal solution of copper, arsenic, mercury, Vichy water, preparations of gold, quinine, iodine, sarsaparilla and bitters. Many of these he tried himself without success. He writes:

Severe dietary measures and purgatives are incapable of curing cancer; and if such a regimen does bring about a diminution of the size of the tumour, as also of the whole body, the cancer rapidly regains its volume as soon as the primitive rigor of the diet has been somewhat relaxed.

Two 18th century French surgeons made important contributions to our concept of the pathology and adequate surgical treatment of breast cancer. Henri Le Dran (1685–1770) of the Charité Hospital, Paris, taught that cancer of the breast was a local lesion in its earliest stage which then would spread through the lymphatics to the regional lymph nodes. Once there was involvement of the lymph nodes in the axilla, the prognosis would be considerably worse. Jean-Louis Petit (1674–1750) (see Figure 6.2), first Director of the French Academy of Surgery, described the basic tenets of an adequate mastectomy – wide excision of the tumour and removal of the axillary lymph nodes. He wrote:

The roots of the cancer were the enlarged lymphatic glands; that the gland should be looked for and removed and that the pectoral fascia and even some fibres of muscle itself should be dissected away rather than leave any doubtful tissue. The mammary gland too should not be cut into during the operation. Where the integuments are also affected and strictly joined to the cancer there is little hope to expect a perfect cure if they are not both clearly extirpated together.

Over the next century, many surgeons advocated complete mastectomy together with removal of the lymph nodes in the axilla. In 1784, Benjamin Bell (1749–1806), surgeon at the Edinburgh Royal Infirmary, in his six volume textbook, wrote: 'Even when only a small portion of the breast is diseased, the whole mamma should be removed. The axillary glands should be dissected by opening up the armpit but as much skin as possible should be preserved'.

In 1825, Sir Astley Cooper (1768–1841) (see Figure 6.26) wrote in his *Lectures on the Principles and Practice of Surgery*:

It will be sometimes necessary to remove the whole breast, where much is apparently contaminated; for there is more generally diseased than is perceived and it is best not to leave any small portions of it, as tubercles reappear in them . . . if a gland in the axilla be enlarged, it should be removed, and with it all the intervening cellular substance. If several glands in the axilla be enlarged, their removal does not succeed in preventing the return of the disease.

Note that, already, the poor prognosis of extensive axillary involvement was well recognised.

By 1844, Joseph Pancoast (1805–1882) (Figure 11.4), Professor of Surgery at Jefferson Medical College, Philadelphia, was advising still more radical surgery: involved muscle should be removed, even affected

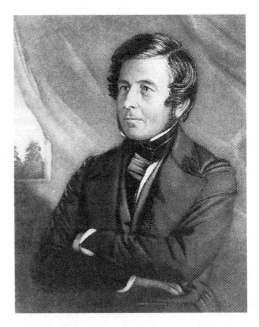

Figure 11.4 Joseph Pancoast.
From Robbins GF: *The Breast*. Austin, Silvergirl, 1984.

portions of ribs should be resected with the cutting forceps or a saw, and 'such of the axillary glands as are supposed to be scirrhous, or are even indurated and enlarged, should be taken away' (Figure 11.5).

Many experienced surgeons, however, appalled at the early recurrences they saw following removal of the breast tumour, wondered whether surgery was indicated at all in many cases and whether, in fact, it often did more harm than good. Robert Liston (1794–1847), Professor of Surgery at University College Hospital, London, and the first surgeon to operate using ether anaesthesia in England (see Chapter 7) wrote:

Recourse may be had to the knife in some cases but the circumstances must be very favourable indeed to induce a surgeon to recommend or warrant him in undertaking any operation for removal of malignant disease of the breast. When the disease has been of some standing there is a considerable risk of the axillary glands having become contaminated. No-one could now be found so rash or so cruel as to attempt the removal of glands thus affected.

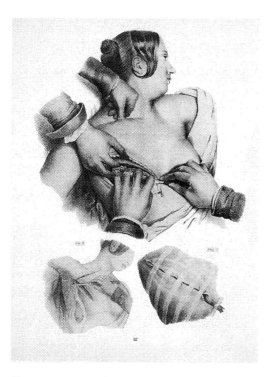

Figure 11.5 Pancoast's mastectomy technique.
From Pancoast J: *Treatise on Operative Surgery*.
Philadelphia, Carey and Hart, 1844.

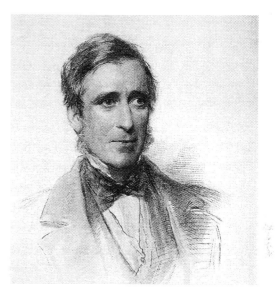

Figure 11.6 Sir James Paget.
Royal College of Surgeons of England.

That wise surgeon Sir James Paget (1814–1899)
(Figure 11.6), of St Bartholomew's Hospital, London,
wrote in his *Lectures on Surgical Pathology* in 1853:

We have come to ask ourselves whether it is probable that
the operation will add to the length or comfort of life
enough to justify incurring the risk for its own consequences. I cannot doubt that the answer may be often in
the affirmative; (1) in cases of acute hard cancer, the
operation may be rightly performed though speedy
recurrence and death may be expected, its performance is
justified by the probability that it will in some measure
prolong life and save the patient from dreadful suffering (2)
on similar grounds the operation seems proper in all cases
in which it is clear that the local disease is destroying
life by pain, profuse discharge or mental anguish, and it is
not accompanied by evidence of such cachexia as would
make the operation extremely hazardous. (3) In all cases in
which it is not probable that the operation will shorten life,
a motive for its performance is afforded by the expectation

that part of the patient's life will be spent with less suffering and in hope, instead of despair, for when they are
no longer sensible of their disease there are few cancerous
patients who will not enjoy the hope of long immunity,
though it be most unreasonable and not encouraged.

   On the other side there are many cases in which the
balance is clearly against operation; (1) In well developed
chronic cancers, especially in old persons, it is so little
probable that the operation will add either to the comfort
or to the length of life that its risk had better not be
incurred. These indeed are the cases in which the operation may be longest survived, but they are also those in
which without operation life is most prolonged and least
burdened. (2) In cases in which the cachexia or evident
constitutional disease is more than proportionate to the
local disease, the operation should be refused; it is too
likely to be fatal by its own consequences or possibly by
accelerating the progress of cancer in organs more
important than the breast. On similar grounds and yet
more certain it should not be performed when there is any
reasonable suspicion of internal cancer [i.e. the presence
of metastases, HE]. (3) If there be no weighty motives for
its performance the operation should be avoided in all
patients whose general health (independently of the
cancerous diathesis) makes its risk unusually great.

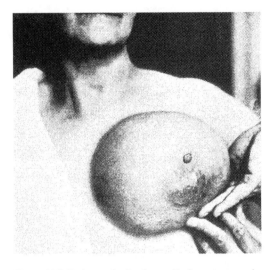

Figure 11.7 Patient submitted to radical mastectomy by William Halsted in 1912. Today this tumour would be regarded as technically inoperable.
From Halsted WS: Developments in the Skin-grafting operation for Cancer of the Breast. *Journal of the American Medical Association* 1913; 60, 416.

Much of this philosophy, written 150 years ago, is relevant to surgical practice today.

Paget went on to show that in 235 cases he had had an operative mortality of 10% and he said that he had not seen a case where recurrence was delayed beyond eight years. He had followed the life histories of 139 patients with scirrhous carcinoma of the breast for as much as nine years and had found that, except for a few cases, those who had had no operation lived longer than those who had had surgery. It must be remembered, of course, that in those days patients would rarely present themselves to the surgeon with the small tumour of one centimetre or less that is so commonly seen in the clinics today; one has only to read the case descriptions or look at the clinical photographs of patients in the last century to realise that the so-called 'early' breast tumours in the 19th and early 20th century were often actually visible, with skin attachment and often actually ulcerated – so-called Stage III tumours (Figure 11.7).

Paget was a remarkable man, eminent as a pathologist, surgeon and teacher. He qualified at St Bartholomew's at the age of 22 and spent the whole of his professional life at that famous medical school. As a student he was the first to observe the parasite *Trichina spiralis* in a patient's muscle. He gave the original description in 1882 of the quite common condition of osteitis deformans, more usually termed 'Paget's disease of bone', which is still of unknown aetiology. He described 15 cases of a disease of the nipple, all of which were followed by cancer in the underlying breast, now termed 'Paget's disease of the nipple', and he also described the rarer pre-malignant condition of 'Paget's disease of the penis'. He served as both Serjeant-surgeon to Queen Victoria and as President of the Royal College of Surgeons of England.

Of course, the early mastectomies were performed without any form of anaesthesia and without the benefit of antiseptic surgery. Once these twin blessings had been introduced, mastectomies could be carried out by means of careful dissection and without the fear of almost inevitable suppuration of the wound. Thus, in 1870, Joseph Lister (see Figure 7.15) wrote:

I have at present a patient about to leave the Infirmary three weeks after the removal of the entire mamma for scirrhous, all the axillary glands having been at the same time cleared out after division of both the pectoral muscles so as to permit the shoulder to be thrown back and the axilla freely exposed as is done in the dissecting room – a practice I have for some years adopted where the lymphatic glands are affected in the disease.

The development of the radical operation

In Germany the concept developed of cancer dissemination via the lymphatics thanks to the work of Richard von Volkmann (1830–1889) of Hale (an early exponent of antiseptic surgery in Germany) and Lothar Heidenhain (1860–1940) of Berlin, who published a detailed study of the spread of breast cancer in 1889. Volkmann himself, by 1875, was advocating routine removal of the fascia over

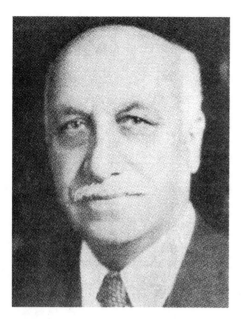

Figure 11.8 Willy Meyer.
From Robbins GF: *The Breast*. Austin, Silvergirl, 1984.

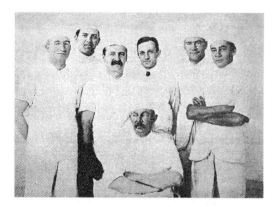

Figure 11.9 William Halsted with his ex-residents in 1904 at the Johns Hopkins Hospital. Halsted is seated. Immediately behind him, without a surgeon's cap, stands Harvey Cushing. To Cushing's left is JMT Finney, wearing an early pair of surgical gloves. Finney was a pioneer abdominal surgeon, who devised the pyloroplasty operation used today. To Cushing's right is Joseph Bloodgood, after whom the 'blue-domed cysts' of the breast are named.
From Fulton JF: *Harvey Cushing, a Biography*. Oxford, Blackwell, 1946.

pectoralis major together with the entire breast and an extensive portion of the overlying skin, together with removal of the entire fatty tissue of the axilla. If the underlying muscle was bound to the tumour a thick layer of muscle was also excised.

Gradually, surgeons were moving to the concept of the radical mastectomy, whose detailed technique was evolved by Willy Meyer (1858–1932) (Figure 11.8) of the New York Hospital and William Stewart Halsted (1852–1922) (Figure 11.9 and see also Figure 7.11). Meyer drew attention to the danger of dissemination of the cancer cells in the wound if the tumour was handled during the operation and in 1894 wrote:

Since Heidenhain has shown that in a great number of cases of cancer of the breast the pectoralis major muscle is also involved by the disease and that, if left in place, the growth is more liable to recur, it has become, I believe, the duty of the surgeon always to remove this muscle with the breast and the axillary contents . . . within the last three years I have operated according to this plan on six female patients.

Meyer included removal of pectoralis minor in his operative procedure, a technique later adopted by Halsted. The large wound defect was treated by skin grafting about eight to ten days after the initial mastectomy.

Halsted did much to pioneer the operation of radical mastectomy which, in the United States, was often termed the Halsted mastectomy. In 1890 he wrote:

About eight years ago I began not only to typically clean out the axilla in all cases of cancer of the breast but also to excise in almost every case the pectoralis major muscle or at least a generous piece of it, and to give the tumour on all sides an exceedingly wide berth. It is impossible to determine with the naked eye whether or not the disease has extended into the pectoral muscle. [Figure 11.10]

By 1898, Halsted was advising dissection of the supraclavicular nodes in the majority of cases and even removal of the mediastinal nodes, although, in later years, he abandoned the supraclavicular part of the dissection. Halsted was also performing immediate skin grafting to the resultant large raw

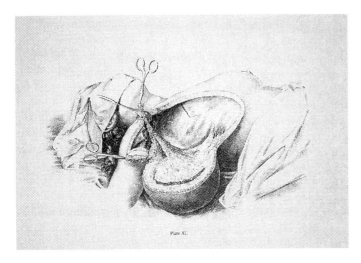

Plate XI.

Figure 11.10 The Halsted radical mastectomy.
From Halsted WS: The results of operations performed for the cure of cancer of the breast performed at the Johns Hopkins Hospital from June 1889 to January 1894. *Johns Hopkins Hospital Bulletin* 1894–5; 4, 297.

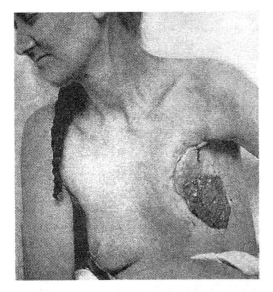

Figure 11.11 A patient operated upon by Halsted. The massive skin defect was allowed to heal by granulation tissue or else grafted.

area, having used the available skin to cover the axillary contents (Figure 11.11). By 1907, Halsted was able to demonstrate the well known relationship between the staging of the tumour and its prognosis. In a series of 210 radical mastectomies, 60 patients had axillary nodes which were shown to be negative for tumour, and 85% of these were alive three years later. In 110 patients with axillary nodes involved, survival dropped to 31%; in 40 patients in whom both axillary and supraclavicular nodes were involved, the survival was only 10%. We have already noted, of course, that many of Halsted's so-called 'early cases' are what we would regard today as locally advanced tumours and it is not surprising, therefore, that there was an overall 64% death rate with local or distant recurrence within three years of mastectomy.

William Stewart Halsted was an extraordinary man. I have already described his contribution to aseptic surgical technique by the introduction of surgical gloves and his work on local anaesthesia (Chapter 7). He also made important advances in other fields: hernia surgery, intestinal anastomosis and a meticulous haemostatic method of operative surgery. However, he was unaware of the

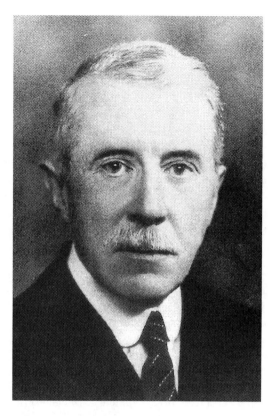

Figure 11.12 W Sampson Handley.
Royal College of Surgeons of England.

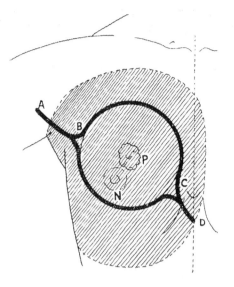

Figure 11.13 Sampson Handley's diagram of the area to be removed for adequate clearance in breast cancer.

habit-forming nature of cocaine and was weaned of his addiction to the drug only by reverting to morphine and was, for the rest of his life, an altered person, often in indifferent health. Harvey Cushing (1869–1939) (Figure 11.9), one of the fathers of neurosurgery, and Halsted's resident for three years in Baltimore, wrote after Halsted's death:

A man of unique personality, shy, something of a recluse, fastidious in his tastes and in his friendships, an aristocrat in his breeding, scholarly in his habits, the victim for many years of indifferent health, he nevertheless was one of the few American surgeons who may be considered to have established a school of surgery comparable, in a sense, to the school of Billroth in Vienna. He had few of the qualities supposed to accompany what the world regards as a successful surgeon. Over modest about his work, indifferent to matters of priority, caring little for the

gregarious gatherings of medical men, unassuming, having little interest in private practice, he spent his medical life avoiding patients – even students when this was possible – and, when health permitted, working in clinic and laboratory at the solution of a succession of problems which aroused his interest. He had that rare form of imagination which sees problems, and the technical ability combined with persistence which enabled him to attack them with promise of a successful issue. Many of his contributions, not only to his craft but to the science of medicine in general, were fundamental in character and of enduring importance.

At about this time, W Sampson Handley (1872–1962) (Figure 11.12) of the Middlesex Hospital, London, published his monograph on *Cancer of the Breast and its Operative Treatment*. His philosophy was to affect the therapy of breast cancer over the next half century and certainly deeply influenced Halsted. This was the cancer permeation hypothesis – that breast cancer spreads centrifugally, primarily in the plane of the subcutaneous tissues and along lymphatics (Figure 11.13). Blood spread was considered to be unimportant; bone spread occurred by way of the lymphatic plexus of the deep fascia, and even intra-abdominal spread was

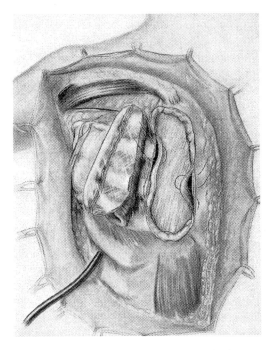

Figure 11.14 The chest-wall defect left by Urban's super-radical mastectomy.

From Urban JA: Radical mastectomy in continuity with en bloc resection of the internal mammary lymph node chain. *Cancer* 1952; 5, 992.

due to permeation along the sheath of the rectus muscle of the abdominal wall. It was this concept that led to the feeling that if only a sufficiently wide sweep could be made around the tumour the chances of a cure could be increased. Handley himself employed not only a very wide radical mastectomy but also, from 1920 onwards, implanted radium needles into the anterior intercostal spaces in order to deal with the internal mammary lymph nodes.

The apparent logical extension of these pathological findings was to attempt to increase the radicality of the radical mastectomy. Erling Dahl-Iverson (1892–1978) at the Rigshospitalet, Copenhagen, in 1951 performed an extrapleural dissection of the internal mammary nodes, as did Mario Margottini

(1897–1970) of the National Cancer Institute, Rome, the following year, while Owen Wangensteen (1898–1981) in Minneapolis advised splitting the sternum to remove the internal mammary nodes and dissection of the nodes above the clavicle. But it was Jerry Urban (1914–1991) at the Memorial Hospital, New York, who perfected a massive operation that combined radical mastectomy with en bloc resection of the internal mammary chain by removal of part of the sternum together with the inner ends of the second to the fifth rib and with repair of the resultant defect with fascia taken from the thigh. This operation took about five hours and required on average a three-pint blood transfusion (Figure 11.14).

So, for the first half of the 20th century, the concept of centrifugal spread of breast cancer held sway and with it the cult of radical mastectomy. Indeed, any progress seemed to depend on developing still more radical ablations of the breast and its surrounds. It has only been in comparatively recent years that the development of controlled clinical trials has shown that survival bears no relationship to the radicality of the surgeon. The permeation theory of spread of the tumour has long since been displaced by the realisation that it is blood-borne dissemination of the tumour that is the vitally important clue to prognosis. This in turn has made us realise that the answer to progress in breast cancer lies not with still more radical mastectomies but has two aims in mind: first, adequate control of the local disease and, second, the prevention or treatment of secondary spread of the tumour.

Even in those early days there were occasional pioneers, usually regarded as dangerous heretics, who were ready to try less mutilating procedures. Robert McWhirter (1904–1994) (Figure 11.15), Professor of Radiotherapy at the Edinburgh Royal Infirmary, treated a series of 757 patients between 1941 and 1945 by simple mastectomy followed by radiotherapy. He compared these cases with 411 patients treated by radical surgery together with post-operative radiotherapy between 1935 and 1940 and showed, if anything, that survival was

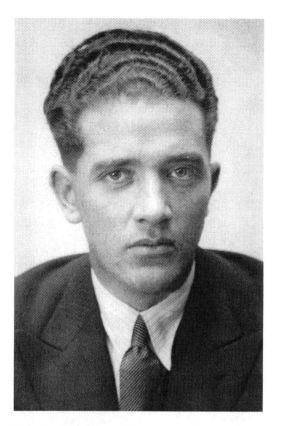

Figure 11.15 Robert McWhirter.
Royal College of Surgeons of England.

greater in the more conservatively treated group. I remember well, as a young surgeon, just not believing that anyone would dare not to do a radical mastectomy on a patient with breast cancer and, if he did, that he should have the temerity to claim that his results were at least no worse than could be obtained by the radical operation.

Meanwhile, David Patey (1899–1977), at the Middlesex Hospital, was experimenting with preservation of pectoralis major, except in those few cases where it was invaded by the tumour. In 1948 he reviewed his mastectomies performed between 1930 and 1943. Comparing his radical mastectomies with patients treated by his modified operation, now often called the Patey mastectomy, he

showed there was no difference in the survival rate or local recurrence rate between the two groups. Prophetically, he wrote:

Until an efficient general agent for the treatment of carcinoma of the breast is developed, a high proportion of cases are doomed to die of the disease whatever combination of local treatment by surgery and irradiation is used, because in such a high proportion of cases the disease has passed outside the field of local attack when the patient first comes for treatment.

Long before these clinical experiments, however, a still more unconventional form of treatment was being developed at St Bartholomew's Hospital, London. After the First World War, Geoffrey Keynes (1887–1982), who we have already met as a pioneer of blood transfusion (Chapter 9), returned to Bart's and investigated the use of the newly developed radium needles in the treatment of advanced and inoperable breast cancer. By 1927, he was able to report a five year experience in which he had shown that good local control of the disease could often be obtained. To quote his own words:

Having satisfied myself that radium could be used successfully when the disease was beyond surgery, I began to wonder whether it might not be used, perhaps in combination with conservative surgery, for treating cancer of the breast in its earlier stages. [Figure 11.16]

Keynes' results were entirely comparable with those obtained by mastectomy but unfortunately his work was interrupted by the outbreak of the Second World War, when he joined the Royal Air Force, and the supplies of radium were dispersed because of the dangers of air raids on London. Interestingly enough, after the war, a review of the late results of his cases showed that these were comparable to those obtained by radical surgery. However, of course, there was a significant gain in the quality of life of these patients (Figure 11.17).

Radiation therapy in the treatment of early breast cancer was pioneered at the Curie Institute in Paris around 1936. In recent years published results from many major centres have encouraged surgeons and radiotherapists around the world to

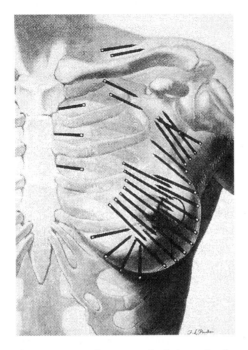

Figure 11.16 Geoffrey Keynes 'technique of radium implantation'.
From Keynes G: The radium treatment of carcinoma of the breast. *British Journal of Surgery* 1931–2; 19, 425.

(a)

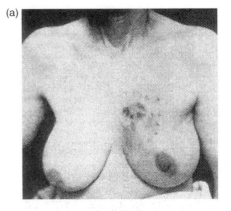

Fig. 312.—*Case* 1. Before excision of scar.

(b)

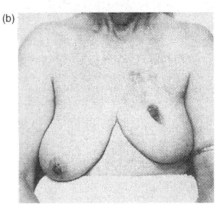

Figure 11.17 Patient treated by Keynes with radium implantation: (a) early result; (b) seven years after treatment.
From Keynes G: The radium treatment of carcinoma of the breast. *British Journal of Surgery* 1931–2; 19, 425.

use local excision of the tumour combined with radiotherapy as a substitute for mastectomy. The survival rate for women treated by this technique has been shown, in numerous trials, to be exactly comparable to that which is achieved by mastectomy, and this is not difficult to understand. Death from breast cancer results not from the local disease but from the effects of secondary spread of the tumour. Once the primary lesion has been controlled, whether this is by local excision, radiotherapy, or the most radical surgery that surgeons can devise, the patient's fate depends on whether or not sub-clinical dissemination of the disease had taken place before the primary lesion was removed. The means by which the tumour is treated locally can in no way decide this vital issue (Figure 11.18).

The treatment of the advanced disease

Breast cancer shares with prostatic tumours the strange phenomenon that, in many cases, the growth is sensitive to changes in the sex hormone environment. George Beatson (1848–1933) in Glasgow reported regression of advanced breast cancer in patients in whom he had removed the ovaries. Hugh Lett (1876–1964) of the London Hospital reviewed 99 patients thus treated; in spite

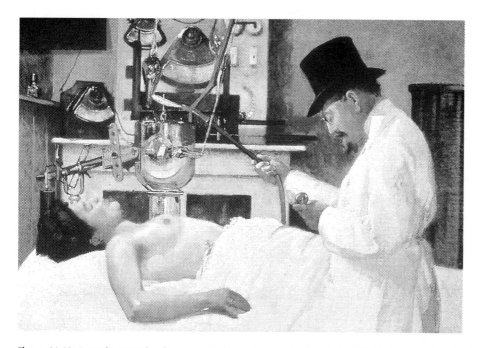

Figure 11.18 An early example of treatment of breast cancer by irradiation (1908). The French radiotherapist wears no protection from the X-rays. Many of these early pioneers, including Madame Marie Curie herself, developed serious complications which included skin cancer and aplastic anaemia.

of spectacular early response to oophorectomy in several, only one patient had a relatively long and complete response. The isolation of cortisone as replacement therapy allowed Charles Huggins (1901–1997) to perform bilateral removal of the suprarenal glands (adrenalectomy) together with oophorectomy in 1952. The rationale of this procedure is that, after removal of the ovaries, the suprarenal cortex is a source of the female sex hormone oestrogen. Huggins received the Nobel Prize in 1966, one of only nine surgeons ever to receive this award. Later, removal of the pituitary gland was employed. In large series of cases, regression of disseminated breast disease would be found in about a third of cases following these procedures, some with quite dramatic responses. In recent years, however, the development of new hormonal agents and of cytotoxic anti-cancer drugs has made these major surgical procedures obsolete.

12

Cutting for the stone

The three 'elective' operations (that is to say, those carried out for reasons other than the emergency care of wounds and injuries) performed from the earliest days of surgery were trephination of the skull, circumcision and cutting for the bladder stone. The first two were considered in Chapter 1, circumcision as a ritual, religious, fertility or initiation rite and trephination, certainly in many cases, performed for somewhat mystical reasons. Cutting for bladder stone may therefore safely be pronounced as the most ancient operation undertaken for the relief of a specific surgical condition.

The oldest bladder stone so far discovered was obtained from the grave of a boy aged about 16 years in the prehistoric cemetery at El Amrah in Upper Egypt and was dated at about 4800 BC. It was presented by its discoverer, Professor Elliot Smith, to the museum of the Royal College of Surgeons of England (Figure 12.1). Sad to relate, this unique specimen was destroyed when the college was bombed in 1941.

Descriptions of means to relieve the patient of the agonies of his bladder stone have come down to us in ancient writings. Indeed, specialists must have already been in existence in Ancient Greece in the 4th and 5th centuries BC since in the Hippocratic oath it is mentioned that the treatment of patients with stone is to be left in their hands. 'I will not covet persons labouring under the stone, but will leave this to be done by men who are practitioners of this work'.

There are three possible surgical approaches to remove a stone from the bladder: first by cutting down on to the base of the bladder through the perineum, immediately in front of the rectum; second by passing crushing instruments into the bladder along the urethra; and third by opening the bladder through the lower abdomen. Each of these approaches has a long history studded with both successes and failures.

Perineal lithotomy

Opening the bladder through the perineum to remove a bladder stone (*lithos*, stone, *otomy*, to make an opening into) was practised by the ancient Hindu surgeons, the Greeks, the Romans and the Arabians. Ammonius of Alexandria carried out the operation about 200 BC. The Roman encyclopaedist Celsus (25 BC–50 AD) gave an excellent description of the operation in the 1st century AD. He advised that the operation should only be performed on children between the ages of 9 and 14. Several days were first spent on a light or fasting diet. The patient was then instructed to walk and jump about so that the stone would descend to the neck of the bladder. The child was held in the lap of a strong and intelligent person who steadied the patient by pressing his chest against the child's shoulder blades (Figure 12.2). The operator stood or sat facing his patient and inserted two fingers of the left hand (well dipped in oil) into the anus. The right hand was pressed on the lower abdomen, pushing the bladder and thus forcing the stone into the grip of the left index finger within the rectum so as to produce

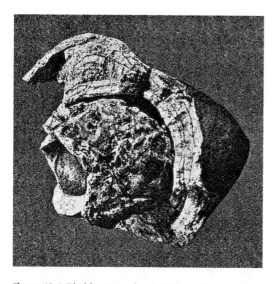

Figure 12.1 Bladder stone dated 4800 BC. The specimen was destroyed when the Hunterian Museum at the Royal College of Surgeons of England was severely damaged by a bomb in 1941.

a bulge in the perineum. An incision was made in front of the anus and carried deeply into the region of the bladder base; the stone was then pushed out by the finger in the rectum. It might be necessary at this stage to use a hook to dislodge the stone. The wound was then dressed with wool and warm oil (Figure 12.3).

The Hindu surgeon Susruta of Benares gave a good description of this operation. Unfortunately, there is still controversy concerning the period when he thrived and his works have been attributed to dates which range from the 6th century BC to the 6th century AD. His instructions were very similar to those of Celsus but he went into meticulous detail, such as that the surgeon should first ensure that his fingernails were closely cut. After extraction of the stone, the patient was to be placed in a bath of warm water and haemorrhage treated by irrigation of the bladder by means of a syringe.

This simple operation, which involved the use of no special instruments, merely a knife and perhaps a pair of forceps or a hook to help extract the stone,

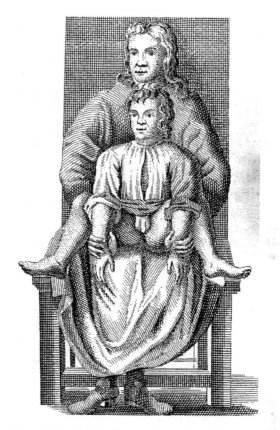

Figure 12.2 A child held in the lithotomy position. From Ellis H: *A History of Bladder Stone*. Oxford, Blackwell, 1969.

became known as the lesser operation or the apparatus minor. Anatomically, it involved opening the base of the bladder immediately above the prostate and it was for this reason that the operation was usually advised only for young boys, since these subjects would have only a small prostate gland.

About 1520, a new technique of lithotomy was introduced by the Italian surgeon Franciscus de Romanis of Cremona. This was published by his pupil, Marianus Sanctus (1490–1550), in 1522, so that the procedure came to be described as the Marian operation. It was also termed the greater operation or the apparatus major because of the additional instruments to be employed. The plan of

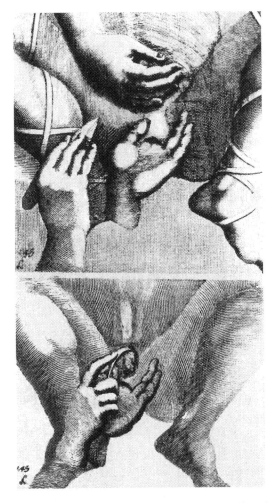

Figure 12.3 The operation of the apparatus minor; the only requirements were a knife and a hook.
From Ellis H: *A History of Bladder Stone*. Oxford, Blackwell, 1969.

the procedure was to pass a grooved staff into the bladder along the urethra and subsequently to cut down upon this instrument, so that yet another name for the operation was 'cutting on the staff'. A vertical incision was made in the mid-line onto a groove in the staff to open the urethra. This wound was then dilated, using a series of instruments which would tear through the prostate and bladder neck (Figure 12.4). Stone-holding forceps with two,

three or four blades were then passed into the wound to remove the stone, or, if this proved to be too large, it was first crushed with large forceps and the fragments removed with the scoop or hook. Those who survived the initial haemorrhage and sepsis were often incontinent of urine with persistent draining and infected sinuses, and impotence following the operation was not uncommon. It seems incredible to us in these days of smooth and potent anaesthetics that anyone could possibly submit himself willingly to such torture. It was, indeed, only the terrible and protracted agonies produced by stone in the bladder that gave men sufficient courage to place themselves under the lithotomist's cruel instruments. Once the patient consented to the operation, there was then the problem, of course, of keeping him still enough to be cut for the stone. This usually meant trussing him up and using three or four strong assistants to hold him still (Figure 12.5). The old surgical writers describe in depth the care and precautions in binding and holding the patient in the lithotomy position. Thus the great Ambroise Paré, in 1575, wrote:

The patient shall be placed upon a firm table or bench with a cloth many times doubled under his buttocks, and a pillow under his loynes and back, so that he may lie halfe upright with his thighs lifted up and his legs and heels drawn back to his buttocks. Then shall his feet be bound with a ligature of three fingers breadth passed about his ankles, and with the heads thereof being drawn upwards to his neck, and cast about it, and so brought downewards, both his hands shall bee bound to his knees. The patient thus bound, it is fit you have foure strong men at hand; that is, two to hold his armes, and other two who may so firmely and straightly hold the knee with one hand, and the foot with the other, that he may neither move his limmes nor stirre his buttocks but be forced to keep the same posture with his whole body.

Could it be that the tradition that has died so hard in our medical schools of selecting students for their ability on the rugby field stems from the days when it was probably necessary to choose one's young assistants for brawn equally well as brain?

The next step in the history of lithotomy is perhaps one of the strangest; it concerns the

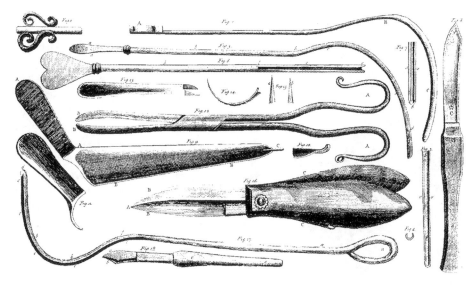

Figure 12.4 The instruments for the operation of the apparatus major.
From Heister L: *General System of Surgery*. London, 5th English edition, 1753.

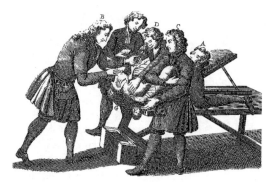

Figure 12.5 The surgeon and his three assistants for the apparatus major operation. The patient is in the lithotomy position. The surgeon's instruments are conveniently at hand in his waist pouch.
From Heister L: *General System of Surgery*. London, 5th English edition, 1753.

development of the lateral perineal approach to the bladder by a medically unqualified Frenchman of humble origin. Jacques Beaulieu was born in 1651, the son of poor peasants, at Beaufort in Burgundy. He was perhaps inspired to surgery when as a boy he fell ill and while in hospital did all he could to

help other patients and begged to be taught how to bleed. After serving in the cavalry as a trooper, he left the army at the age of 21 and became apprenticed to an itinerant Italian surgeon, Pauloni, who cut for the stone. In 1690 he changed his name to Frère Jacques (Figure 12.6), adopted the habit of a monk (although he never trained for the church), and in turn became an itinerant lithotomist. In 1697, at the age of 46, he arrived in Paris and applied for permission to cut for the stone. The surgeons at the Hôtel Dieu ordered that he first demonstrate his skill on a cadaver in whom a stone had been introduced into the bladder via the abdomen. He passed a solid grooveless metal staff into the bladder, then incised the perineum two fingers medial to the tuber ischii, carrying the cut forward from the side of the anus. The stone was felt by a finger in the wound, a dilator was passed into the bladder and the stone removed by forceps. Subsequent dissection by Méry, surgeon to the Hôtel Dieu, revealed that the incision had passed between the ischio-cavernosus and the bulbo-cavernosus muscles, then through the prostate and the whole length of the neck of the bladder and

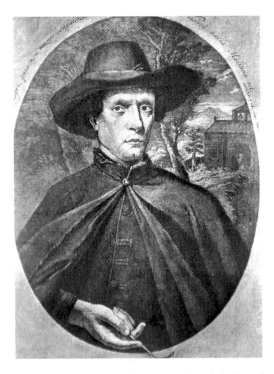

Figure 12.6 Frère Jacques. He wears a priest's habit and carries a bladder sound. This portrait hangs in the Royal College of Surgeons of England.

thence half an inch into the bladder itself. In spite of the satisfactory operation, the Board refused to grant a licence; this was probably because Frère Jacques paid no attention to the ritual of pre-operative bleeding or purging, and used no astrin-gents, but stated that he relied instead on God to heal the wound. Lateral lithotomy, even in this crude form, was safer than the mid-line procedure in adults, since it gave wider access with less tissue trauma. Moreover, the pre- and post-operative treatment used by others at this time probably did more harm than complete conservatism!

Frère Jacques, his licence refused, travelled to Fontainebleau where the court was in residence. Here he was allowed to operate on a shoe-maker with a stone in the bladder. Cure was obtained within three weeks, and Louis XIV was so impressed that he gave instructions that Frère Jacques be lodged with the Royal valet and be given the King's Licence to practise. A short period of success fol-lowed, with its inevitable popularity, so that a guard of soldiers was required to keep the mass of spec-tators who crowded round in some sort of order. However, a series of disasters then befell the surgeon. From April to July 1698 he carried out lithotomies in the Hôtel Dieu and at the Charité: of these 60 patients, 13 were cured and the rest remained in hospital with incontinence, fistulae or other com-plications. No less than seven died in one day at the Charité so that Frère Jacques was actually driven to accusing the monks of poisoning his patients. Post-mortem, however, revealed no evidence of poison but did demonstrate bladders cut through in many places, the rectum injured, the urethra cut off from the bladder base, the vagina lacerated or major arteries divided.

That year Frère Jacques left Paris and resumed his wanderings through France and Holland. Even-tually he returned to Versailles, where he collabo-rated with Fagon, Surgeon to the King, and from whom he probably learned some much needed anatomy. Experiments were carried out on many bodies, as a result of which the original operation was modified and a grooved staff employed; 38 operations were performed at Versailles in 1701 without a death – a remarkable record (Figure 12.7). Fagon was not dispassionate in his interest in this procedure since he himself laboured under a stone in the bladder. His faith in Frère Jacques was demonstrated by his request that his colleague should remove his stone. This was forbidden by the family and the operation was eventually performed by Marechal.

Another crisis occurred in 1703 when he was consulted by the Marechal de Lorges, a cautious man, who first watched Frère Jacques operate upon 22 poor patients, all of whom survived, before submitting himself to lithotomy. All was in vain, since the Marechal succumbed after surgery. Yet again Frère Jacques took to the road, to Amsterdam, Brussels, Geneva, Nancy, Liège, Strasbourg, Vienna, Venice, Padua and Rome. His practice was by no means unsuccessful and he retired to his native

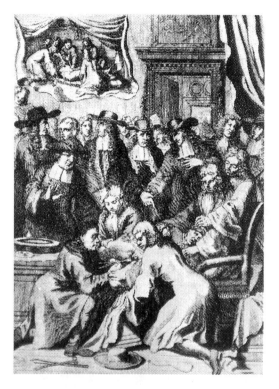

Figure 12.7 Frère Jacques operating.
From Desnos E: *Histoire de L'Urologie*. Paris, Doin, 1914.

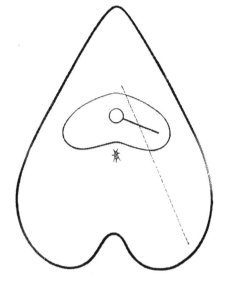

Figure 12.9 The incision in the perineum advised by
Sir Henry Thompson for lithotomy. The dotted line
represents the skin incision and the continuous line the
cut through the base of the prostate. This differs little from
the approach used by Cheselden some 200 years earlier.
From Thompson H: *Practical Lithotomy and Lithotrity*.
London, Churchill, 1863.

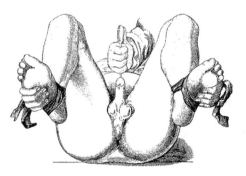

Figure 12.8 Patient in the lithotomy position with sound in
place. The position identical to that used by the early
lithotomists was still employed in the 19th century.
From Thompson H: *Practical Lithotomy and Lithotrity*.
London, Churchill, 1863.

village at 69, dying there in 1714 a wealthy man, and
leaving most of his money to various charities. This
remarkable surgeon is said to have operated upon
4500 patients for bladder stone and another 2000
for hernia.

The operation of Frère Jacques was taken up and
modified by William Cheselden (1688–1752) who was
certainly the greatest lithotomist produced in England, if not in the world, and who we have already met
in Chapter 6 (see Figure 6.10). An expert anatomist,
he made careful dissections and clearly describes
the surgical anatomy of the lateral operation:

This operation I do in the following manner: I tie the
patient as for the greater apparatus, but lay him upon a
blanket several doubles upon an horizontal table three
feet high, with his head only raised [Figure 12.8]. I first
make as long an incision as I can [Figure 12.9] beginning
near the place where the old operation ends, cutting down
between the musculus accelerator urinae and erector

penis and by the side of the intestinum rectum colon. I then feel for the staff, holding down the gut all the while with one or two fingers of my left hand and cut upon it in that part of the urethra which lies beyond the corpora cavernosa urethrae and in the prostate gland cutting from below upwards, to avoid wounding the gut; and then passing the gorget very carefully in the groove of the staff into the bladder, bear the point of the gorget hard against the staff, observing all the while that they do not separate and let the gorget slip to the outside of the bladder; then I pass the forceps into the right side of the bladder, the wound being on the left side of the perinaeum; and as they pass, carefully attend to their entering the bladder, which is known by their overcoming a straightness which there will be in the place of the wound; then taking care to push them no further so that the bladder may not be hurt, I first feel for the stone with the end of them, which having felt, I open the forceps and slide one blade underneath it and the other at the top; and if I apprehend the stone is not in the right place in the forceps, I shift it before I offer to extract, and then extract it very deliberately so that it may not slip suddenly out of the forceps, and that the parts of the wound may have time to stretch, taking great care not to grip it so hard as to break it and if I find the stone very large, I again cut upon it as it is held in the forceps. Here I must take notice, it is very convenient to have the bladder empty of urine before the operation, and if there is any quantity to flow out of the bladder at the passing in of the gorget, the bladder does not contract, but collapses into folds, which makes it difficult to lay hold of the stone without hurting the bladder, but if the bladder is con- tracted it is so easy to lay hold of it that I have never been delayed one moment, unless the stone was very small. Lastly, I tie the blood vessels with the help of a crooked needle, and use no other dressing than a little bit of lint besmeared with blood, that it may not stick too long in the wound, and all the dressings during the cure are very slight, almost superficial, and without any bandage to retain them; because that will be wetted with urine and gall the skin. At first I keep the patient very cool to prevent bleeding, and sometimes apply a rag, dipped in cold water to the wound, and to the genital parts, which I have found very useful in hot weather particularly. In children it is often alone sufficient to stop the bleeding, and always helpful in men. The day before the operation I give a purge to empty the gut and never neglect to give a laxative medicine, or clyster a few days after, if the belly is at all tense, or if they have not a natural stool.

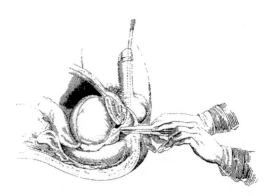

Figure 12.10 Thompson's illustration of lateral lithotomy. The original subtitle reads 'Anatomy of parts interested in lithotomy. Mr Bagg has represented this very carefully for me from a dissection made expressly for the purpose'. From Thompson H: *Practical Lithotomy and Lithotrity*. London, Churchill, 1863.

Cheselden published the following figures: '213 patients cut at St Thomas' Hospital, of the first fifty only three died. Of the second fifty, three; of the third fifty, eight; and of the last sixty-three, six. Several of these patients had the smallpox during their cure, some of whom died, and these are not reckoned among those who had the operation.' The reason why so few died in the two first fifties, Cheselden explained, was that at that time very few bad cases were offered the operation, whereas later, the operation being in great demand, even the most aged and most miserable cases expected to be saved by it. Cheselden ends this remarkable document by saying:

If I have any reputation in this way I have earned it dearly, for no one ever endured more anxiety and sickness before an operation, yet from the time I began to operate, all uneasiness ceased; and if I have had better success than some others, I do not impute it to more knowledge but to the happiness of mind that was never ruffled or discon- certed, and a hand that never trembled during an operation.

Right up to the 20th century perineal lithotomy was still being performed (Figure 12.10), in later years, of course, with the benefit of general anaesthesia.

Suprapubic lithotomy

The suprapubic approach to the bladder via a low mid-line abdominal incision, with the bladder distended to push away the peritoneum, is the usual open method employed in the removal of bladder stone today. It combines simplicity with the advantage that any associated abnormality within the bladder can be dealt with at the same time. Its story goes back over 400 years.

The first recorded operation of this kind was carried out by Pierre Franco (?1500–1561). As a Protestant, he was forced to flee from France and practised his calling in Lausanne in Switzerland, although he eventually returned to Orange in France to practise. In the year of his death he gave an account of an operation on a child of about three years of age who had a stone in the bladder the size of a hen's egg. He was unable to remove the stone via the perineal approach because the enormous stone could not be pushed down into the neck of the bladder. The child's parents begged him to try to relieve the small patient of his sufferings so he therefore pushed the stone up into the groin with his fingers in the rectum, got his assistant to fix the stone in this situation and then cut down immediately above the pubis into the calculus. The little patient recovered, but Franco advised others not to follow his example! Most surgeons did, indeed, take his advice and that of Hippocrates before him, who stated that wounds of the bladder were invariably fatal. Other objections raised to the high operation, as it was called, were that urine from the bladder would flow into the abdominal cavity, that an incision into the bladder would not heal, and that intestines would prolapse through the abdominal wound. Indeed, it was not until the 18th century that Johann Bonnet was reported to have carried out the suprapubic operation frequently and with success at the Hôtel Dieu in Paris.

The third surgeon to operate with success was Jan Groenvelt, a Dutch surgeon who settled in London, changed his name to Greenfield and, in 1710, wrote:

I once had a patient in Long Lane Moorfields, upon whom I was obliged to perform this high operation and very successfully extracted the stone making the incision near the groin, the patient soon recovering; which shows that wounds in the fibrous part of the bladder are not always mortal.

James Douglas, who described the pelvic peritoneal pouch that now carries his name, studied the anatomy of the surgical approaches to the bladder in 1717. His brother, John Douglas (died c. 1742), realised that the bladder could be opened extraperitoneally above the pubis when in the distended state, carried out the operation in 1719 and published a book on the subject in 1720 that rejoiced in the title of *Lithotomia Douglassiana, or an account of a new method of making a high operation in order to extract the stone out of the bladder. This is much easier to the patient, much sooner done by the operator and the cure more certain than after any of the other methods now in use. By which also several of the most dismal consequences of the common operations are entirely prevented, such as incontinency of urine, impotency, fistulae, etc. invented and successfully performed by John Douglas, surgeon.*

Douglas fully reviewed published accounts, both for and against, that preceded his own work, then detailed his suprapubic approach into the distended bladder. He writes:

My patient was between 15 and 17 years of age and was cut two days before last Christmas and in a month's time the wound was perfectly Sicatrize'd, (i.e. healed). The operation was over in one minute and I believe will never be above two.

He now performs all his natural faculties as well as he had never been troubled with the stone. There were two physicians, two surgeons, and an apothecary present at the operation but to save them the trouble of answering every little prig's impertinent question I don't think it is proper to mention them.

The stone is illustrated in Douglas' book and measured about two inches by one and a half inches. Advantages of this new operation as listed by Douglas were: avoidance of impotence, incontinence and fistula, no excessive loss of blood because there was no occasion to cut any of the great vessels, and no considerable force being required to extract the stone because the incision could be made as large as necessary.

Three of the first four patients operated upon by Douglas recovered safely.

Douglas, who had dedicated his monograph to the trustees and medical staff of the Westminster Infirmary, offered his services to that institution on 21st November 1721, and they were gratefully accepted; he became consultant surgeon and the first lithotomist on its staff. At his own expense he got the trustees of the Infirmary to publish the following advertisement on 7th March 1722:

Notice is hereby given to the poor troubled with stone in the bladder that they will be received at the Infirmary in Petty France, Westminster, in order to there cure at all seasons of the year, without any other recommendation than a certificate under the hand of Mr John Douglas, surgeon, in Fetter Lane, Lithotomist to the said Infirmary.

A short but brilliant period of fame now fell to Douglas. He was elected Fellow of the Royal Society in January 1722 and given the Freedom of the Company of Barber Surgeons the following year. Mr John Trustram, clerk to the Worshipful Company of Barbers, has kindly sent me this extract from the Company's minutes of 26th April 1723:

It is ordered that Mr John Douglas Surgeon and fforeigne brother of this Company shall be admitted into the freedom and Livery of this Company and be discharged and acquitted from holding or paying any fine for his freedom or Livery, or for all or any offices to the Parlour door as a Compliment to him for introducing the new method of Cutting for the Stone and to express the sense this Court hath of the usefullness thereof.

In 1724, Douglas was made Freeman of the City of London. However, as we shall soon see, the high operation fell into disfavour, and in that same year he was replaced by Cheselden as lithotomist to Westminster.

The high operation was taken up with enthusiasm by William Cheselden in 1722 and he described the procedure in detail in his *Treatise on the High Operation for the Stone* published in 1723. In this he carefully illustrated how the bladder,

when distended with water, strips the peritoneum above the pubis, thus allowing itself to be opened extraperitoneally (Figure 12.11). To fill the bladder he devised an ingenious syringe attached to a metal catheter by a length of ox's ureter. Before operation the bowel was emptied by ordering a slender diet for about two days, and clysters (enemas) were given a little before the operation. The patient was lain on the bed or on a quilt placed upon a table, with his legs off the bed and his thighs raised. A catheter was passed and as much barley water as would fill the bladder to its utmost distension was injected. An assistant grasped the penis to prevent reflux of water, the catheter was withdrawn and the assistant continued to compress the urethra. The first incision was made with a round-edged knife through skin and fat and continued between the recti down to the bladder. A four inch incision was advised in the adult. The bladder was then exposed with a straight scalpel and opened by means of a crooked knife while the water flowed out of the incision. A finger was introduced into the bladder incision, along which a very thin forceps was directed in order to seize the stone. The wound was dressed with soft compresses, kept on with a loose bandage and changed every six hours until urine ceased to discharge.

Cheselden reports on nine patients cut in this way. All were male, with ages varying from 4 to 19 years. There was only one death – John Clark, of Braintree of Essex, aged 18, who was cut on 12th July 1722 and had two large stones removed. He developed a hectic fever followed by diarrhoea and died 25 days post-operatively. At post-mortem the wound and bladder were healthy but the right kidney contained four ounces of pus and ten stones, with, in addition, one very large stone in the ureter on the same side.

Only a year after the publication of his book, however, Cheselden was no longer enthusiastic for the abdominal operation and he returned to his work on improving the perineal lithotomy as already described. No doubt this was as the result of disasters and near disasters in his own and other hands in which the peritoneum was opened,

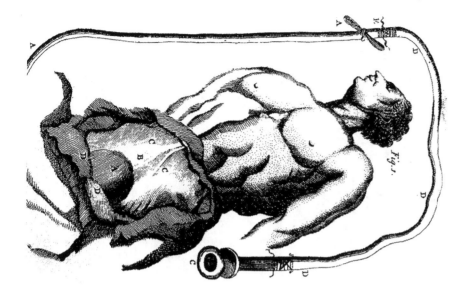

Figure 12.11 Cheselden's dissection to demonstrate that the distended bladder (A) extends extraperitoneally above the pubis. Illustrated also is his catheter (V) with its attached length of ox ureter (D). From Cheselden W: *Treatise on the High Operation for Stone*. London, 1723.

intestine prolapsed and was returned only with difficulty or even lacerated, and sometimes the bladder itself burst from injecting too much water.

In 1737, at the very height of his fame, Cheselden retired from all his previous hospital appointments and became resident surgeon to the Royal Hospital, Chelsea, home, of course, of the Chelsea Pensioners. He died in 1752, his rather sudden death being attributed to drinking ale after eating hot buns. His tomb can be seen to this day in the grounds of the Royal Hospital.

By 1850, Murray Humphry, of Addenbrooke's Hospital, Cambridge, in performing a successful suprapubic operation on a boy of 14, could collect only 104 published cases of this procedure, of which no less than 31 were fatal. The majority had been performed for very large stones.

It was not until the end of the 19th century, corresponding to the blooming of abdominal surgery in general, that the suprapubic operation began to become the routine and safe procedure it is today. For this to happen, the two great boons of modern surgery – anaesthesia and asepsis – were required.

Transurethral lithotrity

Throughout the centuries, patients teased by the agonies of bladder stone and surgeons dissatisfied with the difficulties and dangers of cutting for the stone dreamed of some means of removing the calculus through the natural passage from the bladder – the urethra. The ancient Egyptians would dilate the urethra by means of a wooden tube the thickness of the thumb, pushed in with considerable force alternating with blowing down the urethra. The stone was pressed against the tube by fingers in the rectum and sucked out. Whether this succeeded or not is a matter of conjecture. A number of patients experimented on themselves; one introduced a long nail into his bladder, impinged the end upon the stone and struck hard with a blacksmith's hammer to split it. General

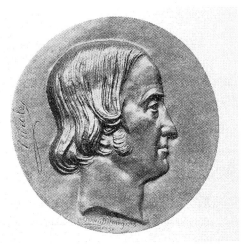

Figure 12.12 Jean Civiale; medallion by David d'Angers.

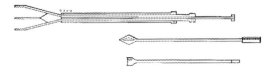

Figure 12.13 Civiale's trilabe. The stone was caught between the three blades and then drilled.
From Ellis H: *A History of Bladder Stone.* Oxford, Blackwell, 1969.

Martin of Lucknow disintegrated the stone in his bladder in 1783 by nine months of steady work using a fine curved file. Sir Astley Cooper, of Guy's Hospital, described how he removed multiple small stones from the bladder, a total of 84, from an elderly priest at repeated sittings using specially designed fine curved forceps.

Over the years, a number of surgeons experimented on corpses using crushing instruments passed along a hollow tube introduced into the bladder, but it remained for a brilliant young surgeon in Paris to carry out the first successful operation in man – surely the historical beginning of minimal access surgery!

Jean Civiale (1792–1867) (Figure 12.12) had already commenced a series of experiments in 1817, when he was still only a second year medical student under Baron Dupuytren in the University of Paris, in an effort to ascertain whether it was possible to crush stone in the bladder without injuring its walls. To him falls the honour of performing the first successful lithotrity, on 13th January 1824, at the Necker Hospital in Paris. Civiale's instrument, the trilabe (Figure 12.13), consisted of two metal cylinders, one within the other, the smaller of which had three branches fixed on its distal end by means of hinges. The inner tube was projected into the bladder, manipulated to seize the stone, and then withdrawn into the outer tube so that its branches fixed upon the stone, which was then perforated by a gimlet. Numerous modifications were made over the next few years (Figure 12.14). Several sittings were required to break up the calculus, which was then passed *per via natura* in the urine.

Baron Charles Louis Stanislas Heurteloup (1793–1864), who became a violent antagonist of Civiale, designed a rather similar instrument called the 'perce-pierre' in which he hollowed out the stone instead of making numerous separate perforations into it (Figure 12.15). Heurteloup travelled from France to England in 1829, lived in Vere Street in London, and was the first to perform lithotrity in this country. The first patient he treated in England was a Mr Wattie, a former seaman aged 64 years, of Upper Ebury Street, Pimlico, who had two calculi destroyed in three sessions on 24th and 25th July and 20th August 1929, using the 'perce-pierre'. The operation was performed in the house of Mr Anthony White, Surgeon to Westminster Hospital. In 1831 Heurteloup published *Cases of lithotrity, or examples of the stone cured without incision* in English.

There now ensued a period of tremendous inventiveness and ingenuity on the part of surgeons and surgical instrument makers; gradually the crushing lithotrite as we know it today was developed, the work being principally carried out by surgeons in France and Great Britain. Eventually the modern instrument was evolved (Figure 12.16) in which the stone, caught between the jaws of the instrument, would be crushed by turning a screw.

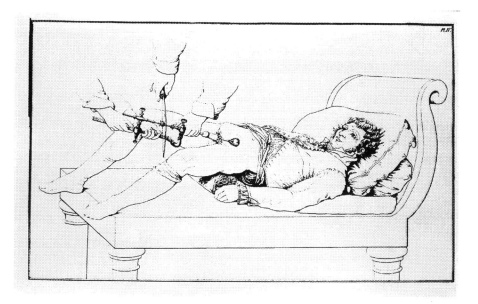

Figure 12.14 'Un malade au moment de l'operation.' The calculus is trapped in the jaws of the trilabe and is being drilled by a gimlet activated by a bow.
From Civiale J: *Traité Pratique et Historique de la Lithotritie*. Paris, Baillière, 1847.

Surgeons became extremely skilled in the use of these instruments and countless patients were, in consequence, relieved of their sufferings.

The surgeon today has a choice of techniques in dealing with a stone in the bladder. He may use the open abdominal approach, especially if there is some co-existent bladder pathology that requires treatment. He may use a lithotrite, but now he need no longer call upon the exquisite sense of touch of his predecessors, who learned how to manipulate the calculus blindly between the crushing blades of the instrument within the bladder. Modern technology allows the surgeon to do this under direct vision by means of a fibre-optic illuminated viewing system. Finally, the stone may be disintegrated within the bladder using a shock wave ultrasonic beam, the fragments of stone being removed with a bladder irrigator.

One of the intriguing mysteries of bladder stone is its frequency throughout medical history of the past and yet its rarity in Europe today. Old surgical writings abound with descriptions of large numbers of victims of the stone, especially children; indeed a common cause of crying in infants at night listed in the old textbooks was bladder stone – hardly the first thing a modern paediatrician would consider! Bladder stone has virtually disappeared from the children's hospitals in this country. Ridley Thomas analysed the total incidence of vesical calculus and its frequency at different age groups at the Norfolk and Norwich Hospital, using three 10-year periods – 1871–1880, 1901–1910 and 1929–1938; in addition he gave the figures for the five years 1943–1947. Figure 12.17 which is based on these statistics, shows vividly how the frequency of both total and infant bladder stone has dropped remarkably in living memory.

Bladder stone is now extremely rare in northern Europe, although it is occasionally seen in southern parts of Europe, such as Sicily and Greece. However it persists as a major problem in Turkey, India and China.

One might attribute the high incidence of stone in adults in the past to the ravages of untreated or

(a)

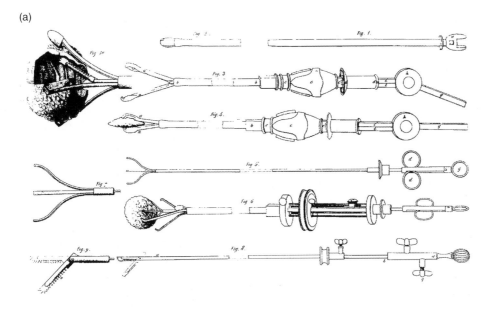

(b)

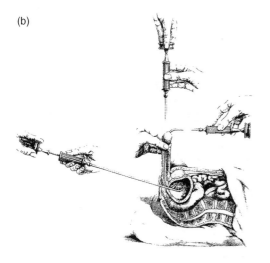

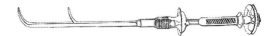

Figure 12.16 Lithotrite used by Sir Henry Thompson and made by Charrière.

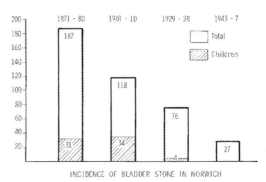

INCIDENCE OF BLADDER STONE IN NORWICH

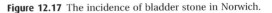

Figure 12.15 Baron Charles Heurteloup's instruments: (a) on display; (b) in use.
From Heurteloup C: *Cases of Lithotrity or Examples of the Stone Cured without Incision*. London, Underwood, 1831.

Figure 12.17 The incidence of bladder stone in Norwich.

badly treated urinary obstruction from stricture of the urethra and enlargement of the prostate, together with superadded infection. However, the epidemic proportions of the disease in those days suggest some other factor, perhaps dietary, which is not yet fully understood.

Bladder stone was no respecter of social position – kings or their poorest subjects, generals or their humblest troopers, savants or their idlest students, all might fall victim to its ravages; famous patients with definite or putative bladder calculi fill the pages of history. The philosopher Francis Bacon, scientist Isaac Newton, physicians William Harvey and Hermann Boerhaave, the anatomist Antonio Scarpa, the writer Horace Walpole, Peter the Great, Louis XIV, George IV and Oliver Cromwell have all been said to have had bladder stone. Thomas Sydenham (1626–1689), who started his career fighting with the Puritan Army in the Civil War and who rose to become the 'Prince of Practical Physicians', suffered from stone. He wrote with personal feeling when he described the symptoms thus: 'He suffers until at last he is worn out by the joint attack of age and disease, and the miserable wretch is so happy as to die'.

Surely the best known stone is that of Samuel Pepys, who suffered from the calculus from infancy. 'I remember not my life without the pain of the stone in the kidneys (even to the making of bloody water upon any extraordinary motion) until I was about twenty years of age.' There seemed to be a family tendency for the disease; his mother voided a large stone which, to his disappointment, she threw into the fire. An aunt also passed a calculus and his brother John at Cambridge 'hath the pain of the stone and makes bloody water with great pain in the beginning just as mine did'.

At the age of 20, while a student at Trinity Hall, Cambridge, in the summer of 1653, Pepys had a violent attack of renal colic. This he attributes to a long walk with his friends to Aristotle's well, where they slaked their thirsts with great draughts of cold water. It appears that following this attack the calculus passed from the kidney to the bladder and

henceforth he was to be subject to violent attacks of vesical pain.

In spite of this, his courting abilities remained apparently unaffected, and he married Elizabeth St Michel on 1st December 1655.

The cold weather always aggravated Pepys' sufferings and the particularly bad winter of 1658 brought matters to a head; it was obvious that surgery had now become inevitable. He was cut for the stone by Thomas Hollier (1609–1690) of St Thomas' Hospital, on 26 March 1658 at the home of his cousin, Mrs Jane Turner, being fortified for the procedure by a draught containing liquorice, marshmallow, cinnamon, milk, rose water and white of eggs. The stone was the size of a tennis ball, weighed about two ounces and apparently was composed mainly of urates.

Fortunately this was a successful year for Hollier, since, of the 30 patients cut for the stone during those 12 months, all lived, but Hollier was not always so successful; indeed, in September 1659, Pepys attended the Jewish synagogue and there heard 'many lamentations made by Portugal Jews for the death of Ferdinando the merchant who was lately cut by the same hand with myself of the stone'.

His delivery from his calculus was a turning point in Samuel's life and left a deep impression. In after years he gave a dinner each 26th March to those who had stood by him on that momentous day; 'my solemn feast for the cutting of the stone', he called it. The stone itself was carefully preserved and in 1664 Pepys went 'to look out a man to make a case for to keep my stone, that I was cut of in 1658'. This cost twenty-five shillings and was duly produced whenever any of his friends needed encouragement to undergo a similar operation.

Benjamin Franklin, although not formally trained as a physician, was particularly interested in medicine and indeed invented the flexible catheter. Towards the end of his long life (he died at the age of 84), he remarked 'only three incurable diseases have fallen to my share, viz, gout, the stone, and old age'. Symptoms of bladder stone appeared in his middle seventies and in 1784, when he was 78, he wrote:

It is true as you have heard that I have the stone, but not that I had thoughts of being cut for it. It is as yet very tolerable. It gives me no pain but in a carriage, on a pavement, or when I make some quick movement. If I can prevent its growing larger, which I hope to do, by abstemious living and gentle exercise I can go on pretty comfortably with it to the end of my journey which can now be of no great distance.

Unfortunately, in spite of all sorts of remedies, the symptoms did indeed progress so that the following year Franklin wrote that he was 'disabled by the stone, which in the easiest carriage gives me pain, wounds my bladder and occasions me to make bloody urine'. By the end of the autumn of 1789 he was 'afflicted with almost constant and grievious pain to combat which I have been obliged to recourse to opium, which indeed has afforded me some ease from time to time, but then it has taken away my appetite, and so impeded my digestion that I am become totally emaciated and little remains of me but a skeleton covered with skin'.

Although he was advised by his friends to be cut for the stone he refused their advice and he died, bed-bound, as a result of pneumonia complicated by a lung abscess.

Napoleon Bonaparte suffered with urinary frequency and dysuria for many years. The fact that he would often sleep for no more than two to three hours at a time was attributed by Constant, his valet, not to any superhuman power but to the desire to get up and pass his water. At the battle of Borodino in the Russian Campaign of 1812 he had to dismount from his horse frequently; he had persistent thirst, swelling of the legs and great difficulty passing his urine, which was no less than one third sediment. Further attacks of dysuria occurred in later years. In exile on St Helena he had difficulty with micturition and was seen at times leaning with his head against a wall or tree and passing urine in small, painful dribbles. 'This is my weak spot, it is by this that I shall die.'

The post-mortem following Napoleon's death at the age of 51 on 5th May, 1821, was carried out by Dr Dominique Antommarchi in the presence of sixteen others. As well as a scirrhous ulcer of the stomach, adherent to the left lobe of the liver, and a hepatomegaly, Antommarchi reported that 'The bladder, which was empty and much contracted, contained a certain quantity of gravel, mixed with some small calculi. Numerous red spots were scattered upon its mucous membrane, and the coats of the organ were in a diseased state.'

Who can say to what extent history has been altered by these strange concretions of the bladder? Who can say what might have happened in the Russian Campaign in 1812 if modern surgical skill had been available in those days, to relieve Napoleon of his stones? How many personalities have been altered, decisions changed, judgements affected or genius thwarted by the torturing pains, the chronic sepsis and uraemic renal damage resulting from bladder stone?

On the other hand, without this strange centuries-long epidemic of bladder stone, how far might the progress of surgery have been delayed? After all, it was upon this pathology that the art of surgery evolved, from the first primitive cuts into the perineum up to the sophisticated instrumentation of the lithotritists and to some of the earliest assays on the surgical breaching of the abdominal cavity.

Bladder stone will no doubt eventually die out, to become a surgical rarity throughout the world, just as it has already done in this country. Its countless victims through the ages, however, might derive some post-mortem satisfaction from the thought that their sufferings have contributed in some small way to the progress and good of humanity.

13

Thyroid and parathyroid

The thyroid gland was known to Galen, who thought it produced fluid to lubricate the larynx. It was described by Vesalius (1514–1564), who called it the glandulae laryngis and agreed with Galen about its function. It was named the thyroid (Greek *thyreos*, shield) by Thomas Wharton (1614–1673) of London (who also described the duct of the submandibular salivary gland), who believed it was designed by Nature to give women a beautifully rounded neck! Astley Cooper (1768–1841) (see Figure 6.26) appears to have been the first to believe that the organ performed some definite function. He noted the large lymphatics which passed from it to the thoracic duct and postulated that they conveyed the secretion from the gland.

Enlargement of the thyroid gland produced such an obvious physical change in the neck that it has been observed since early times. Old names applied to such a swelling were struma (Latin for a swollen gland), bronchocele (a cystic mass in the neck) and goitre (from the Latin *gutta*, throat); this last term is often used today.

One common cause of thyroid enlargement is iodine deficiency. Iodine is found in sea water and it is not surprising that iodine deficient areas in the world are far removed from the sea and particularly occur in elevated inland zones. Goitre is said to have been known in China as far back as 2700 BC, where it was found in mountainous regions. As long ago as the 4th century AD, Chinese physicians recommended the use of seaweed for this condition and, of course, seaweed is rich in iodine. In the United Kingdom, Derbyshire is as far away from the sea as one can get, and as a young resident surgical officer in Sheffield, the author became well acquainted with 'Derbyshire neck', so named in the 18th century. Medical visitors to Northern India, Nepal and to the Ethiopian highlands will be struck by the high incidence of large thyroid masses, and this was certainly my experience as examiner many years ago in the University of Addis Ababa and also in visits to Nepal for the British Council. Although goitre was not common along the shores of the Mediterranean, it was well recognised even by non-medical Roman authors to be a feature of residents in the Alps; thus Juvenal, in the 1st century AD wrote 'Who wonders at a swelling in the neck in the Alps? ' Celsus, also in the 1st century AD, defined bronchocele and described cystic goitre in mountainous regions. Goitre was so common in Switzerland that it is often seen in paintings and statues from that country. Indeed, a standard technique to kill a Swiss prisoner was to slit open his goitre (Figure 13.1). Here, as in other civilised areas, iodine deficient goitre has been all but abolished by iodination of table salt but it was in Switzerland that so much of the surgery of the thyroid gland, as we shall see, was developed. In the United States goitre was endemic in the mid West and it is to this that we owe the expertise in thyroid surgery of the Mayo brothers of Rochester, Minnesota, and of George Crile in Cleveland, Ohio.

Shakespeare gives a characteristically concise description of goitre and its geographical association:

When we were boys,
Who would believe that there were mountaineers,
Dewlapp'd like bulls, whose throats had hanging at 'em
Wallets of flesh?

(*The Tempest* III.3, 43–47.)

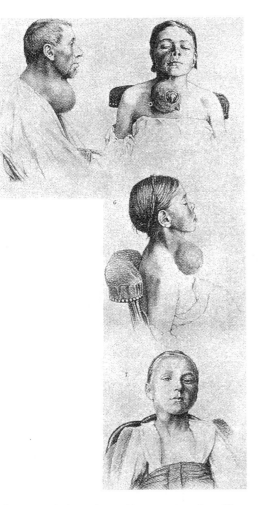

Figure 13.1 Swiss patients with enormous goitres. The thyroid mass of the girl on the right has ulcerated through the skin. The lowermost picture is of the same child after thyroidectomy.

From Kocher T: Zur pathologie and therapie der Kropfres. *Deutsche Zeitschrift für Chirurgie* 1874; 4, 417.

Surgery

The surgical treatment of goitre has an ancient, although in its early stages rather uninteresting history. Celsus, the Roman encyclopaedist of the 1st century AD, reported that operation for removal of such a mass was dangerous. Albucasis, the 11th century surgeon of Cordoba (see Chapter 4), also speaks of extirpation of the gland. Certainly, the surgeons of Salerno in the 12th century were transfixing large goitres with setons, threads passed through the mass to produce suppuration, as well as treating these patients with seaweed, either dried or burned. Guy de Chauliac (see Chapter 4) in the 14th century used the cautery and setons for goitre treatment. Lorenz Heister (see Figure 6.7), in his *General System of Surgery* of 1753, pointed out that these masses were painless and, indeed, regarded among the Tyrolese as an ornament rather than a disfigurement. It is unlikely that patients would have offered themselves for radical treatment unless the mass compressing the trachea was causing asphyxiation.

The first well documented partial thyroidectomy was carried out by Pierre-Joseph Desault (see Figure 6.3) in 1791. He removed a 4 cm diameter mass from the thyroid through a vertical incision, tying off the superior and inferior thyroid arteries and then dissecting the gland from the trachea. The wound suppurated but healed within a month. Baron Guillaume Dupuytren (1777–1835) attempted a total removal of the thyroid in 1808, tying all four arteries; the patient died of shock.

In the 19th century the mortality of thyroid surgery was over 40% and many leading surgeons advised against operation. Thyroidectomy was condemned by the French Academy of Medicine in 1850. Theodor Kocher collected reports of 146 operations on the thyroid carried out world-wide between 1850 and 1877 and noted an operative mortality of 21%.

Even when anaesthetics became available, many surgeons believed that operations on the thyroid gland were too hazardous to be attempted. Thus Samuel D Gross (1805–1884), Professor of Surgery at Jefferson Medical College, Philadelphia, wrote in his *System of Surgery* in 1866:

In a word, can the thyroid gland, when in a state of enlargement, be removed with a reasonable hope of saving the patient? Experience emphatically answers, no. This conclusion is not invalidated by the fact that the operation has, in a few instances, been successfully performed . . . every step he takes will be environed with difficulty, every stroke of his knife will be followed by a torrent of blood, and lucky will it be for him if his victim lives long enough to enable him to finish his horrid butchering. Should the patient survive the immediate effects of the operation, if thus it may be called, death will be almost certain to overtake him from secondary haemorrhage, or from inflammation of the cervical vessels, oesophagus and respiratory organs. When the tumour is large, the wound is of frightful extent, involving all the most important and delicate structures of the neck and rendering it almost impossible, from the constant motion of the windpipe and oesophagus, that much of it would unite by first intention. Thus, whether we view this operation in relation to the difficulties which must necessarily attend its execution, or with reference to the severity of the subsequent inflammation, it is equally deserving of rebuke and condemnation. No honest and sensible surgeon, it seems to me, would ever engage in it.

Theodor Billroth (see Figure 8.5), while Professor of Surgery in Zurich between 1861 and 1867, performed 59 thyroid operations, including 20 enucleations, mostly for solid nodules. Of these cases, eight patients died, seven from sepsis. Disturbed by these figures, Billroth practically abandoned the operation when he moved to Vienna except in cases of patients threatened with asphyxia, carrying out only 16 operations over the next ten years with five deaths. He only started elective thyroid surgery again in 1877 after he had been convinced by, and had adopted, the antiseptic technique.

Thyroid surgery as we know it today owes much to one man, the Swiss surgeon Theodor Kocher (1841–1917) (Figure 13.2). He was born in Berne, the son of an engineer. He attended medical school there and, apart from a year after graduation touring the great medical schools of Vienna, Berlin, Paris and London where, among others, he visited the clinics of Billroth and Lister, he spent the whole of his professional life in that city. He was appointed Professor of Surgery at the University of Berne at the age of 31 and died, still in office, at the age of 76. He was a quiet, serene, rather austere man and, apart from an interest in painting, dedicated his life to surgery. As a teacher, technical surgeon and investigator, he made numerous contributions. He described his well known subcostal

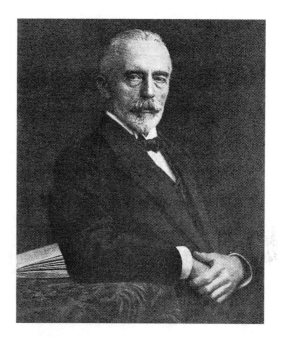

Figure 13.2 Theodor Kocher.
From Zimmerman LM, Veith L: *Great Ideas in the History of Surgery*. New York, Dover, 1961.

incision for exposure of the gall bladder, which is frequently used to this day. He popularised the collar incision for thyroidectomy which bears his name and which replaced the ugly vertical mid-line incision used by previous surgeons. He described the technique for mobilisation of the duodenum by division of its lateral peritoneal attachments, for which American surgeons have invented the phrase 'Kocherisation of the duodenum'. In 1870, he wrote a long article in which he described his method of reduction of a dislocated shoulder, still popular today, which could be carried out almost painlessly, without anaesthesia or assistance: 'Bend the arm at the elbow, press it against the body, rotate outwards 'til a resistance is felt, lift the externally rotated upper arm in the sagittal plane as far as possible forwards, and finally turn inwards slowly'.

He wrote a popular, beautifully illustrated and widely translated *Operative Surgery* (Figure 13.3) in which his profound knowledge of anatomy is

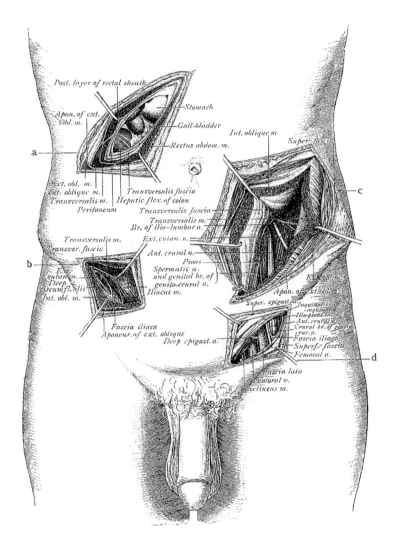

Figure 13.3 Illustration of various incisions from Kocher's *Textbook of Operative Surgery* (2nd edition, London, Black, 1903). The uppermost incision is Kocher's incision for gall bladder surgery.

demonstrated by its details of surgical approaches to every joint.

However, it was Kocher's contributions to the surgery of the thyroid gland which constitute his greatest claim to fame and earned him the Nobel Prize for Medicine in 1909.

We have already mentioned that Switzerland, being mountainous and land-bound, is an iodine deficient region. Before iodination of table salt was introduced, enormous goitres, often associated with cretinism, were endemic. Kocher's first challenge was to deal with these gigantic nodular enlargements of the gland, which, apart from their cosmetic disfigurement, often produced respiratory obstruction. Kocher taught precise anatomical dissection as the basis for thyroid surgery with preliminary ligation of the two principal arteries of the gland on each side, which greatly reduced the

(a)

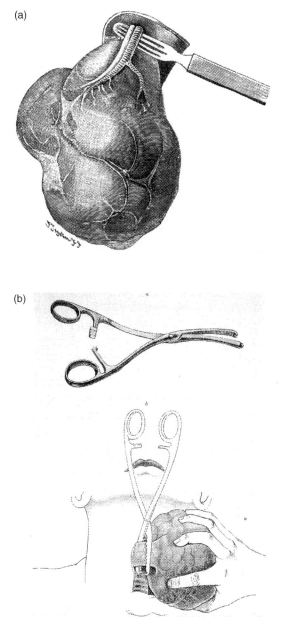

(b)

Figure 13.4 Kocher's thyroidectomy technique.
(a) Isolation of the superior thyroid vessels; the instrument is Kocher's gland dissector. (b) Application of Kocher's crushing forceps to the thyroid isthmus before ligation.
From Kocher T: *Textbook of Operative Surgery*. London, 2nd English edition, Black, 1903.

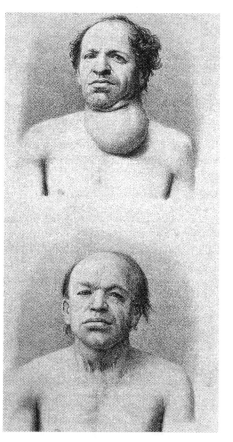

Figure 13.5 Goitre patient of Kocher before and after thyroidectomy.
From Kocher T: Uber kropfextirpation und ihr folgen. *Archiv für Klinische Chirurgie* 1883; 29, 254.

amount and danger of bleeding (Figure 13.4). His successive reports of his results showed progressive improvement from a mortality rate of 12.8% in 1883 to a level of less than 0.5%. In one series of cases, reported in 1898, there was only a single death in 600 consecutive cases, and this was due to an anaesthetic complication (Figure 13.5).

Radical removal of the thyroid gland may damage the recurrent laryngeal nerve with consequent hoarseness, remove the parathyroid glands with resultant tetany, or result in hypothyroidism if insufficient functioning thyroid tissue remains.

Kocher pointed out that great care must be taken to avoid the recurrent nerve and wrote: 'Since we have adhered strictly to this procedure, the hoarseness, formerly so frequently observed after operation, has now become exceptional'.

When Kocher commenced his thyroid surgery, the function of the gland was poorly appreciated and it was not until 1882 that the consequences of its radical removal were first understood. The parathyroid glands were not even recognised at this stage, and the symptoms of tetany that follow their removal were confused with the features of myxoedema. This will be discussed further in the section on the parathyroid glands. It is a fascinating reflection on the operative techniques of the two early pioneers of thyroid surgery, Billroth and Kocher, that Billroth did not encounter hypothyroidism in his cases but had a high incidence of tetany, whereas Kocher had the opposite experience. William Halsted (see Figure 7.11), who was a friend of Kocher and had watched him operate on many occasions, explained this anomaly in his *The Operative Story of Goitre* (1919):

I have pondered this question for many years and conclude that the explanation probably lies in the operative methods of the two illustrious surgeons. Kocher, neat and precise, operating in a relatively bloodless manner, scrupulously removed the entire thyroid gland, doing little damage outside its capsule. Billroth, operating more rapidly, and, as I recall his manner, with less regard for the tissues and less concern for haemorrhage, might easily have removed the parathyroids or at least have interfered with their blood supply, and have left fragments of the thyroid.

Hypothyroidism

The story that brings together the complex threads of thyroid deficiency – cretinism, myxoedema, the malign results of radical thyroidectomy and the treatment of these conditions with thyroid extract – is long in years and fascinating in content.

Cretinism (Figure 13.6) was described in Switzerland in the 16th century by Josias Simmler (1530–1576) and Johannes Stumpf (1500–1558). Felix

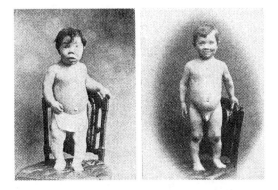

Figure 13.6 Cretinous infant before and after treatment with thyroid extract.
From Singer C, Underwood EA: *A Short History of Medicine.* Oxford, 2nd edition, Oxford University Press, 1962.

Platter (1536–1614), who qualified in Montpellier and then returned as Professor of Medicine to Basle, his native city, described in 1602 the deaf, dumb, mentally defective cretins seen in the canton of Valais:

Many infants are affected, who besides their innate simple mindedness, the head is now and then misformed, the tongue immense and tumid, a struma often in the throat, they show a deformed appearance; and seated in solemn stateliness, staring, and a stick resting between their hands, their bodies twisted variously, their eyes wide apart, they show immoderate laughter and wonder at unknown things.

Thomas Blizzard Curling (1811–1888), surgeon at the London Hospital, published a report in 1850 entitled *Two Cases of Absence of the Thyroid Body Connected with Defective Cerebral Development* in which he described two children, one aged six months and the other ten years, who, at postmortem, proved to have absence of the thyroid gland and commented 'which may be regarded as tending to confirm the more modern opinion respecting the connection between cretinism and bronchocele'.

Hypothyroidism in adults was first described by Sir William Gull (1816–1890), physician at Guy's Hospital, who published a paper in 1873 entitled *On a Cretinoid State Supervening in Adult Life in*

Women. He reported five cases, two in detail and three others seen on only one or two occasions. These are perfect descriptions of what was a newly discovered disease. It was a fine piece of observation to recognise, on clinical grounds only, that in reality this and cretinism were one and the same disease, for none of his cases were fatal and he states that 'from the folds of fat about the neck I am not able to state what the exact condition of it (the thyroid) was'.

In passing, we should note that Sir William Gull was a remarkable clinical observer who described the features of tabes dorsalis, syringomyelia and anorexia nervosa, the last of which he named. He insisted on following his fatal cases to a post-mortem examination, and Sir William Hale-White, in his *Great Doctors of the Nineteenth Century*, relates:

A patient of his left the hospital; one Saturday afternoon, Gull heard that this patient had died at his home 20 miles from London. Gull at once sent a note to his house physician at Guy's asking him to breakfast on Sunday and telling him to bring tools to make a post-mortem examination. This he did, the two drove to the patient's house and, after much opposition, which Gull overcame, the post-mortem examination was made and the diagnosis established.

It was William Miller Ord (1834–1902) of St Thomas' Hospital, London, who used the term 'myxoedema' in 1877, to describe the jelly-like swelling of connective tissues seen in this condition. Perhaps it is unfortunate that this name is so often used to describe hypothyroidism since many patients do not have this classical feature.

Meanwhile, important experimental studies were being carried out by Morritz Schiff (1823–1896) in Geneva. In 1859 he showed that total removal of the thyroid in dogs resulted in death after a week although guinea pigs would survive a little longer. Fatality was not related to infection or to damage of the recurrent laryngeal nerve. He went on in 1884 to demonstrate that transplant of thyroid tissue intra-abdominally prevented this fatal effect.

The first well documented occurrence of hypo-thyroidism following thyroidectomy was made by

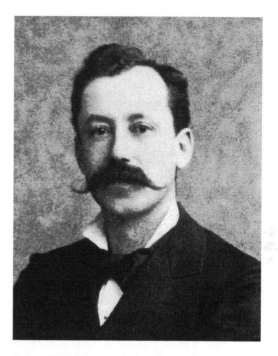

Figure 13.7 Jacques-Louis Reverdin. Photograph provided by Dr Guy Saudan, Lausanne.

Jacques-Louis Reverdin (1842–1929) (Figure 13.7), who reported to a meeting of the Medical Society of Geneva on September 15th, 1882, hitherto undescribed symptoms following goitre surgery:

Two or three months after the operation the patients have presented for the most part with a state of weakness, pallor, anaemia and, in two of them, oedema of the face and hands with albuminuria; in one case there was pupil contraction, melancholy and prostration and in another facies resembled that seen in cretins.

At the same meeting it was recorded that Theodor Kocher reported that he had seen a case of depression and weakness following thyroidectomy.

The following year, Reverdin, together with his cousin and personal assistant, Auguste Reverdin (1848–1908), documented in meticulous detail the results of his first 22 goitre operations. No less than five of their patients developed these unto-ward symptoms. All of them had undergone total thyroidectomy. Reverdin pointed out that these

(a)

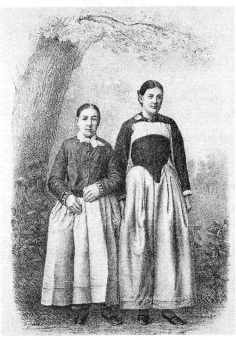

(b)

Figure 13.8 Kocher's first patient noted to have post-operative myxoedema. (a) The patient and her younger sister before her operation. (b) Nine years after surgery. The younger sister is now fully grown, in contrast to the stunted patient.
From Kocher T: Uber kropfextirpation und ihre folgen. *Archiv für Klinische Chirurgie* 1883; 29, 254.

features resembled the syndrome described by Sir William Gull and made the important recommendation that only partial removal of the thyroid gland should be performed.

Kocher, after the Geneva meeting, went back to study his own cases and reported a similar phenomenon at the Twelfth Congress of Surgeons in Berlin in 1883. Of the 34 patients upon whom total removal of the gland had been performed, 18 returned for examination and all but two of these revealed the evidence of myxoedema. Those with partial resections had escaped (Figure 13.8). He wrote:

As a rule, soon after discharge from the hospital, but in occasional cases, not before the lapse of four or five months, the patients begin to complain of fatigue and especially of weakness and heaviness in the extremities . . . in addition there is a sensation of coldness. The mental alertness decreases. Children who were formerly among the brightest pupils suddenly fall back. There is gradually increasing slowness of speech and of all other movements . . . if we are to give a name to this picture we cannot fail to recognise its relation to idiocy and cretinism; the stunted growth, the large head, the swollen nose, thick lips, heavy body and clumsiness of thought and speech undoubtedly point to a related evil.

Kocher termed this syndrome the rather bizarre name of 'cachexia strumipriva' while Reverdin introduced the much more apt title of 'operative myxoedema'.

In November 1883, Sir Felix Semon (1849–1921), laryngologist at St Thomas' Hospital, suggested at a meeting of the Clinical Society of London that the three conditions of myxoedema, cretinism and cachexia strumipriva were all caused by loss of function of the thyroid gland. His opinion was ridiculed at the time, and publication in the transactions of the Society was refused. However, his paper was published later that year in the *British Medical Journal*.

To settle the matter, the Clinical Society appointed a committee to investigate the whole subject. A member of this committee was Victor Horsley (1857–1916) who we have already met as a pioneer of neurosurgery (Chapter 8). At that time he was Superintendent of the Brown Institution in

London. Between 1884 and 1886, Horsley carried out a series of crucial experiments on monkeys. Thyroidectomy in these animals resulted in death within one to two months with features of myxoedema, including infiltration of the subcutaneous tissues with sticky and jelly-like material. It is interesting that the clinical picture was somewhat obscured since some of the features, such as tremors which followed five days after surgery, we now know were due to concomitant removal of the parathyroids. Horsley mistakenly concluded that the thyroid must secrete some substance needed for the proper nutrition of the central nervous system.

At this time, as we have already noted, Morritz Schiff was treating animals by grafting the thyroid into the abdomen after thyroidectomy and Horsley repeated these studies. The results were only temporarily successful since the transplanted thyroid tissue was absorbed. In 1891 George Redmayne Murray (1865–1939), a pupil of Horsley who was then Professor of Pathology in Durham and later became Professor of Medicine in Manchester, employed subcutaneous injections of glycerine extract of sheep's thyroid in a woman of 46 with obvious myxoedema, with dramatic results. In fact, under thyroid treatment this patient lived to the age of 74. The next year, 1892, Hector Mackenzie (1856–1929) and, independently, Edward Lawrence Fox (1859–1938) reported successful cases in which thyroid extract was given by mouth instead of by injection. On Christmas Day, 1914, Edward Kendall (1886–1972) at the Mayo Clinic isolated the active principle, thyroxine, from the thyroid, making the treatment of hypothyroidism one of the simplest, safest and most rewarding in the whole field of therapeutics. Interestingly enough, Kendall went on to discover cortisone and was awarded the Nobel Prize for Medicine in 1950.

Hyperthyroidism

At the end of the 18th century a strange association between enlargement of the thyroid, palpitations of the heart and protrusion of the eyes began to be

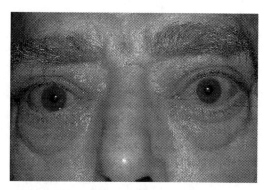

Figure 13.9 Exophthalmos in hyperthyroidism. Patient of the author at Westminster Hospital.

reported (Figure 13.9). The first classical description of this was given by Caleb Hillier Parry (1755–1822), physician at the General Hospital in Bath. In 1786 he observed a patient with a goitre, palpitations and protrusion of the eyes. He collected seven further cases in which enlargement of the thyroid was associated with palpitations but not exophthalmos. His account of these eight patients, entitled *Enlargement of the Thyroid Gland in Connection with Enlargement or Palpitation of the Heart*, was published after his death in 1825. He states: 'My attendance on the three last patients first suggested to me the notion of some connection between the malady of the heart and bronchocele' (i.e. thyroid enlargement).

The next important contribution was made ten years later by Robert Graves (1796–1853) of the Meath Hospital, Dublin, who, together with his colleague, William Stokes (1804–1878), is acknowledged as the Founder of the Dublin School of Medicine. In 1835 he published a short paper *Palpitation of the Heart with Enlargement of the Thyroid Gland* in which he described three cases of palpitation associated with goitre, in one of whom exophthalmos was present. Of this patient he wrote:

A lady aged 20 became affected with some symptoms which were supposed to be hysterical . . . after she had been in this nervous state about three months, it was observed that her pulse had become singularly rapid. This rapidity existed apparently without any cause and was constant, the pulse being never under 120 and often much higher. She next complained of weakness upon exertion and began to look pale and thin. Thus she continued for a year ... it was now observed that her eyes assumed a singular appearance for the eyeballs were apparently enlarged, so that when she slept or tried to shut her eyes they were incapable of closing. When the eyes were opened, the white sclerotic could be seen to a breadth of several lines around the cornea.

Graves was convinced that the enlargement of the thyroid gland was caused by hypertrophy, in contrast to the usual type of goitre which comprises a mass of nodules. He writes:

I have lately seen three cases of violent long continued palpitations in females in each of which the same peculiarity presented itself, viz., enlargement of the thyroid gland. The size of the gland, at all times considerably greater than natural, was subject to remarkable variations in every one of these patients. When the palpitations were violent, the gland used notably to swell and became distended, having all the appearances of being increased in size ... the swelling immediately began to subside as the violence of the paroxysm of palpitation decreased and during the intervals the size of the gland remained stationary.

A fourth case, a female patient providing another example of association with exophthalmos, was observed by Graves in 1838. It was in his honour that Armand Trousseau (1801–1867), the distinguished Parisian physician, used the term 'Graves' disease' in 1860.

In 1840, Karl von Basedow (1799–1854) of Merseburg described three females and one male with exophthalmos, palpitations and enlargement of the thyroid gland and described the hypertrophy of the cellular tissues of the orbit. He also noted emaciation, amenorrhoea, excessive sweating, diarrhoea, tremor and local myxoedema of the legs.

It is interesting that in Germany the disease is frequently called Basedow's disease, whereas Graves' disease is used in English speaking countries. Another rather old fashioned term still in common use is 'thyrotoxicosis', suggesting some toxic product of the thyroid gland, used in the days before it was realised that the features of the disease, apart from the exophthalmos, can be

explained by excessive production of thyroxine. The term 'hyperthyroidism' was introduced by Charles Mayo (1865–1939) in 1907; it is certainly the most sensible name for this condition and the one I will always personally use.

It should be remembered that until the early 20th century, the whole concept of a ductless system of glands (the endocrine system) producing internal secretions was only vaguely understood, indeed the term 'hormone' was first used by the physiologist Sir Ernest Starling (1866–1927) in 1907. This was in spite of the fact that as long ago as 1690, Frederik Ruysch (1638–1731), a celebrated anatomist of Amsterdam, suggested that organs such as the thyroid poured into the circulation substances which were of importance. Graves himself ascribed the thyroid enlargement in his patients to overaction of the heart.

An important observation was published in 1884 by Ludwig Rehn (1849–1930) of Frankfurt-am-Main who reported three patients cured incidently of their palpitations when the thyroid gland was removed for dyspnoea. He proposed, therefore, that it was overaction of the thyroid that was responsible for the condition and that thyroidectomy was thus the logical method for treatment.

Thyroidectomy is a technically demanding procedure. Operating on the thyroid in a patient with advanced hyperthyroidism in the days before effective drugs were available to control the metabolic complications of the overactive gland was hazardous indeed. Patients were not considered for surgery until already extremely ill and many died immediately after the operation with hyperpyrexia, uncontrolled tachycardia and heart failure. The mid-West states of the USA have a particularly high incidence of goitre, and hyperthyroidism seems especially common there. It is not surprising, therefore, that it was two mid-West surgeons who made important contributions to the problem of surgery in this condition.

George Crile (1864–1943) (Figure 13.10), founder of the Cleveland Clinic, Cleveland, Ohio, performed his first thyroidectomy in 1898. Dismayed by the high mortality following operations on

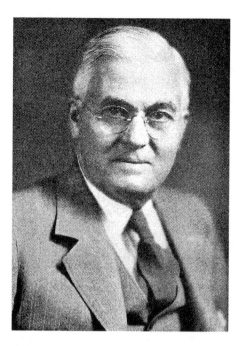

Figure 13.10 George Crile.
Royal College of Surgeons of England.

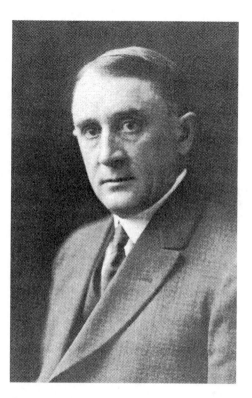

Figure 13.11 Charles Mayo.
Royal College of Surgeons of England.

patients with advanced hyperthyroidism, he introduced his technique of 'stealing the goitre' in 1907. The patient was heavily sedated for several days, not informed of the time or even date of the operation, but anaesthetised in the ward before being taken to the operating theatre (or even operated upon in the ward itself), with a gratifying improvement in results. Crile also carried out important work on surgical shock and in the development of radical block dissection of the neck in cancer of the head and neck.

Meanwhile, in Rochester, Minnesota, Charles Mayo (1865–1939) (Figure 13.11) had performed his first thyroidectomy in 1890 with his brother Will (1861–1939) (Figure 13.12). The patient was a 60-year-old man with a goitre that hung down onto his chest and forced his head backwards as far as it would go. He was suffering from severe breathing difficulties. By 1908 Charles Mayo could report 234 thyroidectomies for hyperthyroidism with a

mortality of 11.5%. He advocated the technique of staged surgery introduced by Kocher: at the first stage, the blood vessels to the thyroid gland were tied on one or both sides, at a second stage one lobe might be removed and at the third stage the other. A dramatic advance was made by Mayo's medical colleague, Henry Plummer (1874–1937), who showed that administration of iodine in the form of potassium iodide rapidly brought the toxic symptoms of hyperthyroidism under control. This rendered the multiple stage operation no longer necessary because most patients could be made ready for a one stage operation in from ten days to three weeks. The dreaded post-operative crisis was averted, and mortality dropped to less than 1%. After thorough testing of this method for a year, Plummer reported the remarkable results to a meeting of the Association of American Physicians in 1923.

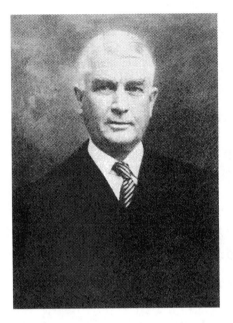

Figure 13.12 William Mayo.
Royal College of Surgeons of England.

The introduction of the antithyroid drug thiouracil in 1943 and then of the safer carbimazole in 1960, and the use in recent years of beta-blocking drugs which allow rapid control of the palpitations and tachycardia in this condition, have made the pre-operative preparation of patients with hyperthyroidism a straightforward procedure. Nowadays, surgery in this condition is associated with minimal mortality and morbidity. Moreover, in 1942, radioactive iodine was first used to treat the condition. Today, many patients are managed by what, to them, is the simple business of drinking a glass of water which contains this tasteless and colourless material, a miracle of modern therapeutics!

I cannot mention the Mayo brothers in a book on surgical history without a word of that medical phenomenon, the Mayo Clinic, which is undoubtedly the best known medical centre in the USA, if not in the world. The story begins in the year 1845, when William Worrall Mayo (1819–1911) emigrated from Salford, then a village outside Manchester, to

the United States of America. Mayo first practised as a pharmaceutical chemist in New York but soon turned to the study of medicine. After qualifying in 1854, he worked in various cities until the opportunities afforded by the development of the North-West Territories induced him to settle in Rochester, Minnesota, then very much a frontier town. Indeed, in 1862, Dr Mayo was one of the leaders involved in quelling a rising of the Sioux Indians.

William Mayo was born in 1861 and his brother, Charles, in 1865. The two boys helped their father in his surgical practice and, in after years, they were wont to recount how Charles used to stand on a biscuit box in order to assist in operations. Long before the boys entered their formal training, they had been receiving practical instruction from their father. William graduated at the University of Minnesota in Minneapolis in 1883 and Charles at the North-Western University in Chicago in 1885.

In August 1883, Rochester was devastated by a tornado. Dr William Mayo senior took charge of an improvised hospital with such efficiency that it was suggested that he should establish a permanent hospital in Rochester. In 1889, therefore, old Dr Mayo, then aged 70, and his two sons opened St Mary's Hospital with 27 beds and five nurses. Other physicians and surgeons joined the staff and this was the beginning of the Mayo Clinic, a brilliant experiment in group practice. In 1919, the Mayo brothers turned over their personal assets to establish the Mayo Foundation with an entirely salaried staff. A graduate medical school had already been opened in 1915 and this was followed by an undergraduate school in 1972.

Incredibly, this little town of some 50 000 people in the middle of the farming mid West remains a 'medical mecca' – the whole industry of the town, for practical purposes, being the pursuit of medicine, with patients and students coming from all over the world. I first visited the clinic in 1972, arriving in a small commuter plane from Chicago. It was met by a group of porters with stretchers and wheelchairs to deal with the passengers leaving the plane in plaster casts, with nasogastric tubes or bandaged heads. I was the only person to walk off

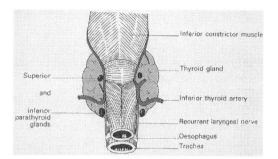
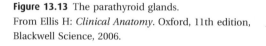

Figure 13.13 The parathyroid glands.
From Ellis H: *Clinical Anatomy*. Oxford, 11th edition,
Blackwell Science, 2006.

that plane and one porter said to me 'as you can
walk, you must be a visiting doctor'. Of course, he
was right.

The parathyroid glands

The parathyroids are four (sometimes three, sometimes five) small nodules, about half a centimetre in
length, found two on each side on the posterior
aspect of the thyroid gland (Figure 13.13). Occasionally, one or more of the glands may be found
elsewhere in the neck or even in the superior part of
the thorax. Anatomically, they were only fully recognised in man at the beginning of the 20th century
and several more decades passed before their
physiological importance was fully understood.

In 1862 Sir Richard Owen (1804–1892), then
conservator at the Royal College of Surgeons in
London, reported in the *Transactions of the
Zoological Society of London* his dissection findings
in the body of an Indian rhinoceros that had died
at the London Zoo (Figure 13.14). He described
'a small, compact, yellow glandular body attached
to the thyroid at the place where the veins emerge'.
These glands were also noted in man by Rudolph
Virchow (1821–1902), pathologist at the Charité
Hospital in Berlin. No attention was given to either
of these descriptions. In 1880 Yvar Sandström
(1852–1889), while a medical student at Uppsala,
Sweden, dissected 50 human bodies, made animal

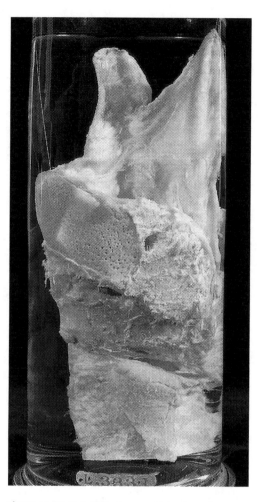
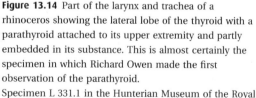

Figure 13.14 Part of the larynx and trachea of a
rhinoceros showing the lateral lobe of the thyroid with a
parathyroid attached to its upper extremity and partly
embedded in its substance. This is almost certainly the
specimen in which Richard Owen made the first
observation of the parathyroid.
Specimen L 331.1 in the Hunterian Museum of the Royal
College of Surgeons of England.

studies, carried out histological examination and
reported his findings of two glands, one on each
side, in 43 out of his 50 human subjects. He named
these 'glandulae parathyroideae' but again this
study was all but ignored.

In 1891 Eugène Gley (1857–1930) of Paris noted the parathyroid glands in the rabbit and showed them to be essential to life although he concluded, wrongly, that their function was the same as that of the thyroid. It was Gley who rediscovered and gave due recognition to Sandström's description. By 1909, numerous workers, including Giulio Vassale (1862–1912) of Modena, Italy, David Welsh (1865–1948) in Edinburgh and William Halsted (see Figure 7.11) in Baltimore had shown that removal of the parathyroids resulted in tetany, was associated with a drop in the serum calcium and was relieved by injection of either calcium salts or parathyroid extract. It was now realised that the phenomenon of 'tetania thyreopriva', not infrequently fatal, that followed the early thyroidectomies – first reported from Billroth's clinic in 1880, then by Reverdin in 1882 and by Theodore Kocher in 1883, as well as occurring in the experimental thyroidectomies performed by Schiff and by Horsley around 1885 – was simply the result of damage to the parathyroid glands at the time of thyroid surgery. Careful operative technique, with preservation of the posterior aspect of the thyroid lobe on each side, all but obviated this post-operative complication.

Tumours of the parathyroid are usually benign adenomas. They are not common, but when they do occur they produce their effects by excess secretion of parathyroid hormone. This mobilises calcium from the skeleton, producing bone rarefaction and cyst formation and, as a more frequent manifestation, results in stone formation in the renal tract from the excess secretion of calcium in the urine.

Generalised decalcification of the skeleton associated with cyst formation (osteitis fibrosa cystica) was first studied systematically by Friedrich von Recklinghausen (1833–1910), Professor of Pathology successively at the universities of Konigsberg, Würzburg and then Strasbourg. In 1891 he gave an accurate description of three patients with this condition although, at that time, he had no idea of its aetiology. In 1903 Max Askanazy (1865–1940), a pathologist in Geneva, discovered a parathyroid tumour in a patient with this condition, although, interestingly enough, he did not associate the two

pathologies. Further reports of the association of the two conditions led to the suggestion that removal of the tumour would be the correct treatment for this condition, now often called von Recklinghausen's disease of bone, but it was not until 1925 that Felix Mandl (1892–1957) performed the first removal of a parathyroid tumour. His patient was a man with advanced osteitis fibrosa cystica who complained of generalised bone pain, fatigue and muscle weakness. Mandl explored the neck and found a tumour measuring 2.5 cm by 1.5 cm lying on a branch of the inferior thyroid artery. A pathological examination proved this to be an adenoma of the parathyroid gland. The patient immediately lost his symptoms and remained well for six years. The symptoms recurred in 1932, with the development now of renal stones. Mandl explored the neck once again but found no parathyroid abnormality; the patient died from renal failure. At autopsy it was found that death was due to renal disease and no abnormal parathyroid tissue could be found. However, by now, enough successful operations had been performed to establish this procedure. In 1932, also, Fuller Albright (1900–1969) in Boston diagnosed a parathyroid adenoma in a female patient with renal stones who was found to have a greatly raised serum calcium level. The neck was explored, a parathyroid adenoma removed, and the calcium level returned to normal. Today, sophisticated imaging techniques make it possible to localise the parathyroid tumour pre-operatively in the majority of cases with a great degree of accuracy.

A few words about the pioneer of parathyroid surgery – Felix Mandl (1892–1957) was born in Brno, then in Austria, now in the Czech Republic, the son of an industrialist. His medical studies at the University of Vienna were interrupted by the First World War, during which he served on the Austrian front as an ambulance man. He qualified in 1919. Four years later he was appointed assistant to Julius von Hochenegg, a distinguished but autocratic and cantankerous chief at the University Clinic, and it was here that the parathyroid work was performed.

In 1932 Mandl was appointed surgeon to the newly opened Canning Child Hospital and Research Institute for the Study of Cancer, a prestigious promotion, but his time there was to be all too short. In 1938 came the Anschluss – the Nazis marched into Austria. Mandl, a Jew, was dismissed from his post and, indeed, his life was in danger. He was fortunate in being able to escape to what was then Palestine, under the British Mandate, and was promptly appointed Professor of Surgery at the prestigious Hadassah Hospital in Jerusalem. After the war, he was invited back to Vienna to become Director, in 1947, of the rebuilt Emperor Franz-Josef Hospital. He died suddenly of heart failure in 1957, in his 65th year; a remarkable career.

14

Thoracic and vascular surgery

Lung surgery

The early history of chest surgery, as with so many other fields of surgical endeavour, is the story of the treatment of trauma and infection. In the first part of this chapter, we shall meet in this context, once again, a number of the surgical pioneers who have appeared in previous chapters.

Pneumothorax and collapse of the lung, as well as frequently severe haemorrhage from large vessels and from the heart itself, made open wounds of the chest particularly lethal injuries. Thus, that doyen of trauma surgery Ambroise Paré (see Figure 9.4) wrote in 1585:

We may know that the lungs are wounded by the foaming and spumous blood coming out both at the wound and cast up by vomiting. He is vexed with a grievous shortness of breath and with a pain in his side. We may perceive the heart to be wounded by the abundance of blood that cometh out of the wound, by the trembling of all the whole body, by the faint and small pulse, paleness of the face, cold sweat, with often swounding, coldness of the extreme parts and sudden death.

The first written report of chest injuries is to be found in the Edwin Smith papyrus (see Figure 2.4), which dates from about 1550 BC but is almost certainly a copy of a much more ancient Egyptian text. Of its 48 case reports, three involve chest wounds.

In the 13th century, Theodoric and his pupil, Henri de Mondeville, both advocated suturing wounds of the chest in order to prevent air entering through the thoracic cavity. Others, such as Guy de Chauliac (see Figure 4.7), opposed immediate closure in order to allow the escape of blood. Ambroise Paré was also against immediate suture of chest wounds although he agreed that this was a controversial topic. He describes an interesting case of chest injury that he dealt with in the campaign in Turin in 1537:

While in Turin in the service of the late M de Montejan, I was called to treat a Parisian soldier named L'Evesque, under command of Captain Renouart, who was wounded with three severe sword thrusts. One great wound under the right breast penetrated the chest cavity. A great quantity of blood collected on the diaphragm, which impeded respiration and he could speak only with great pain. He had a high fever and with it all he spat blood and had severe pain in his wounded side. The surgeon who first treated him had sewn up his wound so nothing could come out. The next day I was called to see the patient, and seeing the complications and death approaching, I was constrained to open the wound, at the orifice of which I found blood clot. Then I had the patient's legs lifted, with the head and upper part of the body leaning over the bed, resting one hand on a stool lower than the bed. Being so placed I had him close his mouth and nose and inflate the lungs. The diaphragm, intercostal and epigastric muscles contracting, caused the blood collected in the chest to jet through the wound. And to help him do it better, I put my finger deep in the wound to break up the coagulated blood and seven to eight ounces of fetid and corrupt blood drained. Then I put him in bed and injected the wound with barley water in which rose, honey and sugar candy had been boiled. Then I had him turn from side to side and finally to lie head down as before. Then one saw little thrombi and clots of blood come out with the irrigation. This done, the complications diminished and little by little ceased . . . to conclude, this injury was so well handled that beyond my expectation, the patient recovered.

Both leading surgeons on the French and British sides in the Napoleonic wars, from their own experience, became convinced that closure of thoracic wounds was beneficial. During the Egyptian campaign of 1798 to 1801, Baron Larrey (see Figure 9.7) wrote:

The number of soldiers that died of haemorrhage in consequences of wounds penetrating the chest and injuring the lungs induced me to attend minutely to such accidents.

A soldier was brought to the hospital of the fortress of Ibraym Bey immediately after a wound of this kind made by a cutting instrument that penetrated the thorax between the fifth and sixth true ribs, and followed their direction; it was about eight centimetres in extent; a large quantity of frothy and vermilion blood escaped from it with a hissing noise at each inspiration. His extremities were cold, pulse scarcely perceptible, countenance discoloured, and respiration short and laborious; in short, he was every moment threatened with a fatal suffocation.

After having examined the wound, and the divided edges of the parts, I immediately approximated the two lips of the wound and retained them by means of adhesive plasters, and a suitable bandage round the body.

In adopting this plan, I intended only to hide from the sight of the patient and his comrades the distressing spectacle of a haemorrhage which would soon prove fatal and I therefore thought, that the effusion of blood into the cavity of thorax, could not increase the danger.

But the wound was scarcely closed when he breathed more freely, and felt easier. The heat of the body soon returned and the pulse; in a few hours he became quite calm and to my great surprise grew better. He was cured in a very few days and without difficulty. At the hospital of the imperial guard, we had two cases exactly similar.

George Guthrie (see Figure 9.10), a veteran surgeon of the Napoleonic wars, described several cases of open wounds of the chest treated successfully by deep interrupted suture, compress and bandage. He summed up his experience in his monograph *On Wounds and Injuries of the Chest*, which he published in 1848 and which represents the first book in the English language devoted entirely to the surgery of the chest. His general conclusions were that all wounds of the chest should be closed as quickly as possible, but that if the pleural cavity fills with blood and produces respiratory distress, the wound should be re-opened and the blood evacuated. Serous collections of fluid in the chest should be drained and for this the trocar and cannula can be used.

In spite of this experience, treatment of wounds of the chest remained controversial and, indeed, in the early years of the First World War, chest wounds were treated conservatively under the care of the physicians. Not surprisingly, many of the injured developed an empyema and, of these, 50% died. By 1916 it was realised that chest wounds needed to be treated in the same manner as wounds elsewhere, by excision of damaged tissue, haemostasis, removal of foreign bodies and then closure. Drainage was not used at this time since the underwater drain had not yet been devised, as we shall discuss later. By the end of the War, George Gask (1875–1951), later to become the first Professor of Surgery at St Bartholomew's Hospital, was able to report a large series of penetrating chest wounds associated with injury to the lung with a total mortality of 20%. This compared with a mortality of 79% for chest wounds in the Crimean War.

Empyema, denoting a collection of pus in the pleural cavity, is an old term dating back to the Ancient Greeks (Greek *en*, in, *pyon*, pus), and still commonly used today in preference to the more scientific term of pyothorax. Its clinical features were well described in the Hippocratic writings of the 4th century BC:

In the first case the fever does not go off but is slight during the day and increases at night, and copious sweats supervene, there is a desire to cough and the patient's expectorate nothing worth mentioning, the eyes become hollow, the cheeks have red spots on them, the nails of the hands are bent, the fingers are hot, especially their extremities, there are swellings in the feet, they have no desire of food and small blisters occur over the body.

Note the description 'the nails of the hands are bent', which surely refers to the clubbing of the fingertips that may occur with chronic lung sepsis. A test of great antiquity is Hippocratic succussion, a splashing sound produced by shaking the patient, who should be in the sitting position. It occurs only when fluid and air are present within the chest cavity.

With regard to treatment, Hippocrates advises drainage by the use of the cautery or by incision, while Celsus advises 'on the side where there is the greatest swelling a hot iron must be pushed in until it reaches the pus and the matter is drawn off'. Occasionally, the abscess would point and drain spontaneously through the chest wall; on other occasions it might rupture into the bronchial tree. An example of this is described by Ambroise Paré:

Benedict de Vallé, native of Turin, aged 25 years, fell ill of pleurisy which suppurated and made an empyema. He coughed severely, expectorating fetid pus for six weeks, then it ceased for 20 days, at the end of which when he bent over or shook himself, one heard a sound in his body like a half-filled bottle . . . finally he called me and having studied his illness, I advised him to have a rib opened to drain the pus. He agreed to do this when he was a little stronger. Some days later nature drained the pus by great vomiting, following which he recovered completely by the grace of God and of nature. At present he is as well as if he had never been ill.

Lorenz Heister (see Figure 6.7) in his *General System of Surgery* of 1743 illustrates a trocar and cannula very much like the instrument used today to be employed for the evacuation of pleural collections. The use of a wide bore needle for aspiration was introduced by Thomas Davies (1792–1839) of London in 1835, and by 1844 a report from the newly opened Brompton Hospital in London reported nine cases treated by this method with only one death.

Surgical drainage of a chronic empyema was carried out either by an intercostal incision or by trephining a rib. It was William Arbuthnot Lane (see Figure 10.7), while House Surgeon to the Victoria Hospital for Children in Chelsea, who showed the importance of rib resection in this operation. He published five cases in children with four successes. It took some years before this became standard procedure when experience showed that there was no increased risk of severe infection or necrosis of the cut ends of the ribs.

In the majority of cases of empyema, certainly in chronic disease, the pleura is thickened and the lung fixed by adhesions to the chest wall. However,

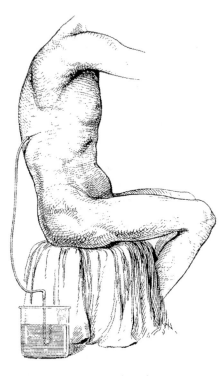

Figure 14.1 Underwater chest drainage.
From Sauerbruch F, O'Shaughnessy OL: *Thoracic Surgery*. London, Arnold, 1937.

if the normal chest is opened, either by trauma or by the surgeon's knife, the negative pressure in the pleural space which keeps the lung held to the chest wall is abolished, air rushes into the pleural cavity and the lung collapses. Moreover, the mediastinum may swing with each respiratory movement, producing the shock of mediastinal flutter. Gotthard von Bülau (1836–1900) of Hamburg solved this problem with his underwater drain (Figure 14.1). When the patient breathes out, the intrapleural pressure rises and the air, blood or pus in the pleural cavity drains through the tube below the underwater seal. When the patient inspires, the water in the chamber rises in the tube and maintains the seal, preventing air entering the pleural cavity. This simple apparatus is used today routinely after chest surgery, thoracic trauma or in drainage of intrapleural collections. The immense value of the underwater drain was

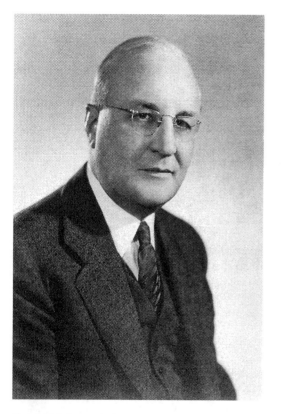

Figure 14.2 Evarts Graham.
Royal College of Surgeons of England.

underlined by the work of Evarts Graham (1883–1957) (Figure 14.2), Professor of Surgery at Washington University in St Louis. During the influenza epidemic of 1918, there were numerous cases of acute streptococcal empyema among the American troops. In this condition, the pus is thin, compared to the thick material seen in chronic empyema and in the more common acute staphylococcal empyema. Open drainage was associated with an extremely high mortality, as much as 70%. Graham used closed drainage with the underwater system and reduced the mortality to 15%. We shall meet Graham again later in this chapter as a pioneer of lung resection, but in addition to his contributions to chest surgery he is remembered as the inventor of cholecystography, the radiological demonstration of

the gall bladder using iodine-labelled phenophthalein. This substance is excreted by the liver into the gall bladder where it is concentrated, and, being radio-opaque, outlines the cavity of the gall bladder. This method has only recently been replaced routinely by ultrasonography.

Tuberculosis

It is difficult for health workers today to realise the enormous impact of tuberculosis, especially of the lungs, in the pre-antibiotic era before the 1950s. As a young student, I was only too aware of the sanatoria being full of young men and women of my age, incarcerated for years, with a significant risk of dying, and of seeing my contemporaries – medical students, young doctors, nurses – afflicted by this disease (Figure 14.3). At the end of the 19th century, surgical means were introduced to collapse, and therefore to rest the diseased lung, as well as to obliterate cavitating disease. In 1882, the same year that Robert Koch (1843–1910) announced the discovery of the bacillus of tuberculosis, Carlos Forlanini (1847–1918), a physician in Turin who later moved to Padua, suggested the use of an artificial pneumothorax in order to collapse the lung and began to perform the procedure in 1888. He used oxygen at first but, because of its rapid absorption, switched to nitrogen. The procedure was taken up with enthusiasm in Chicago by J B Murphy (see Figure 14.22). Other methods of lung collapse were division or crushing of the phrenic nerve, in order to paralyse the diaphragm, and pneumoperitoneum. A more radical method of collapsing the lung was the operation of thoracoplasty, in which the ribs on the affected side were resected, usually in staged procedures. This was first performed by Edouard de Cérenvelle (1843–1913) of Lausanne in 1885 and popularised by Ferdinand Sauerbruch (1875–1951) of Berlin and by many other thoracic surgical pioneers. All these techniques were employed until the introduction of effective anti-tuberculous drugs and we still see the occasional elderly patient who has undergone thoracoplasty (Figure 14.4).

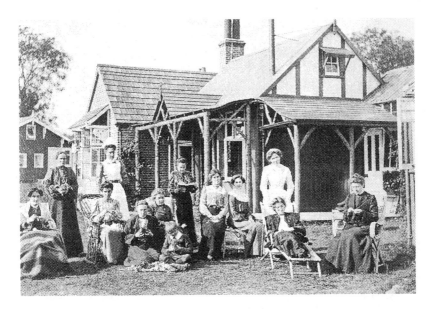

Figure 14.3 A tuberculosis sanatorium; the Maitland Sanatorium in Berkshire, 1910.
Photograph provided by the late Mr Roger Parker FRCS (ENT surgeon, Reading).

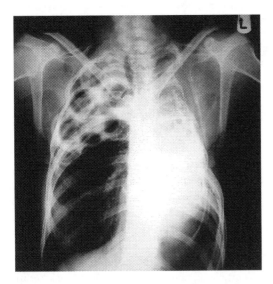

Figure 14.4 Chest X-ray of a patient after extensive
surgery for pulmonary tuberculosis; thoracoplasty on
the left, plombage on the right using lucite spheres.
X-ray provided by Mr Jules Dussek FRCS, Guy's
Hospital.

Resection of the lung

Early attempts at removing all or part of a lung
were carried out for chronic infection – tuberculosis, bronchiectasis and lung abscess. M H Block
(died 1883) of Danzig carried out pneumonectomies in rabbits in 1881, showed that the animals
could survive and considered, therefore, that the
operation would be possible in the human. He then
operated on his female cousin who had tuberculosis of the apices of both lungs. She died post-
operatively and Block, in despair, shot himself,
cutting short what would probably have been a
brilliant career. Domenico Biondi (1855–1914),
Professor of Surgery in Padua, soon afterwards
published extensive animal studies of pneumonectomies in a number of species and in 1884 reported
successful removal of the lung in animals in which
he had previously induced tuberculosis. Theodore
Tuffier (1857–1929) in Paris successfully resected
a tuberculous apex of the lung in 1891 and this
procedure was soon followed by a number of other
surgeons.

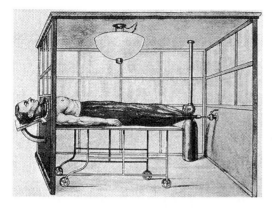

Figure 14.5 Sauerbruch's low-pressure chamber for thoracic surgery.
From Sauerbruch F: Zur Pathologie des offenen Pneumothorax. *Mitteilungen aus den Grenzgebieten der Medizin und Chirurgie Jena*, volume 14, 1904.

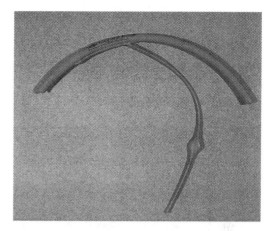

Figure 14.6 A rubber cuffed endotracheal tube. Nowadays these are made of plastic. Westminster Hospital.

The first surgeon to remove an entire lung, the operation of pneumonectomy, was Sir William Macewen (see Figure 10.16) who, in 1895, simply scooped out a lung that had been almost destroyed by tuberculosis. Four weeks later, he obliterated the great space left behind by performing a two-stage thoracoplasty and the patient was well 11 years later.

The pioneers of lung resection faced two severe technical problems. The first was how to deal with the pedicle of the lobe or of the hilum of the lung with its large pulmonary vessels and the divided bronchial stump. Initially, a tourniquet was used at the hilum to produce necrosis of the lobe, with subsequent removal of the dead tissue. Later the hilum was clamped and a mass ligature was used, followed later still by suturing the hilum over a tourniquet, with the eventual development of the modern technique of dissecting out each of the main structures and closing them individually by ligation or suture.

The second, and even more difficult, hazard was anaesthetising the patient for chest surgery, since opening the thorax resulted in collapse of the lung. The standard technique was simply to use a tightly fitting mask over the patient's mouth and nose. Rudolph Matas (1860–1957) of New Orleans used a bellows system through a tracheostomy tube to inflate the lungs and in 1899, his colleague, F W Parham, used the apparatus to remove a growth from the chest wall with success. Ferdinand Sauerbruch (1875–1951), while an assistant to Johann von Mikulicz in Breslau, introduced a negative pressure chamber which contained the body of the patient plus the surgical team. The patient's head projected through an opening in the chamber and was available for the anaesthetist. The negative pressure in the chamber overcame the problem of the pneumothorax in the opened chest, but the negative pressure cabinet produced almost impossible conditions for the operative team and the positive pressure through the face mask inflated the stomach as well as the lungs of the patient (Figure 14.5).

It was the development of the endotracheal tube by Ivan Magill and Stanley Rowbotham during the First World War (see Chapter 9) that really paved the way for modern thoracic anaesthesia, while the development of the cuffed endotracheal tube by Ralph Walters (1883–1979) of Maddison, Wisconsin, and Arthur Guedel (1883–1956) of Los Angeles enabled the anaesthetic to be given via the normal lung while the bronchus of the affected lung was sealed off by the cuff (Figure 14.6).

The first successful elective lobectomies were performed by Themistokles Gluck (1853–1942),

Director of the Kaiser and Kaiserin Hospital, Berlin, in 1901. The first case had resections of the left lower and part of the left upper lobe for bronchiectasis; the second was for gangrene of the left lower lobe following a septic pulmonary infarct. In 1907 Gluck resected the right lower lobe of a 5-year-old for tuberculosis. The first dissection lobectomy, the technique used today of dealing individually with the structures of the hilum, was performed in 1912 by Morriston Davies (1879–1965) of University College Hospital, London. The patient, who had a carcinoma of the lung, unfortunately died of empyema but autopsy showed that the bronchial stump was intact. It was not until the 1930s that this method became the treatment of choice.

Hugh Morriston Davies had a remarkable career. A brilliant student, he was appointed to the staff at University College Hospital at the age of 29. He studied under Sauerbruch in Berlin and in 1912 performed the first thoracoplasty in the United Kingdom. In 1916 he suffered a severe infection of his right hand after operating on a septic case and this appeared to be the end of his surgical career. He resigned his hospital appointment and purchased a sanatorium for tuberculosis in North Wales, but, finding that there was nobody there to operate on his patients, taught himself to operate with his left hand and made his sanatorium a centre for the surgical treatment of pulmonary tuberculosis, continuing to work until the age of 80.

The landmark year for the modern dissection pneumonectomy was 1933 when Evarts Graham (see Figure 14.2) operated on a 40-year-old obstetrician with lung cancer (Figure 14.7). The patient survived an empyema and bronchopleural fistula in the post-operative period and outlived his surgeon; Graham himself died of lung cancer in 1957.

In the same year as Graham's success, 1933, William Rienhoff (1894–1980) of the Johns Hopkins Hospital, Baltimore, performed two successful dissection pneumonectomies. His first was for a benign lung tumour in a child of three and his second for a carcinoma of the lung. It was Rienhoff who laid down the modern principles of dealing with the hilum; he ligated the pulmonary vessels indivi-

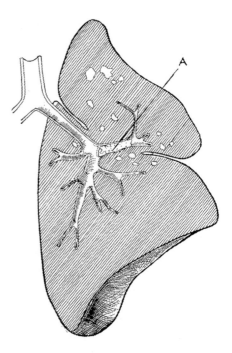

Figure 14.7 The first pneumonectomy for lung cancer. Diagram of the resected lung, showing (A) the location of the tumour in the upper lobe bronchus. The location of numerous small abscesses is also demonstrated. From Graham EA, Singer JJ: Successful removal of an entire lung for carcinoma of the bronchus. *Journal of the American Medical Association* 1933; 101, 1371.

dually, divided the bronchus with the knife and not the cautery, thus avoiding damage to its blood supply, closed the bronchus with interrupted sutures, drained the chest, and showed that the opposite lung will expand to obliterate the dead space within the thorax.

Cardiac surgery

To the lay public, an operation on the heart seems to be the ultimate mystery. Indeed, even to the surgeons who had already conquered the other major organs, the concept of operating on this constantly beating and vital muscle seemed a distant dream, especially when arrest of the blood circulation for more than a few minutes, under normal conditions, was known to be fatal. Even that great pioneer of modern scientific surgery, Theodor Billroth (see Figure 8.5) wrote in 1893: 'Any surgeon who would attempt an operation on the heart should lose the respect of his colleagues'.

The surgery of the heart and its great vessels can be divided chronologically into four rather overlapping phases: the first is the surgery of the pericardium, the fibrous sac surrounding the heart, and of the adjacent great vessels; the second, 'blind' surgery of the beating heart itself; the third, open heart surgery using either hypothermia, a heart by-pass or combination of the two; and finally transplantation of the hopelessly damaged heart. This fourth topic is dealt with in Chapter 15.

Extracardiac surgery

A small stab wound of the heart may prove fatal, not from the cardiac haemorrhage itself, but from the pressure on the heart from the blood collecting in the pericardial sac. This condition, haemopericardium, was first described by Giovanni Morgagni (1682–1771) in 1769. Dominique Jean Larrey, Napoleon's surgeon (see Figure 9.7), in 1810 operated on a soldier with tamponade following a self-inflicted knife wound of the chest. Operating 45 days after the injury, Larrey opened the left chest through the fourth intercostal space, opened the pericardium with a bistoury and evacuated a tin basin-full of serous fluid mixed with old blood clots. The patient's condition improved considerably but unfortunately he died three weeks later from the almost inevitable post-operative infection. By the end of the 19th century, it was well recognised that this condition should be treated by aspiration or surgical drainage, and some 400 cases were recorded with a 10% survival.

Constrictive pericarditis

A condition of gross fibrous or calcific thickening of the pericardium, often due to tuberculosis, was first described by Richard Lower (1631–1691) of Oxford, who performed early animal experiments in blood transfusion. He wrote of an autopsy in 1669: 'The pericardium of the whole heart was everywhere closely adherent, so that with the finger it was scarcely possible to separate it from the heart; further this membrane was thick, opaque and as if transformed into callus'.

Ludwig Rehn (1849–1930), of Frankfurt am Main, who we shall meet shortly as the first surgeon successfully to deal with a stab wound of the heart, published a report in 1920 of four patients with constrictive pericarditis, one of whom had been operated on seven years previously. The following year Viktor Schmieden (1874–1945) published a detailed description of the operation, which he compared to the peeling of an orange. By 1937 he was able to report on 22 cases that he had operated upon with eight operative deaths, six patients returning to full activity and the remainder having had a marked improvement.

Persistent ductus arteriosus (Figure 14.8a)

The ductus arteriosus, between the pulmonary artery and the aorta, is one of the shunts present in the fetal circulation. Normally it closes a few hours after birth and is completely obliterated within a few weeks, leaving a persistent fibrous strand, the ligamentum arteriosum, as its relic. Persistence of the ductus is one of the common forms of congenital heart disease. If small, it may remain symptomless, the only risk being of later infection – subacute bacterial endarteritis. If large, however, it results in progressive pulmonary hypertension as blood at high pressure in significant amounts is pumped into the pulmonary circulation. The technique of dealing with this condition surgically was worked out by John Monroe (1858–1910) at Tufts Medical School in Boston and published in the *Annals of Surgery* in 1907. He showed, in newborn cadaver dissections, how the heart could be approached through a median sternotomy and how the ductus could be ligated, but never had a case referred to him. Surprisingly, therefore, it was not

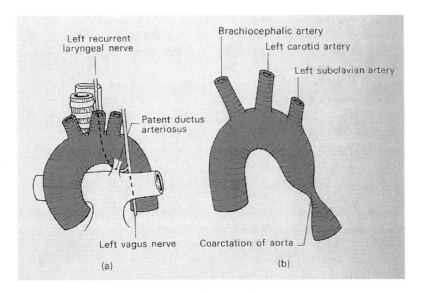

Figure 14.8 (a) A diagram of a persistent ductus arteriosus. (b) Coarctation of the aorta. From Ellis H: *Clinical Anatomy*. Oxford, Blackwell, 11th edition, 2006.

until 1938 that the operation was successfully performed by Robert Gross (1905–1989) while chief resident at the Boston Children's Hospital. The patient was an undernourished girl of 7 who had become breathless after moderate exercise and whose physical activities had thus been considerably limited. The mediastinum was approached through the left chest and the short ductus was tied with a braided silk ligature. A sterile stethoscope was used at the operation and this confirmed that the extremely loud continuous murmur had disappeared. The operation was uneventful, the blood taken from a donor prior to the operation was not used, and the girl made an uneventful recovery. In 1940, Gross reported another three successes and over the next 20 years no fewer than 1500 cases of persistent ductus were treated by ligation at this centre, with a mortality of only 3%. In his 1940 report, Gross was doubtful whether patients already affected by bacterial endocarditis could be regarded as suitable for operation, however Oswald Tubbs (1908–1993), at St Bartholomew's Hospital, London, using the sulphonamide sulphapyridine, first ligated

an infected ductus in 1939 and by 1943 reported six survivors in nine cases.

Coarctation of the aorta (Figure 14.8b)

Coarctation of the aorta is a congenital anomaly in which the aorta in the region of the ductus arteriosus is grossly narrowed. One theory of its aetiology is that it represents an extension of the fibrosing process that closes the ductus soon after birth. The problem may present as heart failure in infancy, but more often becomes manifest some years later as gross hypertension, the subject having survived because of the development of an extraordinary system of collateral channels between the branches of the aorta above and below the constriction. The high blood pressure, incidentally, is the result of poor perfusion of the kidneys.

It fell to Clarence Crafoord (1899–1984) of the Karolinska Institute in Stockholm to carry out the first resection of a coarctation in 1944. The aorta was cross-clamped above and below the stenosis, the segment excised and direct suture of the divided

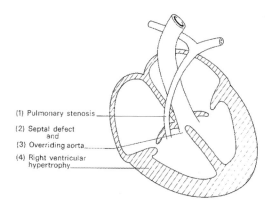

(1) Pulmonary stenosis
(2) Septal defect
     and
(3) Overriding aorta
(4) Right ventricular
     hypertrophy

Figure 14.9 The tetralogy of Fallot.
From Ellis H: *Clinical Anatomy*. Oxford, Blackwell, 11th edition, 2006.

ends carried out. The first patient was a boy of 12 and the second patient, a few days later, a 27-year-old farmer. Both operations were successful. The following year, Robert Gross, who was probably unaware of Crafoord's successes, (carried out, remember, during World War II), resected a coarctation in a 5-year-old boy who died of heart failure. The following week he operated successfully on a 12-year-old girl. Gross went on to show, in 1948, that a preserved segment of aorta could be used as a homograft to restore continuity after resection of a long coarctation.

Fallot's tetralogy

In 1884, Etienne-Louis Fallot of Marseilles described three cases of a tetralogy of congenital anomalies of the heart, now recognised to be one of the commonest causes of 'blue babies' – infants who are cyanosed from birth because of defective oxygenation of the blood. This results either from shunting of the blood through a defect in the septum between the right and left sides of the heart, or because of obstruction of the pulmonary trunk, with resultant deficiency of lung perfusion, or a combination of the two. Fallot's tetralogy (Figure 14.9) comprises

stenosis of the pulmonary trunk, hypertrophy of the right ventricle, a ventricular septal defect and the aorta over-riding both the ventricles. The first operations to deal with this problem represent one of the major steps in the development of modern heart surgery. Russell Brock wrote: 'It showed that cyanotic congenital heart disease, previously incurable and always fatal, could be cured by surgery. This inspired and stimulated the enormous advance in cardiac surgery that followed with almost breathless rapidity within a very short time'.

The story starts with Dr Helen Taussig (1898–1986), Professor of Paediatrics at the Johns Hopkins Hospital, Baltimore, who is regarded as the 'mother' of paediatric cardiology. She had noted that babies with Fallot's tetralogy who had an associated persistent ductus arteriosus were in better condition and survived longer than children without this additional defect. She realised that the ductus was acting as a shunt, allowing oxygenated arterial blood from the aorta to enter the pulmonary artery distal to the stenosis. This suggested to her that a man-made shunt might serve the same purpose. She put the proposition to Robert Gross, with his expertise on the surgery of patent ductus arteriosus, but he regarded children with Fallot's tetralogy as being inoperable. She therefore turned to Alfred Blalock (1899–1964), who was appointed to the staff of her hospital in 1941 and who had already carried out some experimental studies in which he had performed an end-to-end anastomosis of the sub-clavian artery to the pulmonary artery in dogs in order to study pulmonary hypertension. Blalock as a youngster had had pulmonary tuberculosis treated by a pneumothorax and his early education was severely disrupted. After training at Baltimore, he spent three years as Professor of Surgery at Vanderbilt University, where he carried out important studies on shock, showing how closely the clinical picture could be correlated with blood loss. Inspired by Taussig, he produced experimental pulmonary hypertension in dogs and showed that the cyanosis was relieved by subclavian to pulmonary artery anastomosis. The first patient to be submitted to the procedure, in 1944, was a 15-month-old baby whose condition was greatly improved but who died following a further shunt operation that was required a few months later. The following year two further operations were performed on children aged six and 11. In these cases, the brachiocephalic artery was anastomosed end-to-side into the pulmonary artery. Both cases were successful and, by 1952, no less than 1000 of these Blalock–Taussig operations had been performed at the Johns Hopkins Hospital with an operative mortality of just over 15%.

In 1947 Taussig and Blalock lectured and demonstrated their operation in London, Paris and Stockholm and it was rapidly taken up by the European surgeons, particularly Russell Brock (Figure 14.13) at Guy's Hospital and Charles Dubost (Figure 14.28) at the Broussais Hospital in Paris.

Something of the excitement engendered by this operation is caught by this description of the visit of Blalock and Taussig to London by Russell Brock:

Alfred Blalock and Helen Taussig gave a combined lecture in the Great Hall of the British Medical Association; the huge hall was packed. Dr Taussig delivered her address impeccably, followed by Dr Blalock who presented his surgical contribution. The silence of the audience betokened their rapt attention and appreciation. The hall was quite dark for projection of his slides which had been illustrating patients before and after the operation, when suddenly a searchlight beam traversed the full length of the hall and unerringly picked out on the platform a Guy's nursing sister dressed in her attractive blue uniform, sitting on a chair and holding a small cherub-like girl of two and a half years with a halo of blond curly hair and looking pink and well; she had been operated on at Guy's by Blalock a week earlier. The effect was dramatic and theatrical and the applause from the audience was tumultuous.

Not all cases were suitable for this procedure, especially very small infants in whom the subclavian artery was too small for the surgical techniques available at that time. In 1946 Willis Potts (1895–1968) of Chicago, using an ingenious clamp, performed direct side-to-side anastomosis between the aorta and the pulmonary trunk.

In subsequent years, many of these patients, who would otherwise have died, had definitive reconstructions of their cardiac defects once open heart surgery became possible and the shunt operations have now passed into history.

Surgery on the beating heart

Over the centuries, from the time of Galen, wounds of the heart were considered fatal. With the advent of anaesthesia and of antiseptic surgery, the latter part of the 19th century saw an explosion in the surgery of the abdominal cavity, of the chest, skull and the limbs, yet the heart was considered to be a 'no go' region of the body. Theodor Billroth himself, that father of modern surgery from Vienna, stated, 'The surgeon who would attempt to suture a wound of the heart should lose the respect of his colleagues,' while in London Stephen Paget wrote, in 1896, 'No new method and no new discovery can overcome the natural difficulties that attend a wound of the heart. It is true that heart suture has been vaguely proposed as a possible procedure and has been done in animals, but I cannot find that it has ever been attempted in practice'.

However, just a year later, Ludwig Rehn (1849–1930), Professor of Surgery at Frankfurt am Main, reported the case of a young man who had been stabbed in the left chest through the fourth intercostal space and was admitted to hospital breathless, pale and shocked. Rehn opened the chest through the left fourth interspace, resected the fifth rib and opened the pericardium. Blood was seen to be emerging through a pericardial laceration, enlargement of which revealed a large amount of clot and a 1.5 cm wound in the left ventricle. He wrote:

I used a fine needle with silk thread. At the beginning of diastole the needle was passed deeply through the muscle about the wound and at the next diastole the thread was tied . . . after the first suture the bleeding was diminished. By pulling up on the first suture a second was easily applied. It was frightening to note that the heart stopped after each suture was tied in place. After insertion of the third suture, which was specially difficult to insert because of the movement of the heart, the bleeding stopped completely. The heart now seemed to function well and we could breathe again.

The pericardial cavity was packed with iodoform gauze. The patient developed an empyema, which was drained, and, in spite of this, went on to make a full recovery. Rehn reported his success both in the *German Archives of Clinical Surgery* and in *The Lancet* under the title 'The successful treatment of a wound of the heart'.

Soon after Rehn's success, Parrozzani in Rome recorded a second success, which was also reported in *The Lancet* by GS Brock, who added as a comment:

Happily it is only in Italy that surgeons have many opportunities of practicing cardiac surgery – opportunities that they owe to the terrible frequency to which the dagger is resorted to in this country in the quarrels of the lower orders.

What would Brock have thought of the scene in our streets in this country today?

In 1907, ten years after his success, Rehn was able to review no less than 124 recorded cases of operations on cardiac stab wounds, with a recovery rate of 40%. Of the fatal cases, 44% died of haemorrhage and shock and 40% from infection. He advised that the weapon, if still present, should be left in place until the pericardium could be opened fully. He advocated a single intercostal incision carried outwards from the sternal edge and passing through the external wound rather than the large flap used by some other surgeons. If more room was needed, the skin incision was enlarged by converting it to an L-shape along the outer margin of the sternum, dividing the exposed costal cartilages and forcibly retracting the flap of skin and bone.

Rehn's successful operation and the subsequent successes of other surgeons showed that there was nothing 'sacred' about the heart – putting sutures into it was difficult but not impossible.

At the beginning of the 20th century there were a number of suggestions that stenosed valves of the heart might be treated surgically. Sir Thomas Lauder Brunton (1844–1916), Physician at St Bartholomew's Hospital, London, perhaps best known for introducing amyl nitrate in the treatment of angina, wrote a letter to *The Lancet* in 1902 headed *A Preliminary Note on the Possibility of*

Treating Mitral Stenosis by Surgical Methods which followed experiments on dead dogs with instruments passed through the heart wall. Arbuthnot Lane (see Figure 10.7) wrote enthusiastically to *The Lancet* in response to this and was keen to try cutting the valve with a long knife passed down the jugular vein. None of the physicians at Guy's would ever refer a patient to him! Most remarkably of all, Alexis Carrel (1873–1944) (see Figure 15.4) in 1909 and 1910 performed experimental procedures on the dog's heart which included digital exploration of the inside of the heart chambers, dilatation of the mitral valve, incision and suture of the ventricular wall and preparation of a coronary artery for anastomosis. In his paper *On the Experimental Surgery of the Thoracic Aorta and the Heart* he anticipated coronary by-pass surgery by many years, writing:

In certain cases of angina pectoris, when the mouth of the coronary artery is calcified, it would be useful to establish a complementary circulation for the lower part of the arteries. I attempted to perform an indirect anastomosis between the descending aorta and the left coronary artery. It was, for many reasons, a difficult operation. On account of the continuous motion of the heart, it was not easy to dissect and suture the artery. In one case I implanted one end of a long carotid artery, preserved in cold storage on the descending aorta. The other end was passed through the pericardium and anastomosed to the peripheral end of the coronary artery. Unfortunately the operation was too slow. Three minutes after the interruption of the circulation fibrillary contraction appeared but the anastomosis took five minutes. By massage of the heart the dog was kept alive but died two hours later.

As we shall see, direct coronary artery surgery did not become established until the late 1960s!

In the 1920s, two surgeons performed operations for mitral stenosis with recovery of the patient. In Boston, Elliott Cutler (1888–1947), who was to succeed Harvey Cushing as Chief of Surgery at the Brigham Hospital, inserted a narrow knife through the wall of the right ventricle in an 11-year-old girl and blindly cut the stenosed mitral valve. The child recovered and survived for four years, although she remained disabled by repeated episodes of heart failure and can hardly be regarded as a success.

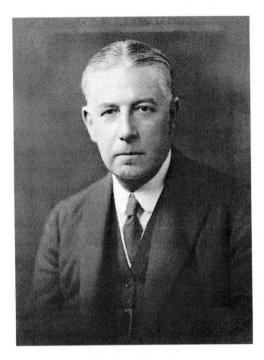

Figure 14.10 Henry Souttar.
Royal College of Surgeons of England.

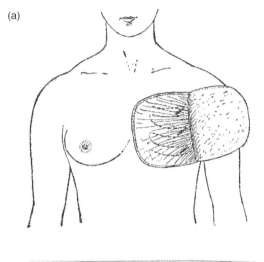

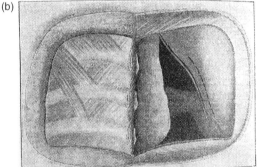

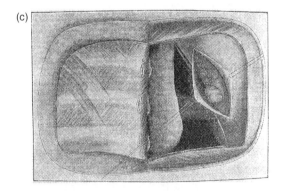

Two further patients submitted to the same procedure died post-operatively.

It was Sir Henry Sessions Souttar (1875–1964) (Figure 14.10), of the London Hospital, who in 1925 carried out the first trans-auricular mitral valvotomy, an operation that would not be revived until 1948. His patient was a girl of 15, under the care of Lord Dawson, who was admitted in a parlous state with cyanosis and heart failure. The heart was approached by turning a large skin flap on the left chest outwards, and a flap of three ribs inwards (Figure 14.11). The mitral valve was dilated by a finger passed through the left auricular appendage (Figure 14.12) which was then closed with a silk ligature. The girl made a smooth recovery and lived in very fair health for five years. She then had a cerebral infarct, probably from a clot in the left auricular appendage, from which she died. Souttar wrote: 'It appears to me that the method of digital

Figure 14.11 Souttar's mitral valvotomy, the approach. (a) Skin flap raised. (b) Chest wall flap with pleura turned inwards. (c) Pericardium opened to reveal the left auricular appendage.

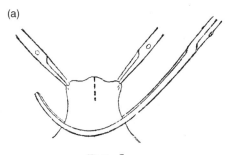

FIG. 5.

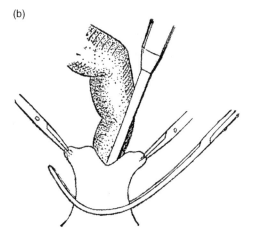

Figure 14.12 Souttar's mitral valvotomy; the procedure. (a) Soft clamp applied to the base of the left auricular appendage. Antero-posterior incision made. (b) Left forefinger inserted into the incision. Clamp was then removed to allow finger to enter the left atrium. From Souttar, H: The surgical treatment of mitral stenosis *BMJ* 1925; 2, 603.

exploration through the auricular appendage cannot be surpassed for simplicity and directness. Not only is the mitral orifice directly to hand, but the aortic valve itself is most certainly within reach, through the mitral orifice'.

Souttar was keen, of course, to repeat the procedure but never did so. He lived long enough, however, to see his operation revived by others. In his eighty-third year he wrote: 'I did not repeat the operation because I couldn't get another case.

Though my patient made an uninterrupted recovery the physicians declared that it was all nonsense and in fact that the operation was unjustifiable'.

The current medical opinion of that time was that the symptoms of valvular disease of the heart were produced by 'exhaustion of the heart muscle' rather than the obstructing effects of the valvular disease.

Progress in direct surgery of the heart now had to wait until the Second World War. A number of examples of successful removal of foreign bodies lodged in the heart were reported during the First World War, for example by the French surgeons Pierre Duval (1874–1941) and Henri Hartmann (1860–1952) and by Berkeley Moynihan (see Figure 8.16). Duval incidentally also pioneered the removal of foreign bodies of warfare lodged in the lung. However, it was the Second World War that provided extensive experience of this type of surgery. At the time of the Normandy Landings in 1944, a young surgeon, Dwight Harken (1910–1993) of the Brigham Hospital, Boston, who had been a surgical registrar at the Brompton Hospital in London before the war, was appointed Chief of Surgery at the United States Army Chest Center in England. In 1946 he published his astonishingly good results of surgery performed for missile wounds of the mediastinum. These comprised 78 missiles located in and around the great vessels, 56 in the heart wall or pericardium and 13 within the heart chambers themselves. Every patient recovered.

After the war, there was renewed interest in the possibility of operating on patients with stenosis of the heart valves. In 1947 Thomas Holmes Sellors (1902–1987) of the Middlesex Hospital operated on a 20-year-old patient with Fallot's tetralogy. He found that the stenosed pulmonary valve projected into the pulmonary trunk with each beat of the heart. He passed a tenotomy knife through the infundibulum of the right ventricle, divided the stenosed valve and the patient did well. Russell Brock (1903–1980) (Figure 14.13), early in the next year, and probably unaware of Sellors' success, used a specially designed dilator in three cases of pulmonary stenosis. Later in the same year, he designed a punch

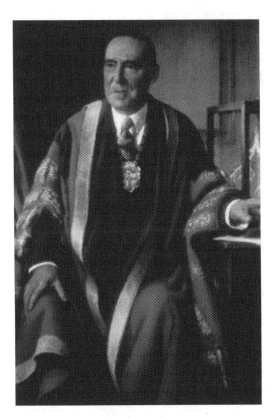

Figure 14.13 Russell Brock.
Portrait in the Gordon Museum, Guy's Hospital.

to resect the infundibular muscle stenosis which is often associated with Fallot's tetralogy.

Also in 1948, and indeed within a few months of each other, four surgeons carried out successful operations for mitral stenosis resulting from rheumatic fever. Horace Smithy (1914–1948), of Charlotte, revived the Cutler operation using a punch passed through the right atrial appendage to remove a portion of the mitral valve. Charles Bailey (1910–1993) at the Hahnemann Hospital, Philadelphia, Dwight Harken in Boston and Russell Brock at Guy's all adopted the finger fracture technique used by Henry Souttar in 1925. It was this technique that was widely adopted although later modifications included using a finger knife, a mechanical dilator or fine scissors. Many thousands

of these 'blind' operations were performed until the introduction of heart by-pass made direct surgery on valves possible.

Russell Brock was one of the great names in post-war thoracic surgery. He was a student at Guy's and spent the whole of his surgical career there and at the Brompton Hospital for Diseases of the Chest. It was the year he spent with Evarts Graham (see Figure 14.2) in St Louis with a Rockefeller fellowship in 1929 that developed his interest in chest surgery. He made important contributions to the detailed anatomy of the lung – so important in segmental resection – and in the treatment of lung abscess, as well as his cardiac work described above. He was a shy man with a brusque manner but was entirely dedicated to his work. In 1965 he was appointed Lord Brock of Wimbledon.

Open heart surgery

By 1950, operative procedures performed either blindly through the heart walls or by shunting of major blood vessels had reached their limits of achievement. Further progress depended on being able to open the heart chambers and carry out direct surgery, for example to suture or patch a septal defect – a 'hole in the heart'. In 1951, Robert Gross, a superb technician, described his ingenious technique in which he sutured a plastic well on to the right atrium through which he opened this chamber; blood would rise up in the well but not overflow from this low pressure cavity. Through the well, he could pass a finger into the atrium to palpate the septal defect and, with his great skill, could suture it through the pool of blood. Obviously this was a difficult operation and any error in diagnosis – if the defect, in fact, involved the ventricular septum for example – would render the procedure impossible.

How then to stop the heart and allow surgery on the now quiet and empty pump? The problem of course, is that, deprived of its circulation, the brain is irreparably damaged in four to five minutes. Two possibilities were now explored, hypothermia or a heart by-pass pump. Cooling the body prolongs the time that the circulation can be interrupted, since cold tissues require less oxygen than normal. Hypothermia was induced by placing the anaesthetised patient in an ice-water bath, giving chlorpromazine to prevent shivering. A temperature of 30°C allows the surgeon a ten-minute period of cardiac arrest; enough to carry out a simple atrial defect repair, for example. Initial experimental work by W G Bigelow (1913–2005) of Toronto, published in 1950, reported that dogs cooled to 20°C allowed 15 minutes of cardiac arrest; in 11 dogs upon whom sham operations were performed on the heart, six survived after recovery. Two years later, John Lewis, assisted by Richard Varco (contemp.) and Walton Lillehei (1918–1999) at the University of Minnesota in Minneapolis cooled a 5-year-old girl to 27°C and repaired an atrial defect with survival. Hypothermia remained the sole method of open heart surgery from 1952 until 1954, when cardiopulmonary bypass became available.

The story of the development of the heart pump is one of great endeavour on the part of a handful of pioneers. The problems were immense, particularly how to oxygenate the blood without filling it with dangerous bubbles of gas and how to pump the blood without the pump itself damaging the blood corpuscles. Much of the early work, in fact, was carried out by one man, John Gibbon (1903–1973), assisted by his wife, who was a laboratory technician. They commenced work in 1934 when Gibbon was a surgical research fellow at the Massachusetts General Hospital in Boston. He started with a second-hand air pump to circulate the blood and an oxygenator which comprised a rotating drum to produce a thin film of blood exposed to oxygen across a mesh screen. It was not until 1939 that the Gibbons could achieve long-term survival of cats subjected to complete interruption of their circulation. The work was interrupted by the war, but recommenced in 1945, by which time Gibbon was Professor of Surgery at Jefferson Medical College in Philadelphia. By 1948, he was able to repair artificially produced ventricular septal defects in dogs. In 1953, Gibbon and his team used the pump to operate on five patients with septal defects. Only one, the first, an 18-year-old girl, survived after her atrial defect was repaired with a continuous silk suture during a 26-minute cardiac arrest period. Discouraged by the disasters of the succeeding four patients, Gibbon abandoned further cardiac surgery at the age of 53.

A year later, in 1954, Walton Lillehei (1918–1999) in Minneapolis introduced a revolutionary idea; he used a donor (usually the child's parent) as the 'pump oxygenator', linking the donor's circulation to that of the patient, and utilising the donor's lungs as the means of oxygenation (Figure 14.14). Assisted by Richard Varco (contemp.) he carried out closure of a ventricular septal defect in a child under cross circulation from the father. The operation went well, but the child died of pneumonia on the 11th day. The second and third patients survived, and a total of 45 complex congenital heart anomalies were repaired with reasonable results. For example, five out of ten children with reconstruction of their Fallot's tetralogy survived. Not surprisingly, the operation came under serious criticism from the moral point of view; it was called an operation with a potential mortality risk of 200%, with the distinct danger that both the patient and the donor might perish. Indeed, one mother potential donor had a difficult anaesthetic induction with cardiac arrest. She recovered, although suffering partial paralysis, and the operation was cancelled. Apart from this, there was, in fact, no donor morbidity. However, the successes did revive interest in the use of a by-pass pump.

Indeed Lillehei himself, with Richard de Wall, developed an effective pump using the technique of bubbling oxygen through the blood and then removing the bubbles in a chamber containing a silicone antifoam substance. This apparatus was first used clinically in 1955 (Figure 14.15).

Meanwhile, at the Mayo Clinic in Rochester, Minnesota, John Kirklin and his team invested heavily in improving the Gibbon pump. The initial results were frankly terrible; all five of Kirklin's patients died immediately or soon after surgery. Of the next ten, five survived, but within two years the mortality was below 10%.

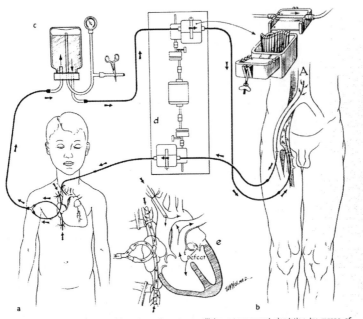

Figure 2 Method for direct vision intracardiac surgery utilizing extracorporeal circulation by means of controlled cross-circulation. **a** Patient, showing sites of arterial and venous cannulations. **b** Donor, showing sites of arterial and venous (superficial femoral and great saphenous) cannulations. **c** Gravity venous drainage reservoir (set on floor below patient). **d** Sigmamotor pump (single motor, two pumping heads) with multi-cams massaging the tubing seen in inset. **e** Close-up of the patient's heart showing the vena cava catheter positioned so as to draw venous blood from both the superior and inferior venae cavae during the cardiac bypass interval. The arterial blood from the donor was circulated to the patient's body through the catheter inserted into the left or right subclavian artery. A, aorta

Figure 14.14 Intracardiac surgery on a child using cross circulation from the parent.
From Lillehei CW: The birth of open-heart surgery. *Cardiovascular Surgery* 1994; 2, 308.

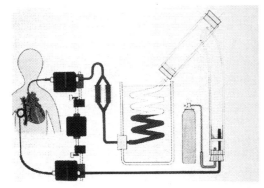

Figure 14.15 Schematic diagram of the De Wall–Lillehei bubble oxygenator.
From Naef AP: *The Story of Thoracic Surgery*. Bern, Hans Huber, 1990.

Now an amazing situation existed. Throughout 1955 to 1956 there were only two places in the world, some 90 miles apart, where it was possible to observe avant garde surgeons of the day performing open heart surgery. Visitors from all over the world commuted between Rochester and Minneapolis to watch Kirklin and Lillehei perform what seemed to be miraculous surgery. Of course, over the next few years the machines and the techniques spread throughout the world.

Artificial heart valves

As early as 1949, Charles Hufnagel (1917–1989) developed a prosthetic caged ball valve and carried out the first human valve implant by inserting his apparatus into the descending aorta, leaving the damaged valve in situ. By 1952, now at the Georgetown University in Washington, he was able to report 23 operations with 17 survivors. Once open heart surgery had been made possible, the way was open for direct valve replacement and the first successful subcoronary aortic valve implant was carried out by Dwight Harken in 1963.

Valve surgery was undoubtedly popularised by Albert Starr (contemp.) in Portland, Oregon. He constructed his own patent of ball valve with an engineer, Lowell Edwards (who had designed the fuel pump used in American fighter planes in World War II) and, by 1967, 1800 Starr–Edwards valves had been implanted world-wide (Figure 14.16).

Other forms of valve replacement were the tilting disc or hinge valve (Figure 14.16), pioneered at the Karolinska Hospital in Stockholm by Viking Bjork (contemp.), and the use of heart valves taken from the pig and calf developed by Donald Ross (contemp.) at the National Heart and Guy's Hospitals in London. These 'biological valves' have the advantage that the patient does not require subsequent anticoagulation therapy to prevent clotting. However, they have a more limited life-span compared with mechanical values and are therefore used in the older age group of patients.

The surgery of coronary artery disease

Attempts to revascularise the heart muscle, the myocardium, in coronary artery disease (now, of course, one of the commonest causes of death in the Western world) commenced in the 1930s. Indeed, Claude Beck (1894–1971), Professor of Surgery at the Western Reserve University, Cleveland, devoted most of his professional life to this. After extensive animal experimentation, he performed the first human operation in this field in a 48-year-old man with severe angina in 1935. Beck abraided the surface of the left ventricle with a burr and sutured to it a pedicled graft of pectoralis major muscle. Seven months later the patient returned to work as a gardener. Over the next two years, Beck

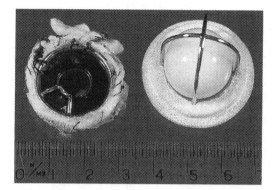

Figure 14.16 Prosthetic heart valves. Flap valve on the left, ball valve on the right.
Guy's Hospital.

carried out a total of 20 such operations. Of the first 16 cases, eight died, although the last five patients in the series all survived.

In 1941, Beck introduced the use of asbestos powder to produce adhesions between the heart muscle and pericardium. Others used talc, carborundum powder and other irritants and, until the advent of coronary bypass surgery, this procedure remained the commonest operation for coronary disease. In 1955 Beck reported 75 such operations with clinical improvement in 90% of cases. He also went on to devise a vein graft between the descending aorta and the coronary sinus, the main venous drainage of the heart, in order to perfuse the heart muscle in a retrograde manner.

Meanwhile, in London, Lawrence O'Shaugnessy (1900–1940) (Figure 14.17) was carrying out dog experiments and clinical studies on the use of the omentum as a vascular graft to the ischaemic heart (cardio-omentopexy). O'Shaugnessy was a New-castle graduate who had worked as a surgeon in the Sudan. While on leave from there, he visited Sauerbruch in Berlin and was inspired to take up cardiac surgery. On returning to England, he set up a cardiovascular clinic at the Lambeth London County Council Hospital. He showed that grey-hounds who had undergone coronary artery ligation had a normal exercise tolerance following an omental graft. By 1938 he could report 12 human

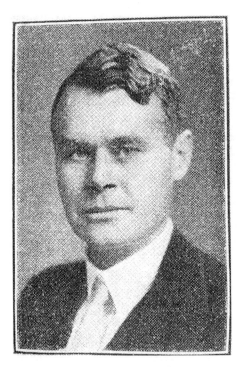

Figure 14.17 Laurence O'Shaugnessy.
Royal College of Surgeons of England.

omentopexy operations; there were three operative deaths but the rest of the patients, all with severe cardiac disease, showed dramatic clinical improvement. At the outbreak of the war, he joined the RAMC and was killed at the evacuation of Dunkirk in 1940, a tragic loss to surgery.

Not surprisingly, the operations of Beck and O'Shaugnessy met with considerable criticism on the grounds that adhesions normally become avascular and that any improvement observed in the patients would be purely subjective. I was particularly interested in this because in 1958, while carrying out experimental studies on post-operative abdominal adhesions for my doctorate thesis, I showed that adhesions between the omentum and devascularised intestine could produce such extensive vascular anastomoses that the ischaemic intestine could survive with its new blood supply. I suggested that the same phenomenon may well

have taken place in these operations on ischaemic hearts.

Another approach to myocardial revascularisation was devised by Arthur Vineberg (1903–1988) at McGill University in Montreal. In this operation, the internal mammary (thoracic) artery was mobilised and implanted into the heart muscle in an effort to produce collateral anastomoses. After extensive animal experiments, he carried out the first human operation in 1950 and in 1964 combined this procedure with omentopexy. He was able to show evidence in post-mortem injection studies of the development of new vascular communications into the hearts.

All these procedures were, of course, to be replaced by direct surgery on the coronary vessels themselves – a procedure, it should be remembered, suggested as long ago as 1910 by Alexis Carrel (see Figure 15.4 and p. 221).

It was to be half a century before Carrel's experimental work would be realised clinically. In 1956, Charles Bailey (1910–1993) at the Hahnemann Hospital, Philadelphia, first performed a coronary artery endarterectomy, removing a localised block in the vessel. This was performed successfully without cardiopulmonary bypass. The first operation of this nature using by-pass was carried out by Charles Dubost (1914–1991) in Paris (see Figure 14.28), who relieved a syphilitic obstruction at the mouth of the right coronary artery. The first coronary by-pass, using a segment of vein, much like the Carrel operation, was first performed by David Sabiston (contemp.) in 1962 (Figure 14.18) but the patient died three days later of a cerebro-vascular accident. Michael de Bakey (1908–2008) of Houston achieved the first success at this operation in 1964.

The other technique used to by-pass an obstructed coronary artery is to employ the distal end of the internal mammary (thoracic) artery as a shunt from the subclavian artery (Figure 14.18). This was first performed by Vasilii Kolesov (1904–1992), Chairman of Surgery at the First Leningrad Medical Institute. The patient was a 44-year-old man with severe angina who had his left internal mammary artery anastomosed to the circumflex coronary

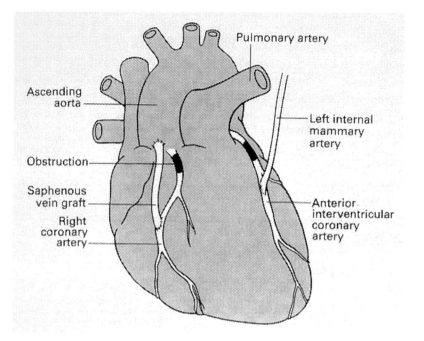

Figure 14.18 Diagram of coronary by-pass graft procedures. A reversed saphenous vein graft is shown on the right coronary artery and an internal thoracic artery (mammary) shunt on the anterior descending branch of the left coronary artery.
From Ellis H, Calne RY, Watson C: *Lecture Notes in General Surgery.* Oxford, Blackwell, 11th edition, 2006.

artery without using by-pass. There was no recurrence of his symptoms at three years. Kolesov went on to devise a circular mechanical suturing device for coronary surgery in 1967, carried out the procedure on a patient with an acute myocardial infarct in 1968 and performed a bilateral graft in 1969. Indeed, between 1964 and 1968, Leningrad was the only centre in the world performing this operation. Poor Kolesov! His pioneer work was not recognised in his own country, let alone in the rest of the world. At the All Union Cardiological Society meeting in Leningrad in June 1967, where he presented his work, a resolution was adopted which stated 'that the surgical treatment of coronary heart disease was impossible and without prospects for the future'. The following year, Charles Bailey performed the first internal mammary by-pass graft in the USA. Today, the coronary by-pass graft operation, often using both saphenous vein and internal mammary

artery, is far and away the heart operation most commonly performed.

Arterial surgery

For nearly two thousand years, arterial surgery consisted of ligation of major arteries for trauma and for aneurysm, and we have given examples of this in several previous chapters. Mentioned by the Roman encyclopaedist Celsus in the 1st century AD, arterial ligation for haemorrhage was popularised by Ambroise Paré in the 16th century (see Chapter 9) to replace the crude and cruel use of the cautery. The first mention of ligation in the treatment of aneurysm is attributed to Aetius who flourished in the 2nd century AD. His works have been lost but fragments are found in later Byzantine compilations. He advised ligation above and below

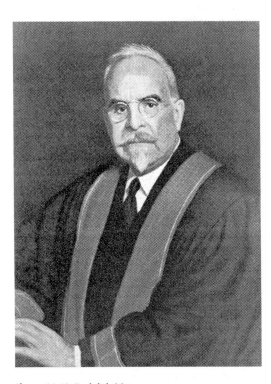

Figure 14.19 Rudolph Matas.
Royal College of Surgeons of England.

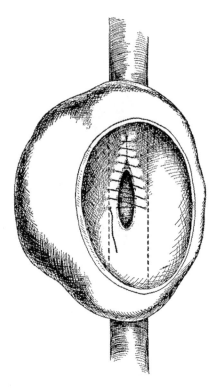

Figure 14.20 The Matas operation for saccular aneurysm; the communication with the sac is sutured from within without obliteration of the main artery. The sac is then closed by a series of sutures from within. Matas R: An operation for the radical cure of aneurysm based upon arteriorrhaphy. *Annals of Surgery* 1903; 37, 161.

the aneurysm, then opening and evacuating the clot from within the sac. Famous names associated with this type of surgery include John Hunter (Figure 6.15) who tied the femoral artery in the subsartorial (Hunter's) canal for popliteal aneurysm and Astley Cooper (Figure 6.26) who performed successful carotid ligation for aneurysm, described an approach to the iliac vessels and tied, sadly unsuccessfully, the abdominal aorta for a massive iliac aneurysm. This latter operation was to be performed with success by Rudolph Matas (1860–1957) (Figure 14.19) of New Orleans in 1925, a century later.

It was Rudolph Matas who took the first steps in reconstructive arterial surgery. In 1888 he performed the first cure of an aneurysm by opening the sac and obliterating it with sutures without obstructing the lumen of the artery (Figure 14.20). In 1903, in an extensive article in the *Annals of*

Surgery, he showed that this technique could be applied with success to saccular aneurysm. When the sac was fusiform, the orifices of the feeding vessels were sutured from within the lumen of the aneurysm and the sac was then obliterated (Figure 14.21). This remained the only method of conservative treatment of aneurysm until the 1950s when, as we shall see, graft replacement of the aneurysm was introduced.

Today, the routine treatment of a wound of a major artery is repair rather than ligation. Yet ligation was the commonly performed operation in the Second World War and vascular repair only became relatively common in the Korean conflict

RDIOVASCULAR SURGERY

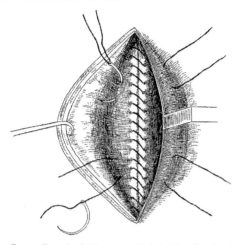

FIG. 5.—Shows the details of the method of obliteration after the

Figure 14.21 The Matas procedure for fusiform aneurysm. The sac is obliterated from within by successive rows of sutures.
Matas R: An operation for the radical cure of aneurysm based upon arteriorrhaphy. *Annals of Surgery* 1903; 37, 161.

(1950–1953). This is somewhat surprising, since the first repair of a gunshot wound of the femoral artery was successfully performed in Chicago in 1897 by J B Murphy (1857–1916) (Figure 14.22). His case report comes at the end of a 15-page description which details experiments he performed in dogs, calves and sheep, and in which he describes his studies on lateral repair, end-to-end suture and apposition by invagination of the carotid and the aorta. Fine silk on small needles was the suture most often used. The patient was an Italian pedlar aged 29 who had been shot in the groin. Two days after the injury, the pulsations in the arteries below the femoral were extremely weak and at the groin a thrill could be felt and a bruit could be heard. The following day, Murphy explored the groin and found an arterio-venous aneurysm of the femoral vessels (Figure 14.23). The vein was repaired; one half inch of the damaged femoral artery was resected and the proximal end invaginated into the distal for one third of an inch with four double-

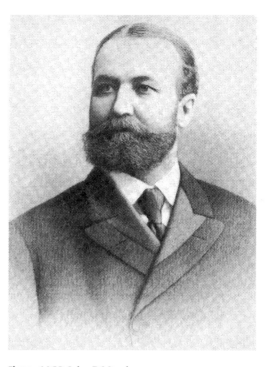

Figure 14.22 John B Murphy.
From Davis L: *Surgeon Extraordinary, the Life of JB Murphy*. London, Harrap, 1938.

needled sutures. A row of sutures was then placed around the edge of the overlapping distal end (Figure 14.24). Pulsation was immediately restored in the artery below the line of suture and could be felt in the pulses at the ankle. The time for the operation was approximately two and a half hours. A month later the patient was able to walk about the ward and had no disturbance of the circulation.

J B Murphy was undoubtedly one of the most colourful characters of American surgery. Even his name reflects something of his character; he was born of humble Irish immigrants on a farm in Wisconsin and was christened plain John Murphy. However, when he went to school, he noticed that the majority of the other boys had at least two initials and so, determined not to be inferior, he added the 'B' to his name. He studied medicine at Rush Medical College in Chicago and spent the rest

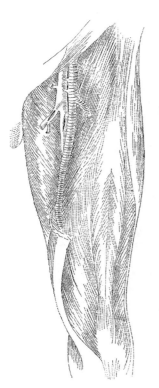

Figure 14.23 Murphy's repair of a gun-shot wound of the femoral artery; the sites of arterial and venous injury. From Murphy JB: Resection of arteries and veins injured in continuity – end to end suture – experimental and clinical research. *Medical Record* 1897; 51, 74.

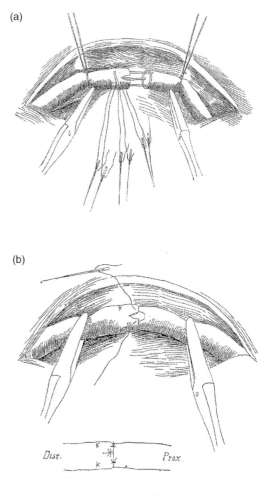

Figure 14.24 Murphy's repair of gun-shot wound of the femoral artery; steps in the vessel repair. Murphy JB: Resection of arteries and veins injured in continuity – end to end suture – experimental and clinical research. *Medical Record* 1897; 51, 74.

of his career in that city apart from two years in Vienna studying under Billroth. Most of his work was carried out at the Mercy Hospital.

Murphy advanced surgical knowledge of almost every region of the body. He was interested in the surgery of the lung and was the first in America to carry out artificial pneumothorax. He was interested in the surgery of bones and joints, and he advanced our management of peritonitis, for which he used fluid replacement by means of a rectal drip. He also invented the Murphy button, an ingenious device for effective intestinal anastomosis which has recently been reintroduced, now in an absorbable form, and did much to popularise

early surgery for acute appendicitis. For this he described the 'Murphy sequence': pain at the umbilicus, vomiting, followed by pain moving to the right iliac fossa – a sequence that is, of course, classical of this condition. After several minor attacks of coronary thrombosis he succumbed to a major infarct at the age of 59. To my mind, it was this case of arterial repair, based on meticulous and extensive experimental studies, which was his most important contribution to surgery.

The next advance was undoubtedly the meticulous experimental work of Alexis Carrel, which commenced in Lyon in 1901 and continued at the Rockefeller Institute in New York, which he joined in 1905. We will describe his techniques for end-to-end suture of blood vessels, which form the basis of modern arterial surgery, in the next chapter (see Figures 15.5 and 15.6).

It is interesting that all this work was carried out before an effective anticoagulant was available so that the surgeon was constantly faced by the problem of clotting within the occluded artery. Heparin was isolated from the liver in 1916 (hence its name – Greek *hepar*, liver). However, it was not put into effective clinical use for a further two decades, a fact that certainly hindered the development of reconstructive arterial surgery.

In spite of the absence of an effective anticoagulant, the operation of embolectomy – the removal of an embolus impacted in, and obstructing, a major artery – was attempted unsuccessfully by Berkeley Moynihan (see Figure 8.16) in Leeds and by Sampson Handley (see Figure 11.12) at the Middlesex Hospital, London, in 1907. The first successes were reported by Ernest Mosny (1861–1918) in France in 1911 and by Einar Key (1872–1954) in Stockholm the following year. The first successful case in the United Kingdom was not achieved until 1934, when Sir Geoffrey Jefferson (1886–1961) of Manchester successfully removed an embolus from the brachial artery. However, even after the introduction of heparin, surgery often failed because of difficulty in removing clots that had propagated down the obstructed artery beyond the embolus. The problem was only overcome in the early 1960s by the introduction of the balloon catheter by Thomas Fogarty (contemp.), which he devised when he was a young surgical resident at the University of Oregon in Portland. This is a fine catheter which is threaded down the lumen of the artery after removal of the embolus. A tiny balloon is inflated at the tip of the catheter which is then withdrawn, removing the obstructing clot with it.

Before reconstructive surgery could be contemplated for degenerative arterial pathology, by far the commonest cause of peripheral arterial disease, it was necessary to delineate the site of the obstruction, its extent, and whether there was vessel patency distal to the obstruction. This was made possible by the development of angiography – X-rays of the vascular tree after injection of radio-opaque contrast material into the artery above the blockage. This was carried out first by the neurologist Antonio Moniz (1874–1955), who performed the first carotid angiogram in Lisbon in 1927, and then by Reynaldo Dos Santos (1880–1970) who performed the first aortogram in the same city two years later. It was his son, Joao Sid Dos Santos (1907–1975) who carried out the first endarterectomy of the femoral artery in 1946, again in Lisbon. This operation utilises the plane of cleavage within the media layer of the arteriosclerotic artery, which allows removal of the central thrombus and the diseased inner layer of the artery with reconstitution of the outer healthy wall of the vessel.

As with so many other basic procedures in vascular surgery, it was Alexis Carrel, with his co-worker Charles Guthrie, who showed experimentally that a segment of vein or a piece of preserved artery could be used as an arterial graft. Indeed, one or two surgeons carried out such procedures in patients. An early pioneer was James Hogarth Pringle (1863–1941) of the Glasgow Royal Infirmary who treated two patients in 1912, one for an aneurysm of the popliteal artery and the second, a boy of 19, for an extensive injury of the brachial artery. The first patient was a male aged 49 whose popliteal aneurysm was syphilitic in origin and who also had a double aortic murmur. The sac was excised and a segment of great saphenous vein was used to replace the arterial trunk (Figure 14.25). The graft remained patent until the patient died three years later of valvular heart disease. In the second case, Pringle replaced six centimetres of the damaged artery with a vein graft and the patient returned to work as a blacksmith two months later. However, it was not until 1948 that Jean Kunlin (1904–1991) of the Hôpital Foch at Suresnes, near Paris,

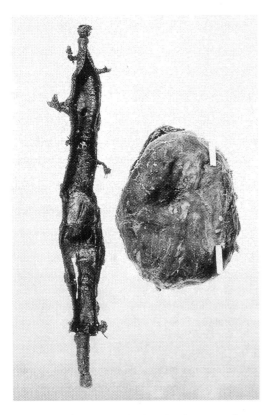

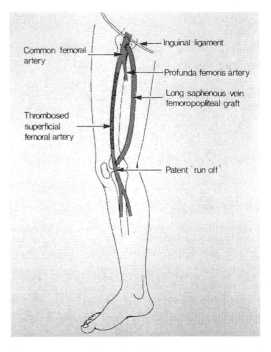

Figure 14.26 A saphenous vein by-pass graft for femoral artery obstruction.

Figure 14.25 The specimen of popliteal artery graft using saphenous vein, Hogarth Pringle's case. On the right is the resected aneurysm.
Museum of the Royal College of Surgeons of Edinburgh.

performed the first by-pass of a blocked femoral artery using the patient's own great saphenous vein. Of course, it was necessary to reverse the vein so that its valves would not occlude the flow of blood. This operation is still popular today (Figure 14.26).

The Korean War proved an enormous incentive to vein grafting and it was rapidly established that many limbs could be saved by such a procedure. For larger vessels, freeze-dried arteries taken from cadavers were used, but their popularity waned as they were found to degenerate with time. They were soon replaced with fabric grafts, made initially from nylon, orlon and Teflon. Knitted or woven dacron is currently used, as is Goretex (expanded polytetrafluoroethylene). In the early days, grafts were home-

made from the surgeon's own nylon shirt-tails. Figure 14.27 shows an aortic graft manufactured by the theatre nurses from my shirt; for all I know it is the only one still in existence.

Aortic aneurysm surgery

In 1951, Charles Dubost (1914–1991) (Figure 14.28) performed the first successful resection of an abdominal aortic aneurysm. This report greatly influenced surgeons throughout the world, who, until then, had regarded this entity as being outside the bounds of surgical removal and reconstruction. Indeed, as a young surgeon myself, I could hardly believe that such an operation was possible, having seen primitive attempts at dealing with this formidable problem by introducing coils of wire into the aneurysmal sac or otherwise having stood by and watched the patient exsanguinate from his ruptured aneurysm. The report of the operation was

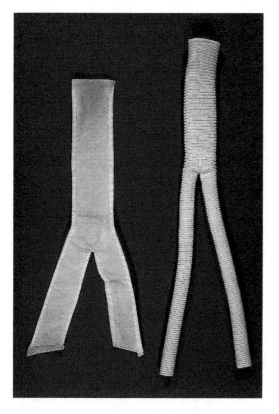

Figure 14.27 An aorto-iliac graft manufactured from the tail of my nylon shirt (left). On the right is a modern Goretex trouser graft used for this purpose.

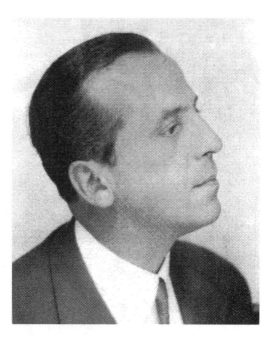

Figure 14.28 Charles Dubost. From Blondeau P: Necrologie de Charles Dubost. *La Presse Médicale* 1991; 20, 397.

published in *La Semaine des Hôpitaux de Paris* in September 1951, six months after the operation had been performed and, very unusually, was reprinted in translation in the USA, in the *Archives of Surgery* in 1952.

The patient was a male aged 50 who presented with a large pulsating mass in the abdomen and with gross vascular disturbance in the legs. One year previously he had had a myocardial infarction. An aortogram showed that the aneurysm commenced just below the kidneys and extended as far as the bifurcation of the aorta. The left common iliac artery was blocked and the right, although patent, had two small aneurysmal dilatations at its origin. The operation was performed through a left thoracoabdominal incision and the aorta exposed

extraperitoneally. An enormous aneurysm was exposed and controlled by clamps proximal to it, immediately below the renal arteries, and by isolating the external and internal iliac arteries. The sac was excised, leaving fragments adherent to the inferior vena cava and the common iliac veins. Reconstruction was performed using a graft taken from the thoracic aorta of a 20-year-old girl removed and frozen three weeks previously. The graft was sutured to the aorta above and to the right common iliac artery below while the stump of the left common iliac artery was anastomosed to the side of the graft (Figure 14.29). Three months after the operation the patient was in good health with strong pulses felt in both legs.

The success of this operation opened the way for elective surgery on similar cases and then as an emergency procedure in what was previously an inevitably fatal situation – rupture of the aneurysm.

Homografts were soon replaced by synthetic grafts and the operation was much simplified

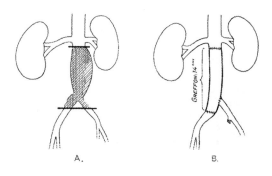
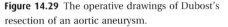

Figure 14.29 The operative drawings of Dubost's resection of an aortic aneurysm.
From Dubost C, Allary M, Oeconomos N: Resection of an aneurysm of the abdominal aorta reestablishment of the continuity by a preserved human arterial graft, with result after five months. *Archives of Surgery* 1952; 64, 405.

when it was realised that the sac itself need not be removed but merely opened, the graft inserted and the sac wall wrapped around the prosthesis.

Charles Dubost was born in Paris, studied in the capital city, qualified just before the Second World War and won the Croix de Guerre as a young medical lieutenant in 1940. He joined the Hôpital Broussais after the war as a general surgeon and in 1947 commenced cardiac surgery in a small special

'blue baby' unit at this hospital. We have already noted that it was that year that Alfred Blalock, on his European tour, demonstrated the Taussig–Blalock operation, and Dubost pioneered the operation in France. He also performed the first coronary endarterectomy under cardiac by-pass.

Dubost was internationally recognised as a leading cardiac surgeon of France. He became an officer of the Légion d'Honneur and was elected both to the Academy of Medicine and Academy of Science.

Endovascular surgery

Recent years have seen exciting advances in the development of minimal access surgery of arterial disease. Andreas Gruntzig (contemp.) in Zurich developed a balloon catheter that could be passed through a stenosed artery, and then blown up to dilate the constricted segment. He carried out the first angioplasties of the iliac and femoral arteries in 1972 and of the coronary arteries in 1977. In the past decade, techniques have been developed to insert prosthetic stents into obstructed arteries after their preliminary dilatation or after reaming out the obstructing segment, and also to repair aneurysms by stenting a graft within the lumen of the sac.

15

Organ transplantation

For centuries men dreamed of the possibility of replacing a diseased or damaged organ by means of a healthy graft. Indeed, in a popular fable, this was actually achieved by the patron saints of medicine, the twins Cosmas and Damian. They practised in Aleppo in what is now Syria, refused to give up their faith and were martyred under Diocletian in the 4th century AD. Visitors to their tomb reported miraculous cures and their bodies were taken to the church of their name in Rome. There a man with a gangrenous leg prayed at their tomb where a miraculous operation took place: the man's diseased leg was removed and that of a blackamoor who had recently died was grafted onto the stump. When the patient awoke in the morning he had two sound legs – one white and one black. This extraordinary graft was the subject of hundreds of paintings, some by the great masters (Figure 15.1).

Mythological surgery apart, it was to be many centuries before organ transplantation as we know it today was to become a reality. Surgeons were faced with a number of important, indeed apparently overwhelming, technical problems. There was the obvious surgical difficulty of maintaining the blood supply of the replaced organ and joining up its various ducts to the recipient. Then there was the difficulty of obtaining a suitable donor organ and the fact that a graft other than from the subject himself would soon die, a phenomenon which we now know is due to immunological rejection.

Some tissues can be transferred from one part of the body to another and will stimulate the blood supply from the host tissues; skin and bone are two examples of this. The bloodless cornea does not set up an immunological reaction in the recipient's tissues, so that corneal grafts can be performed successfully in completely unrelated subjects. Teeth set up a relatively weak reaction; as long ago as 1771, John Hunter (1728–1793) (see Figure 6.15) of St George's Hospital, London, transplanted healthy teeth, obtained at a price from indigent donors, to the gums of wealthier patients, where the graft would 'take' for a considerable time.

Skin grafting

We have already mentioned the work of the Hindu surgeon Susruta who devised a skin flap to replace the nose (see Figure 2.11). This was taken up by Gasparo Tagliacozzi (1546–1599) who, two years before his death, published a book that described his technique in detail. He first fashioned the surface of the stump of the amputated nose then cut a paper pattern of the new nose which he laid on the arm in the area to be chosen for the reconstruction. A skin flap on the arm was then cut to the exact size of the pattern and sutured into the nasal defect. The arm was then firmly splinted against the head (Figure 15.2). The stitches were removed when healing had taken place, about five to seven days after surgery, and the flap was divided from the arm as soon as sound healing had occurred, at about three weeks. Two weeks later, the new nose was trimmed to the desired shape, the nostrils being splinted by packs dipped in egg white inserted into

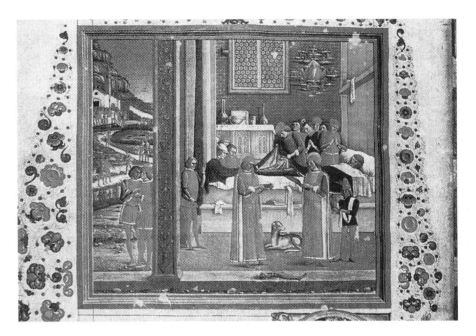

Figure 15.1 The brothers Cosmas and Damian after transplanting the leg of a Moor. Far in the background on the left the crowd inspect the Moor's body. The amputated limb lies in the foreground.
Miniature in a 15th century choir book attributed both to Andrea Mantegna and Guido de Ferrara. Copyright of the Society of Antiquities, London.

their cavities. The final shaping of the nose was carried out by inserting tubes into the nostrils.

Although Tagliacozzi became famous because of his work, his operation was considered by the Church to be sacrilegious, an attempt to improve upon God's handicraft. After his death his body was exhumed and thrown out of the holy ground in which it had been buried. However, later a statue was erected to him in Bologna; appropriately he holds an artificial nose in his hand.

The possibility of transplantation of skin as a free graft without the need to maintain its blood supply was a major advance. Giuseppi Baronio in 1804 showed that various sizes and shapes of pieces of skin could be removed from one area of the sheep's back and grafted successfully into another skin defect in the same animal; the experiment failed if the skin was taken from one animal and grafted to another (Figure 15.3). Felix Guyon (1831–1920) of Paris showed in 1869 that small pieces of skin could

be grafted into a wound and would heal. The same year Jacques Reverdin (1842–1929) of Geneva gave a more refined description of the same procedure and showed that a completely detached piece of skin could continue to live and grow on a raw recipient area if kept firmly in contact. He showed that best results were obtained when a number of small grafts were used, and so-called 'pinch grafts' are still used by this technique to this day. Only comparatively small areas can be thus grafted and the donor sites heal with rather ugly scars.

An important advance was made by Carl Thiersch (1822–1895), who was successively Professor of Surgery at Erlangen and Leipzig. In 1874 he published a paper describing his technique of skin grafting using a wafer-thin film of epidermis and sliver of underlying dermis. Large defects can be thus grafted and the great advantage is that the donor area of skin regenerates and can be used again if necessary – a feature of great value when

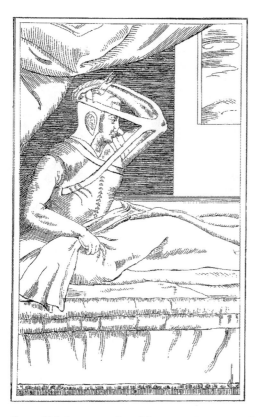

Figure 15.2 Reconstruction of the nose using an arm flap, performed by Tagliacozzi.
From Calne RY: *Renal Transplantation*. London, Arnold, 1963.

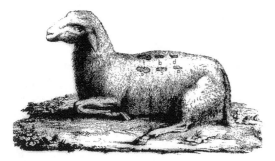

Figure 15.3 Baroni's experiment on skin autografting in the sheep.
From Calne RY: *Renal Transplantation*. London, Arnold, 1963.

extensive skin burns, perhaps involving more than 50% of the body surface, require grafting. The Thiersch graft is the standard procedure used today, now employing specially constructed large razors to cut the graft which can adjust the depth of the graft to the surgeon's requirements (the dermatome).

The First World War of 1914–1918 created vast numbers of casualties with horrible defects of the face which, up until then, would have defied repair. Harold Gillies (1882–1995), a young New Zealand ear, nose and throat surgeon in the RAMC, was designated to set up a dedicated team to deal with these cases and new techniques of skin replacement were rapidly evolved. The most important of these was the tubed pedicle flap. A flap of skin, from the arm, for example, was raised, stitched into a tube and attached to the defect in the patient's face. It derived its blood supply from the donor site, but new blood vessels would grow into it from the recipient area. Once this new blood supply was established, the base of the pedicle could be divided and the skin graft spread out to reconstruct the defect. Obviously this was a lengthy multi-staged procedure, but its results were revolutionary. Indeed, the pedicle flap remained in general use until recent years. Now, using the microscope to anastomose blood vessels, the plastic surgeon can take a flap of skin with its underlying soft tissues, muscle and even bone and transplant this at one stage to repair a massive defect. Indeed, using this technique, severed fingers and even limbs can be sewn back with a very high success rate.

Kidney transplantation

Of the solid organs, the kidney was the first to be used in experimental and then in human transplantation. Indeed, it remains today by far the most common organ to be transplanted. Over the last century a number of vitally important problems were successfully overcome: first the technical details of the transplantation operation; second, the means of improving the condition of the patient dying of renal failure in order to render him fit for surgery; third, and most difficult, the immunological barrier to the transference of tissues from one subject to another.

Emerich Ullmann (1861–1937), a Hungarian surgeon working in Vienna, grafted a kidney of a dog into its neck, joining the renal vessels to the carotid artery and jugular vein by means of tubes of magnesium, and letting urine drain through the ureter on to the skin of the neck. The graft lasted for five days. He showed that grafting a kidney from one dog to another or from a dog to a goat rapidly failed. Early clinical attempts were failures: Mathieu Jaboulay (1860–1913), of Lyon, grafted a pig's kidney to the elbow of a patient in renal failure and used a goat's kidney in another case. Both kidneys failed to secrete urine and were removed. In 1910 Ernst Ungar (1875–1938) of Berlin transplanted both the kidneys of a monkey into the groin of a woman dying of renal failure; the patient died two days later and a post-mortem of the grafted organs showed patchy necrosis. Another attempt, using a monkey kidney, by Schonstadt in 1930 also failed.

The first human kidney allograft was performed by Yu Voronoy (1895–1961) in Kiev in 1933. The kidney of a man who died of a head injury and was blood group B was taken six hours after death and grafted to the thigh of a woman of 26, blood group O, suffering from acute renal failure as a result of a suicide attempt by mercurial poisoning. The graft failed to function and she died two days later. By 1949 Voronoy had performed six such grafts with no substantial renal function in any of them.

It was the work of a remarkable and controversial man, Alexis Carrel (1873–1944) (Figure 15.4), that provided the major advance in the technique of organ transplantation, especially that of suturing small blood vessels together. He qualified in medicine in the University of Lyon in 1893 and studied under Jaboulay, a pioneer in the suture of lacerated arteries and who, as we have already mentioned, performed the first attempts at transplant to human patients. In June 1894, the murder

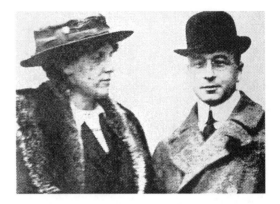

Figure 15.4 Anne Marie de la Meyrie and Alexis Carrel just before their marriage, Paris, 1913.
From Edwards WS: *Alexis Carrel, Visionary Surgeon.* Springfield, Thomas, 1974.

of the President of the French Republic, Sadi Carnet, in Lyon considerably impressed the young Doctor Carrel. Death was due to the transection of the portal vein of this unfortunate man by the knife of his assailant. Carrel insisted that his life could have been saved if surgeons learned to suture blood vessels effectively. Indeed, in the last decade of the 19th century several surgeons in Europe and America experimented with the suture of divided arteries, and the first successful repair of a gunshot wound of the femoral artery was performed in Chicago by J B Murphy (1857–1916) in 1897 (see Figures 14.23 and 14.24).

Carrel, as a young intern, experimented on the suturing of blood vessels, both arteries and veins, using fine needles and thread which he obtained from Lyonnaise lace-workers. In 1904, he moved to the University of Chicago, where he collaborated with the 25-year-old Charles Guthrie. Together, they established a special aseptic animal laboratory which abolished the infections that had dogged previous vascular experiments. They developed the triangulation technique for the anastomosis of fine blood vessels: the two ends were approximated by three separate stitches of fine silk or human hair, placed one-third of the way around the circumference (Figure 15.5). Retraction on each held the vessel ends together to allow insertion of a continuous

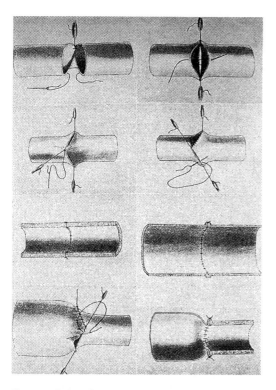

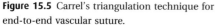

Figure 15.5 Carrel's triangulation technique for end-to-end vascular suture.
From Carrel A: La technique opératoire des anastomoses vasculaires et la transplantation des viscères. *Lyon Médical* 1902; 98, 859–864.

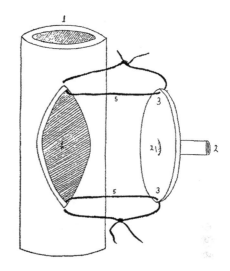

Figure 15.6 The Carrel patch.
From Carrel A: La technique opératoire des anastomoses vasculaires et la transplantation des viscères. *Lyon Médical* 1902; 98, 859–864.

stitch and avoided the possibility of catching the back wall of the artery. In addition, this method avoided picking up the edges of the vessel with forceps, which produced bruising and swelling of the wall, interfered with healing and facilitated thrombosis. Carrel and Guthrie developed grafting of segments of vein into artery, described patch vein grafts, which enlarged the diameter of the artery, and showed that the vein wall thickened to accommodate high arterial pressure. They predicted that the veins could be used for arterial reconstruction but it is surprising that the vein graft and vein patch method was not used in clinical practice until the 1950s. Carrel and Guthrie also demonstrated that a limb could be re-attached after

circulation was interrupted for over an hour, a procedure that was not carried out in human subjects until in 1962 a boy of 12 had his severed arm replanted at the Massachusetts Hospital, Boston.

Carrel had previously grafted a kidney to the neck of a dog in Lyon in 1892. With Guthrie, he now set out to perform numerous renal transplants to the neck in dogs. Together, they developed the Carrel patch – a button of aorta containing the mouth of the renal artery which could be sutured into the excised similar defect in the recipient artery (Figure 15.6). This enabled tiny vessels to be grafted successfully and is a technique used to this day. Other experiments included transplantation of the ovary and the thyroid and even the heart of a small dog to the neck of a large one; the grafted heart survived for two hours. Carrel was soon able to demonstrate that although a dog's kidney transplanted to its own neck could survive, indeed could allow the animal to live in health even when the opposite kidney was removed, transplant of a kidney from one animal to another would fail after a few days. Carrel was clearly aware that although he could overcome technical surgical problems of transplantation, he was defeated by its biology. In a letter to Theodor Kocher, the great Swiss surgeon, in 1914, he wrote 'concerning homoplastic transplantation (from one animal into another) of organs such as the kidney, I have never found positive results to continue after a few months, whereas in autoplastic transplantation the result was always positive. The biological side of the question has to be investigated very much more, and we must find out by what means to prevent the reaction of the organism against a new organ'. This, in fact, was to take almost half a century to achieve.

Before leaving this remarkable man we must just list some of Carrel's other achievements. He was appointed to the Rockefeller Institute for Medical Research in New York in 1906, with its magnificent research facilities. Here he continued his transplant work but in other experiments showed that he could use a graft of the dog's aorta or inferior vena cava kept in ice-cold saline for a week to replace the aorta of a cat. It was not until many years later that this was used clinically; a frozen graft is 'de-natured' and does not set up an immunological reaction. He experimented with lung resection and endotracheal anaesthesia, carried out direct heart surgery in the dog and foretold that it would be possible to operate on diseased heart valves, and carried out fundamental experiments on tissue culture and organ culture (in collaboration with Charles Lindbergh). During the First World War he performed extensive clinical studies on wound healing and infection in specially established military hospitals immediately behind the front line on the Western Front (see Figure 9.28). He was awarded the Nobel Prize for Physiology and Medicine in 1912.

Artificial kidneys

The kidneys function as an ultra-filter: water and small molecules (salts and waste products such as urea) are excreted whereas large molecules are retained or reabsorbed. In order to produce an 'artificial kidney' which will filter out waste products from the blood, a dialysing membrane is required. One such membrane is the patient's own peritoneum. In 1923 G Ganter used peritoneal dialysis to lower the blood urea of animals in renal failure and in 1927 H Heusser and H Werder first attempted to relieve uraemic patients by this means. By 1948, over 100 patients in renal failure treated by this technique were reviewed. The results were poor; there were technical problems with the catheters used, the composition of fluid, and infection, which led of course to peritonitis. However, there were one or two encouraging successes; for example, in 1946 a case was reported of cure of a patient suffering from complete suppression of urine caused by the precipitation of sulphathiazole crystals in the urine by means of peritoneal dialysis.

The modern era commenced in 1959 with the development of intermittent dialysis with a single disposable catheter placed in the peritoneal cavity and with commercially prepared dialysis solutions. In 1968 the first permanent in-dwelling peritoneal catheter was developed and this led to the method of continuous ambulatory peritoneal dialysis (CAPD) which can be carried out in the patient's home. Nowadays some hundred thousand patients world-wide are being treated by this technique, accounting for perhaps one in five of the world's dialysis population.

The term 'artificial kidney' was first used by J J Abel, L G Rowntree and B B Turner in 1913, when they reported successful removal of salicylate from the blood of rabbits by means of an apparatus made up of a series of tubes of celloidin, through which the blood was circulated, immersed in dialysis solution in a bottle. This apparatus allowed toxins to pass through the membrane into the bath while keeping blood corpuscles and plasma within the circulating blood.

The first efficient artificial kidney was constructed by Willem Kolff, and its development is a fascinating story. Kolff was born in Leyden, Holland in 1911, the son of a physician. He qualified in medicine in Leyden in 1938 and joined the university department

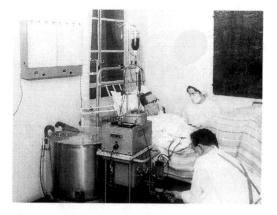

Figure 15.7 Renal dialysis using the 'artificial kidney'. Patient of the author at Westminster Hospital, 1964.

of medicine under Professor Polak Daniels as an intern. With his chief, he discussed the possibility of clearing the blood of toxins in patients dying of renal failure.

When Holland was overrun by the invading German army in May 1940, Polak Daniels and his wife, both Jews, committed suicide. Unwilling to work under the Nazi physician appointed to replace his old chief, Kolff moved to work in the hospital of the small town of Kampen. Here, with the help of an engineering colleague, Kolff built his first dialysis machine in 1943. He realised that the small molecules of urea and other toxic chemicals could cross a semi-permeable membrane, cellophane, and, in addition, that excess of water could be removed from the patient if a more concentrated solution was placed in the dialysis bath.

In wartime Holland, everything needed to build the machine was in short supply or was even unobtainable. The prototype machine was built out of cellophane tubing mounted on wooden drums which were placed in laundry tubs full of the dialysis solution. Plastic tubing was unavailable; rubber tubes were used over and over again. Needles were resharpened and used repeatedly.

The first patient was a 29-year-old female in renal failure – anaemic, breathless and hardly able to see. After her first dialysis she became lucid and her breathing and vision improved. After 12 treatments, all her suitable blood vessels were thrombosed and she died. Autopsy revealed shrunken and scarred kidneys. In all, 17 patients were dialysed in Kampen, with two survivals.

In 1950, the war over, news of Kolff's machine reached beyond Holland. He was invited to the Cleveland Clinic in the USA and here, with more sophisticated equipment, the modern dialysis machine was developed (Figure 15.7). In the Korean War, dialysis was used to treat wounded soldiers in acute renal failure; the mortality dropped from 95% to 35% and the value of renal dialysis was firmly established. The apparatus used today, now miniaturised and provided with disposable dialysis coils, is based on Kolff's original machine (Figure 15.7).

Kolff then stayed on at Cleveland to help develop the heart–lung pump, which made safe open cardiac surgery possible (see Figure 14.15) and, in 1961, devised the intra-aortic balloon for cardiac assist in cases of acute myocardial failure – a device which is now in widespread use. In 1990 he was named by *Life Magazine* as one of the 100 most important Americans (he was by now naturalised) in the 20th century.

The immunological basis of transplantation

The puzzling observations of Carrel, in the early years of the 20th century, of success when an autograft was performed from one part of the animal to another site, and failure when grafts were attempted from one animal to another (heterografts) were solved by the classical studies of Peter Medawar (1915–1987) and his colleagues. Working in Oxford during the Second World War on problems in skin transplantation, he studied a 22-year-old woman who had severe burns on her chest and arm. She received a series of grafts from her brother's thigh to the burned areas, and 15 days later a second set of grafts was applied. Medawar noted rapid degeneration of the second set of skin grafts and realised that this demonstrated acquired immunity by the recipient to the grafts; the so-called 'second set phenomenon'. This led to an extensive series of animal experiments. The 'second set rejection' was more rapid also if the host had first been injected with white cells from the donor. These evidently contained antigens which interfered with the transplant. In 1951, working with Rupert Billingham, it was shown that skin grafts from one rabbit to another could be prolonged by daily injections of cortisone. Medawar's work together with Sir Frank Macfarlane Burnet (1899–1985) of Australia led to their being awarded the Nobel Prize for Medicine in 1960.

Meanwhile, surgeons in a number of centres continued to experiment with renal transplantation in patients dying of advanced kidney failure. Between 1951 and 1953, David Hume (1917–1973) and his team in Boston transplanted kidneys to the thigh in 15 patients, bringing the ureter out to drain onto the side of the leg. Those grafts that functioned continued to do so for from 37 to 180 days, the patients being treated with low dose steroids for immunosuppression. In 1952, at the Necker Hospital in Paris, René Kuss was confronted with a young carpenter aged 16 who had fallen from a scaffolding and ruptured his right kidney. The kidney was removed but after the operation it was discovered that he had a congenital absence of the other kidney. The boy's mother pleaded that she should be allowed to donate one of her kidneys to her son and it was found that the two shared the same major and minor blood groups. The operation was performed on Christmas night of that year; the grafted kidney immediately functioned and the boy's general condition improved considerably, but, as we now would confidently predict, rejection set in after three weeks.

In 1954 there was a major step forward in the story of human organ transplantation – the successful transplant of a kidney from one identical twin to another. Its success proved that, if only the difficult immunological barrier could be overcome by some means or another, then organ transplantation in man could be a feasible proposition. The operation took place on December 23rd, 1954, at the Peter Bent Brigham Hospital in Boston. The patient was a 24-year-old man admitted under the

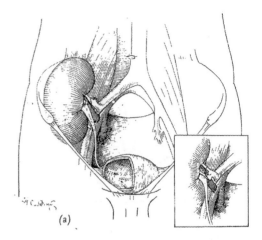

Figure 15.8 Details of the technique of renal transplantation in man as performed by Dr Joseph Murray.
From Merrill JP et al.: Successful homotransplantation of the human kidney between identical twins. *Journal of the American Medical Association* 1956; 160, 277.

care of John Merrill in severe kidney failure. Since the patient had a twin brother, the possibility of a transplant was considered. The patient was dialysed on the artificial kidney, which improved his condition so that further investigations could be carried out. The twins' blood was found to be identical for all the eight blood group systems that were then known. The hospital record of their birth showed that there was a common placenta, and furthermore both twins had the relatively rare Darwin's tubercle of the ears, not possessed by their two siblings. The twins had identical eye colours which, again, were markedly different from those of their siblings. A skin graft was exchanged between the twins: a perfect take was obtained and survived as normal skin for a month. It was decided to go ahead with the operation. Procedures were performed simultaneously on the donor and the recipient in adjacent operating rooms. A normal left kidney was removed from the healthy twin by Hartwell Harrison and grafted into the right lower abdomen of the patient by Joe Murray. The renal vessels were anastomosed to the iliac vessels of the

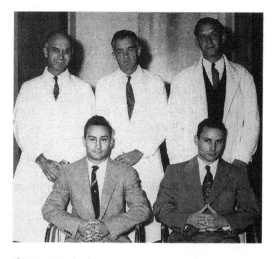

Figure 15.9 The first successful renal transplant between identical twins, 23rd December, 1954. Front row: Richard Herrick, the recipient, on the left, Ronald, the donor, on the right. Back row, left to right: Joseph Murray, surgeon, John Merrill, nephrologist, and Hartwell Harrison, urologist. Courtesy of Dr Joseph Murray.

patient and the ureter implanted into the bladder – a technique which has become the standard practice in all renal transplants (Figure 15.8). The operating time was three and a half hours. When the clamps were released from the blood vessels, the entire kidney became pink and a clear urine flowed copiously from the donor kidney. The post-operative course was smooth for both the patients. A year after the transplantation the patient was well and carrying on unlimited activity. X-rays showed that the graft kidney was functioning well (Figure 15.9).

Surely, if any operation is to receive that much-worn accolade 'a major breakthrough', this was it. By 1961 a couple of dozen more renal transplantations had taken place between human identical twins, of which 17 were performed by the Boston team. Three of their patients died but of the remaining patients, the longest survivor was alive seven years after surgery. Joseph Murray (contemp.) received the Nobel Prize for Medicine in 1990.

There still remained, of course, the tremendous problems of the immunological barrier to trans-

plantation. These successes stimulated world-wide research to make organ transplantation available for patients other than twins. It had already been shown in 1952 by Frank Dixon and his co-workers that the immune reaction could be suppressed in rabbits by using X-ray irradiation. In 1959 John Merrill performed a kidney graft between non-identical twins after irradiating the recipient, and a similar procedure was carried out by the surgical team at the Necker Hospital, Paris, using cobalt irradiation for immune suppression. Apart from an occasional success (the Paris team, for example, achieved the first successful long survivor of a non-twin transplantation), the numerous serious complications of whole-body irradiation led to the eventual abandonment of this method.

In 1959, R Schwartz and W Dameshek, working at Tuft's Medical School, Boston, showed that the treatment of rabbits with 6-mercaptopurine for 14 days produced a long-lasting immunological tolerance to human serum albumin. After seeing this report, a young English surgical registrar, Roy Calne (contemp.), decided to investigate the effect of this drug on renal homograft in dogs. His demonstration that the experimental animal could accept a completely unmatched kidney graft from another donor using this purine analogue provided the basis on which subsequent transplantation of donor organs has depended (Figure 15.10). This was helped considerably by the development of more effective drugs, particularly azathioprine in 1961 and cyclosporin in 1976. Calne went on to become Professor of Surgery in Cambridge, where his unit became a Mecca to surgeons and research workers in this field. He later pioneered liver, pancreas and small intestine transplantation in this country. He has not only been knighted but is one of the few surgeons to have been elected a Fellow of the Royal Society.

Transplantation of other organs

The kidney is the obvious organ for transplantation. It is bilateral, so that, in addition to using a

(a)

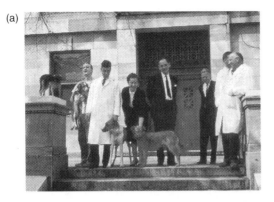

(b)

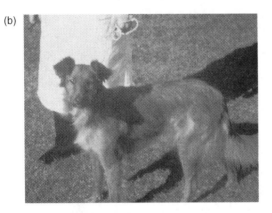

Figure 15.10 (a) Roy Calne, in white coat, with a long-term dog renal graft survivor. (b) – Close-up of the first dog to survive six months after renal transplantation.
Courtesy of Sir Roy Calne.

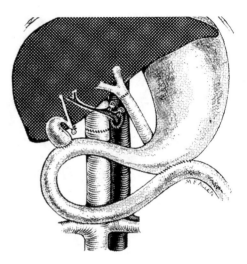

Figure 15.11 The technique of liver transplantation.

proved effective in spite of millions of pounds having been spent on experimental liver dialysis and on the development of implantable or extra-corporeal heart assist machines.

Liver

Liver transplantation represents a formidable technical problem. The patient is desperately ill from advanced malignant disease, cirrhosis, liver poisoning or some other major illness and is deeply jaundiced. There is, at present, no medical means of markedly improving the patient's condition before surgery. Moreover, the technical problems of grafting the vascular and biliary systems of the donor liver into the recipient are complex (Figure 15.11).

C Stuart Welch (1909–1980) in New York in 1955 experimented with auxiliary transplantation of liver in the dog, leaving the original liver in place. After extensive animal experiments, Thomas Starzl (contemp.) of Denver performed the first human liver transplantation in 1963. The patient was a 3-year-old child with congenital biliary atresia; the operation failed. Starzl's first success was not achieved until 1967. This was an 18-month-old

cadaver organ, close relative living donors can volunteer a kidney. In addition, thanks to effective dialysis, the recipient can have his or her general condition improved remarkably and can be maintained for months or years in reasonable health until a suitable graft becomes available. If a kidney graft should fail, the patient can be maintained on dialysis and a subsequent re-grafting can be performed. With other organs, failure can only be rescued by an emergency removal of the donor organ and a re-graft. Other organs present the problems of being single (apart from the lungs) and, to date, long-term support machines have not child with primary cancer of the liver who survived for over a year following transplantation before dying of metastatic disease from the original tumour. The first liver transplant in Europe was performed by Roy Calne in Cambridge in 1968. Further experience, and the introduction of cyclosporin, has greatly improved results, and survivals of 20 years or more are not unusual.

The heart

Carrel and Guthrie, in their classical transplant experiments in the early years of the 20th century, placed a small donor heart into the neck of a dog. The coronary arteries of the donor were perfused through the recipient's carotid artery; venous return from the heart was effected by the pulmonary artery of the graft being anastomosed into the jugular vein of the host.

In the 1950s, a number of groups in the USA and USSR were experimenting with heart transplantation after removal of the recipient heart and using hypothermia. Host survival was obtained for only a few hours. However, the technical difficulties of linking up the pulmonary and systemic circulation were considerable. The advent of the pump oxygenator at this time to take over the host's circulation allowed more time for this complex procedure. An enormous technical advance was made by Norman Shumway (contemp.) and his group at Stanford University in 1961. This rapidly became, and indeed remains, the standard procedure. This modification consisted of dividing the aorta and the pulmonary artery and both the atria transversely in both the donor and the recipient. In this way the entrance of the superior and the inferior vena cava into the right atrium and of the four pulmonary veins into the left atrium remain undisturbed, the left and right atrial walls being sutured to the donor heart at a point anterior to these veins (Figure 15.12). This substantially shortens the time required for the recipient to be on heart by-pass and Shumway's group achieved long-term survivors using immunosuppressive drugs.

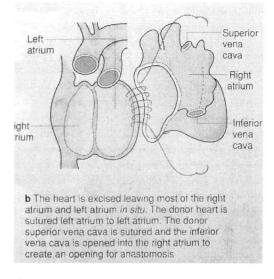

b The heart is excised leaving most of the right atrium and left atrium *in situ*. The donor heart is sutured left atrium to left atrium. The donor superior vena cava is sutured and the inferior vena cava is opened into the right atrium to create an opening for anastomosis

Figure 15.12 The technique of heart transplantation.

The first heart transplant in man was performed by James Hardy and his team at the University of Mississippi in 1964. The patient had terminal heart disease and was given a chimpanzee heart which only supported the patient for approximately an hour before failure occurred. In 1967, Christian Barnard (contemp.) in Cape Town successfully transplanted the heart of a human donor who had died of brain injury into a 54-year-old dentist in chronic heart failure. The patient died of infection on the 17th post-operative day, but a second patient grafted a few weeks later survived for over a year. The heart has always been an organ which engenders great emotion in the public and this operation became perhaps the most publicised in the history of surgery, both the patient and his surgeon becoming what amounted to pop stars with world-wide media coverage.

Isolated lung transplantation in a human was first reported in 1963, again by James Hardy, and combined heart–lung transplantation in 1969 by Denton Cooley in Houston, Texas. Today these procedures have passed into the standard armamentarium of transplant surgery.

Pancreas

Severe diabetes may be complicated by renal failure and so the possibility of pancreas transplantation at the time of renal grafting in such patients is an attractive proposition. Such a graft was first reported by Richard Lillihei in 1966 at the University of Minnesota. Current techniques include implantation of the duct of the pancreas into the bladder or the intestine. Attempts at extracting the islet of Langerhans cells (the cells that produce insulin) from the pancreas and using these as a graft have been subject to intense and expensive research with, at present, only meagre clinical application.

Intestine

Patients who have lost a major part of their small intestine due to injury or disease can be maintained by chronic intravenous feeding – a grim existence. Transplantation of small intestine has been carried out successfully in a small group of patients.

Multiple organ transplantation

Multiple organ transplants are now performed. Roy Calne, for example, has a ten-year survival in a lady who received a heart–lung–liver transplantation for severe lung and liver disease. Another patient with a non-malignant massive intra-abdominal tumour underwent a six-organ transplant of stomach, duodenum, small bowel, liver, pancreas and kidney and was well two and a half years after his operation.

The major problem at present with organ transplantation is a severe lack of donors. This has focused attention on the possibility of xenotransplantation – the use of other species. Much work is being done on modifying donor species by genetic engineering but the problems of rejection and the risks of novel cross-species infections are still to be overcome.

16

Envoi – today and tomorrow

So the time has come briefly to review the present-day surgical scene and to try to peer into the future.

We are living in an age of technological explosion such as has never been experienced before. The older readers, and indeed the author, have lived before television, the space age, the computer and the other wonders that we now take for granted. As a surgeon, I was brought up to make a diagnosis without the help of ultrasound or computerised tomography and to operate without many of the adjuncts now available in the operating theatre, such as vascular grafts, artificial joints, heart–lung machines and the vast array of patient monitoring equipment.

Surgeons have always been quick to adapt to new technology; indeed, they have often been the very first to realise the practical potential of the latest invention. For example, the announcement of the discovery of X-rays by Wilhelm Konrad Roentgen at the Würzburg Physical and Medical Society on the 28th December, 1895, was followed, at almost breathtaking speed, by the first X-ray photograph for clinical purposes being made by Alan Campbell Swinton in London. The newly discovered rays were put to work almost at once by surgeons in the localisation of foreign bodies and the diagnosis of fractures. The first publication I have discovered was published in *The Lancet* on 22nd February, 1896, by Robert Jones and Oliver Lodge of Liverpool. It is quite remarkable that in the space of a couple of months an X-ray machine was built, cases dealt with, a paper prepared and publication achieved. The paper described the localisation of a bullet in the wrist of a 12-year-old boy.

It should perhaps be noted that physicians were rather more tardy. Some even seemed to think that it was an intrusion on the classical clinical methods of inspection, palpation, percussion and auscultation of the thorax to add an X-ray of the chest!

Almost as soon as the newly invented electric light bulb could be miniaturised, Max Nitze (1848–1906), Professor of Urology in Berlin, adapted it to provide illumination so that the interior of the bladder could be inspected with a cystoscope (see Figure 8.24). Other instruments to examine all the other body cavities soon followed.

Harold Hopkins (1918–1994), Professor of Applied Optics at Reading, (who had, by the way, already invented the zoom lens), published an account of his system of flexible glass rods to serve as a medium for the transmission of light from an external source in 1954. This gave much superior illumination compared with that produced by a small electric light bulb. Applied first to rigid endoscopes, it was soon apparent that the system could be adapted for flexible instruments, since the glass fibres were themselves flexible. Sadly, British instrument makers declined to take up this brilliant invention, which was eagerly seized upon by Karl Storz in Germany, whose firm was soon the leading manufacturer of endoscopic instruments in the world. These were being used to examine all the body cavities – bladder, alimentary canal, abdomen, thorax, bronchial tree and so on – before the engineers adapted them to look inside their machinery.

Using the modified original rigid and electrically illuminated cystoscopes, clinicians around the beginning of the 20th century began to examine the insides of the abdominal and thoracic cavities distended with gas (laparoscopy and thoracoscopy, respectively). This was taken up with great enthusiasm by the gynaecologists for pelvic examination and, indeed, for performing simple procedures such as ligation of the tubes for female sterilisation. The fibreoptic system greatly improved the instrumentation for such surgery, and more and more complex operations could be performed. A pioneer of this in England was Patrick Steptoe (1913–1988) of Oldham, Lancashire (he was never on the staff of a teaching hospital). In 1967 he published the first textbook on this type of surgery in the English language entitled *Laparoscopy in Gynaecology*. Incidentally, it was Steptoe, together with the embryologist Robert Edwards, who produced the first 'test-tube baby' by in-vitro fertilisation in 1978.

It was not long before this new technology was applied across the surgical specialties.

Cholecystectomy, removal of the diseased gall bladder, has been a common major abdominal operation since it was first performed in 1882 by Carl Langenbuch (see Figure 8.2), and it was laparoscopic removal of this organ that heralded the use of this instrumentation in general surgery. The first laparoscopic cholecystectomy was carried out by Erich Muhe, of Boblingen, Germany, in September 1985, using a sigmoidoscope, but the operation was met with scepticism. Philippe Mouret, a gynaecologist in Lyons, performed the next cholecystectomy the following year, using his gynaecological laparoscopic instruments, and he must be given the credit for getting the operation accepted. It was taken up with great enthusiasm in the USA by Edward Reddick and Douglas Olsen in Nashville, Tennessee, who began a popular training course, and the operation rapidly spread around the world. It was first performed in Scotland by Professor Alfred Cuschieri in 1987 after extensive studies in the pig model, in England by David Rosin at St Mary's Hospital in London in 1990 and, in the same year, in Asia by Professor Tehempton Udwadia in Mumbai, India.

Today, minimal access surgery, or, to give it its popular name, 'key-hole surgery', with fibreoptic

telescopes, visualisation of the magnified operative field on a television screen, and with brilliantly engineered instruments (Figure 16.1) allows many types of operation to be carried out without the extensive 'surgery of approach' that was previously required to access the diseased organ. Operations on the gall bladder and gynaecological procedures are the most common examples, but many abdominal and thoracic operations – from appendicectomy to major resections of tumours – are now routine. Harvesting a kidney from a living volunteer donor for renal transplantation, for example, has seen a welcomed rise in the numbers of donors, who are spared the need for a long loin incision An emerging and exciting technology which is being developed has been given the label 'natural orifice transluminal endoscopic surgery' ('NOTES'). This uses fibreoptic endoscopic instruments which, instead of being inserted through incisions in the body wall, are introduced through the natural orifices – the mouth, rectum or vagina. For example, the instrument is passed through the mouth into the stomach, then perforates through the gastric wall into the peritoneal cavity. Anthony Kalloo, at the Johns Hopkins Hospital Baltimore, published a successful cholecystectomy in the pig by this technique in 2004. The first human cholecystectomy by the vaginal route has already been carried out.

The explosion in so many fields of technology is seeing astonishing recent advances in surgery. The professional journals, and indeed the newspapers, are full of quite breathtaking advances. A few selected examples, taken at random, include: miniaturised cochlear implants for patients with cochlear deafness; the laser beam to ablate tumours in highly dangerous areas of the body such as the brain with minimal damage to surrounding normal tissues; newer and better synthetic materials as blood vessel conduits and as prostheses to replace resected diseased bones or joints; and computerised muscle stimulation to allow people with paraplegia to walk.

In many examples of stenosis of arteries, whether of the limbs, the neck or the heart itself, dilating

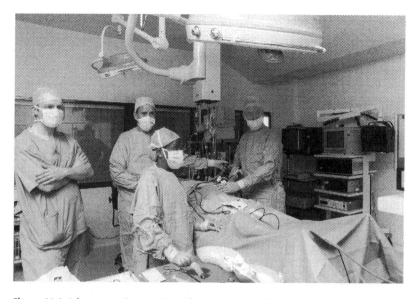

Figure 16.1 A laparoscopic operation. The surgeon and his team watch the procedure, magnified, on the TV screen. (Photograph provided by Mr David Rosin FRCS.)

balloons can now be passed under X-ray control (angioplasty) with or without the insertion of a stent to maintain patency, thus obviating a major surgical exploration. Especially exciting in this respect is a developing technique to pass a graft percutaneously via the femoral artery in order to stent an abdominal aneurysm, a procedure which otherwise involves very major abdominal surgery (see Chapter 14).

In contrast, in other fields, surgery of an extent never dreamed of hitherto can now be performed. A transplant surgeon routinely removes both lungs and the heart and replaces them with a donor graft. Sir Roy Calne's team in Cambridge performed an en bloc transplant of stomach, duodenum, small bowel, liver, pancreas and kidney in a 12-hour operation after removing a massive intra-abdominal tumour.

Guessing the future is something at which surgeons have a particularly bad record. After all, we are pragmatic, practical, down-to-earth doers rather than thinkers. Very few of our predictions have stood the test of time. In 1874, for example, that distin-

guished surgical teacher, John Ericson, at University College Hospital wrote: 'the abdomen, chest and brain, will forever be closed to operations by a wise and humane surgeon'. Worse still, the even more famous surgeon, Theodore Billroth, wrote a few years later: 'a surgeon who tries to suture a heart wound deserves to lose the esteem of his colleagues'.

One question often asked of surgeons, and, of course, discussed among surgeons themselves, is whether the operations of the future will be performed by robots. Will we put our lives into the care of machines that will completely replace their present-day human counterparts, in the way that assembly-line robots have replaced factory workers in many industrial plants?

The following quotation from *The Positronic Man* by Asimov and Silverberg, published in 1993, gives a possible scenario of the future:

He studied the robot surgeon's hand – his cutting hand – as it rested on the desk in utter tranquillity. It was splendidly designed. The fingers were long and tapering, and they were shaped into metallic looping curves of great artistic beauty, curves so graceful and appropriate to their function that one could easily imagine a scalpel being fitted into them and instantly becoming, at the moment they went into action, united in perfect harmony with the fingers that wielded it; surgeon and scalpel fusing into a single marvellously capable tool.

The word 'robot' was first used by Karel Capek in his play *RUR* in 1921, which was an indictment of industrialised society. He used the Czech *robota*, meaning compulsory labour, and *robotnik*, a serf. In the play, Rossum and his son develop humanoid creations to be used as servants by humanity; eventually they become self-willed, revolt against, and then massacre, their masters.

Rather simple industrial robots were first employed in 1961 and since then have become more and more complex and sophisticated. First developed for simple, unpleasant, repetitive or dangerous operations such as die-casting, they can now perform extremely delicate precision manipulations such as building a car or constructing complex electronic components.

The use of robots in the operating theatre is already a matter of fact. As a simple example, the surgeon can use his voice control to adjust the height and slope of the operating table, the theatre illumination and the lighting of his endoscopic apparatus. Of course there are immense problems. Industrial robots perform their work mainly on unchanging items and are allowed trial runs in order to get the procedure right. In surgery, every patient is different and trial runs would have difficulty in finding volunteers!

Already robotic equipment has been introduced in operative procedures, co-operating with, rather than replacing, the surgeon. Thus it can be used to machine the cavity for placement of the prosthesis in hip replacement, for machining of the bone ends in knee replacement, for accurate positioning of a biopsy probe or laser into a cerebral tumour, to carry out surface cutting of the cornea in refraction correction where accuracy has to be measured in microns, and in roboticised transurethral resection of the prostate.

Technology has already developed to allow the surgeon to operate from a remote site, using a

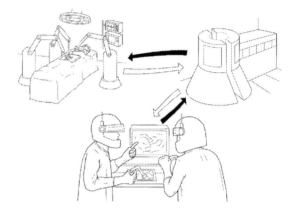

Figure 16.2 Could this be the operating theatre of the future? The surgeons are outside the room with virtual reality, telepresence and robotic manipulator technology. A large central processing unit integrates and controls these sophisticated systems.
From Goh P et al.: Robotics. In Savalgi R, Ellis H, eds *Clinical Anatomy for Laparoscopic and Thoracoscopic Surgery*. Abingdon, Radcliffe Medical Press, 1996.

three-dimensional monitor, to control endoscopic instruments for intra-abdominal and intrathoracic surgery.

Figure 16.2 gives an artist's impression of an endoscopic operating room in the future with virtual reality, telepresence and robotic manipulator technology. A large central processing unit integrates and controls these sophisticated systems.

Peter Goh and his colleagues at the National University of Singapore are developing a robotic 'mouse' to be inserted into the colon and which will be able to drive itself around the curves and corners of the bowel, transmitting pictures to the receiver and being able to perform removal of small polyps or biopsy of larger tumours. The same device could be used in other body cavities, for example, the stomach. Goh predicts:

An endoscopist of the future will insert a dozen of these devices into a dozen patients who will then watch an exciting movie on laser disc as the micro-robot does its job. The endoscopist will return from London to collect the robots (and his fee) and watch the re-runs at his leisure.

The surgeon of tomorrow will certainly explore new frontiers, visit inaccessible parts of the human body and operate where no man has gone before as a result of surgeons and engineers working more closely with each other than ever before to exploit the possibilities of technology.

What other thoughts for the 21st century? Cancer surgery will more or less disappear as effective drug treatments for the disease are developed or, ultimately, its causes found and eliminated. This is very much as the surgery of tuberculosis has disappeared in the Western world. Small uncalcified gall stones can already be dissolved away by prolonged and rather unpleasant treatment with bile salt preparations, or destroyed ultrasonically. More effective biochemical or bioengineering technology may abolish much of gall stone surgery in the future. As cartilage cell implants become developed, degenerative arthritic changes might be controlled at an early stage before joint replacement becomes necessary. The discovery of the causes and then the prevention of arteriosclerosis will eliminate much of current vascular surgery.

So, will surgeons of the next century have to join the dole queue? Not at all. While man remains the most unpleasant and most aggressive of all the earth's creatures, there will always be vast numbers and indeed probably increasing numbers, of victims of trauma, much of it inflicted by man upon man. So the surgeon will revert to the role of his distant forefathers – the man (and now the woman) who binds up the wounds, sets fractures and heals the injuries of mankind.

Index

Note: page numbers in *italics* refer to figures and tables.

Printed in the United States
by Baker & Taylor Publisher Services